I0070156

THROMBOSIS AND STROKE PREVENTION

Third Edition

The Afibber's Guide to Stroke Prevention

Hans R. Larsen MSc ChE

Author of Lone Atrial Fibrillation: Towards a Cure

FOREWORD BY

Patrick Chambers MD

PREFACE BY

Martin Klughaupt MD, FACC

PUBLISHED BY
INTERNATIONAL HEALTH NEWS

Thrombosis and Stroke Prevention 3rd Edition

Published by   International Health News
                                1320 Point Street
                                Victoria BC
                                Canada V8S 1A5
                                E-mail: editor@yourhealthbase.com
                                www.yourhealthbase.com

Thrombosis and Stroke Prevention does not offer medical advice. The information offered is intended to help readers make informed decisions about their health. It is not intended to be a substitute for the advice and care of a physician or other professional health care provider. The author has endeavored to ensure that the information presented is accurate and up to date, but is not responsible for any adverse effects or consequences sustained by any reader using the information contained in this book.

Copyright © 2018 by Hans R. Larsen

All rights reserved. No part of this publication may be reproduced in any form or by any means without permission in writing from the copyright holder, except by a reviewer quoting brief passages in a magazine, newspaper or broadcast.

First Printing – April 2018

ISBN 978-0-9809242-1-3

Also by Hans Larsen

Lone Atrial Fibrillation: Towards a Cure

The Prostate and Its Problems [with William R. Ware PhD]

Thrombosis and Stroke Prevention
Third Edition

The Afibber's Guide to Stroke Prevention

Contents

REVIEWS OF FIRST EDITION

Hans Larsen has delighted us again with this elegant and provocative book on the mechanisms of thrombosis and stroke. He is able to explain the intricate mechanisms involved in the underlying causes of thrombosis leading to strokes, then he provides us the clinical tests for each of these entities, and then offers a rational preventive means to alter this process. This book is a rich document replete with abundant references and will have a profound and enduring impact on patients attempting to understand and modify their risks for thrombosis and stroke, especially those with lone atrial fibrillation. Highly recommended, and a necessary supplemental companion for his *Lone Atrial Fibrillation: Towards A Cure*.
Norman F. Fisher MD, CA, USA

Never before has so much stroke-prevention information been consolidated into one complete, concise, well-referenced, well-researched and very important publication. This book is not just for afibbers, but for all health-conscious individuals looking to avoid blood clots and stroke by understanding who is at risk, how clots form and how to prevent them. The author takes a complex topic and breaks it down into understandable and useful anti-clotting strategies that include a thorough examination of natural alternatives as well as prescription drugs. This is a "must-have" reference everyone needs to own and read.
Jackie Burgess RDH, OH, USA

Hans Larsen's new book *Thrombosis and Stroke Prevention* is extremely valuable for those of us with atrial fibrillation and for all adults. Hans clearly explains the body's pathways to form blood clots and to dissolve them, the medications in common use to affect these processes, and the natural alternatives that can be used to help prevent stroke. His analysis will also help to prevent heart attack and blood clots in the lungs. Read this book; it may save your life!
Sadja Greenwood MD MPH, CA, USA

Hans Larsen's knowledge on thrombosis and stroke prevention far exceeds that of most conventional medical specialists in this area. This simple to read, cutting edge manual on natural alternatives to stroke prevention is a must read for anyone contemplating anti-coagulation therapy or simply wanting to prevent a stroke.
Michael Lam MD MPH, CA, USA

Mr. Larsen guides the AF patient, and his physician, through the basics of blood clotting and how this is affected by the various anti-platelet and anti-coagulant drugs. He makes a particularly valuable contribution in his discussion of "natural", non-pharmaceutical approaches to stroke prevention, which actually has relevance to the general, and not just the AF, population. Those interested in AF and stroke would be hard put to find a more valuable reference on the subject than Mr. Larsen's outstanding little book.
Martin Klughaupt, MD FACC, CA, USA

Foreword
To First Edition

Stroke is the third leading cause of death, behind heart disease and cancer. Risk factors associated with stroke are uniformly on the increase. These include most notably hypertension and diabetes, due primarily to the growing epidemic of obesity.

Deep vein thrombosis (DVT) can lead to pulmonary embolism. Its association with international jet travel has received recent notoriety. Another risk factor, atrial fibrillation, present in nearly five million Americans, is encountered in about 15% of stroke victims. This figure increases with age.

Despite this, those at risk for stroke are not receiving the recommended anticoagulant therapy. This may be due in part to ignorance and in part to medico- legal considerations. Unintended and sometimes unavoidable excessive anticoagulation can lead to a major internal bleed. In addition, some anticoagulant medications require regular monitoring via blood tests. Some can cross-react with numerous other medications. Diet and infection can have a dramatic impact on their efficacy.

Hans Larsen's new book: *Thrombosis and Stroke Prevention* carefully walks the concerned reader through this minefield of strokes, ischemic and hemorrhagic, and how best to avoid them. His well-researched tables comparing the risks and benefits of the various approaches to anticoagulation will not be found in the more traditional books on the topic. They are easily understood by the layman and provide the cold, hard numbers needed for making the difficult decisions involved in selecting the optimum stroke prevention protocol.

Hans Larsen studied with Henrik Dam, the Nobel Prize winning discoverer of vitamin K. Four of the 13 known blood coagulation factors are associated with vitamin K and Hans has well explained the intricacies of their actions as well as the actions of the components of platelet aggregation and the coagulation cascade. His easy style is especially suited to the difficult task of deciphering a topic as complex and tedious as blood coagulation. Like in his earlier book, *Lone Atrial Fibrillation: Towards a Cure*, his approach is comprehensive and unbiased. Recommendations are well reasoned, but at the end readers are left to draw their own now well-informed conclusions.

As the large cohort of baby boomers enters the ranks of seniordom, the topic of this book becomes timelier indeed.

Patrick Chambers, M.D.
Laboratory Director
Torrance Memorial Medical Center
Torrance, CA
April 2004

Preface
To First Edition

In *Thrombosis and Stroke Prevention* Hans Larsen has made an important contribution to the Atrial Fibrillation literature. As a physician and practicing cardiologist I was surprised by his exhaustive research of the relevant medical literature and his ability to glean from this vast body rational and honest conclusions. Mr. Larsen's monograph will be of invaluable help not only to the millions of patients who suffer from AF, but to their physicians as well.

Understanding, and thereby being able to manage, the risk of stroke in AF, has in the past often been difficult and frustrating. From an attitude prevalent in the medical community not so many years ago — that AF is an annoying but essentially harmless disturbance — we have seen a progression of alarm that pronounces that AF is a very common prelude to stroke and must be treated in the most aggressive fashion. Mr. Larsen helps us understand that the AF population is very heterogeneous in terms of stroke risk and that sub-groups of this population should be treated differently: some more and some less aggressively.

On the critical issue of anti-coagulation as prophylaxis against stroke, he has concisely summarized the most extensive recent studies, all of which suggest that for AF patients without identified stroke risk factors (congestive heart failure, hypertension, advanced age, diabetes or a prior history of stroke) anticoagulation with coumarin is not indicated, while for those with stroke risk factors it often is.

Mr. Larsen guides the AF patient, and his physician, through the basics of blood clotting and how this is affected by the various anti-platelet and anti-coagulant drugs. He makes a particularly valuable contribution in his discussion of "natural", non-pharmaceutical approaches to stroke prevention, which actually has relevance to the general, and not just the AF, population.

Those interested in AF and stroke would be hard put to find a more valuable reference on the subject than Mr. Larsen's outstanding little book.

Martin Klughaupt, MD, FACC
The Cardiovascular Institute
Mountain View, California
April 2004

Introduction

Lone atrial fibrillation (LAF), that is atrial fibrillation without underlying structural heart disease, is not a life-threatening disorder and is not associated with fatal arrhythmias such as ventricular fibrillation. It is also generally agreed that LAF, on its own, is not associated with an increased risk of ischemic stroke. However, if LAF is combined with one or more established risk factors for stroke (hypertension, diabetes, heart failure, heart disease, etc.) then the stroke risk is very real and measures are needed to ensure adequate protection.

The standard medical approach to stroke prevention has, until very recently, been pretty well confined to prescribing either aspirin or warfarin. Aspirin, as we shall see, has a negative benefit/risk ratio in preventing a first stroke. The net benefit of warfarin therapy can be substantial when underlying heart disease or a history of stroke or heart attack is present. However, when no additional risk factors for stroke are present, then warfarin therapy is not beneficial and may even be detrimental. Despite this recognized fact, warfarin is often prescribed routinely to AF patients who are unlikely to benefit from it.

There are indeed many myths and misconceptions surrounding stroke prevention in LAF. It is my hope that this book will help dispel at least some of them.

An ischemic stroke occurs when a blood vessel that supplies the brain is blocked and impairs blood flow. The resulting lack of oxygen (ischemia) causes brain cells and tissues to start dying within minutes. There are two types of ischemic stroke – thrombotic and embolic. A thrombotic stroke is caused by the development of a thrombus (blood clot) in the arteries supplying blood to the brain whereas an embolic stroke is caused by a blood clot that forms elsewhere in the body and then travels through the bloodstream to the brain. A cardioembolic stroke is an embolic stroke caused by a clot formed in the heart – often in the left atrial appendage.

The majority of ischemic strokes occurring in the general population are thrombotic in nature; however, when it comes to strokes related to atrial fibrillation they are more likely to be cardioembolic in nature.

Thrombotic and cardioembolic strokes share many risk factors including hypertension, diabetes, heart failure and coronary artery disease. This means that stroke prevention measures known to work in the general population are likely to also benefit atrial fibrillation patients. Thus the whole realm of proven natural stroke prevention agents opens up for the afibber to consider – and what a treasure trove this is! Several natural antithrombotics have been found to be superior to both aspirin and warfarin and have none of their adverse effects.

Selecting a stroke prevention program is, nevertheless, intensely personal and entails making important choices that every afibber needs to make early in their "career". There is no easy way to go about making these choices; a great deal of research and soul-searching is required. This, hopefully, is where my book will help.

The first edition of *Thrombosis and Stroke Prevention* not only provided in-depth discussions of both natural and pharmaceutical stroke prevention agents, it also covered in detail the underlying causes and mechanism of thrombosis (blood clot formation) and stroke. Blood clot formation is a very complex process involving platelet aggregation, coagulation and fibrinolysis. In order to rationally select a stroke prevention program, it is necessary to have at least a rudimentary understanding of the mechanisms and factors involved in these three stages of the thrombosis process. The first two chapters of the book are designed to provide this understanding. Chapters 3 and 4 deal with natural and pharmaceutical antithrombotics and chapter 5 provides detailed questionnaires and tables for estimating stroke risk. Chapter 6 compares the effectiveness of all the agents discussed in previous chapters with some surprising results.

The second edition of *Thrombosis and Stroke Prevention* updated the information presented in the first edition and added a chapter on how to live with warfarin and one providing details on warfarin interactions with other drugs and herbs.

This third edition adds new information about stroke risk factors and schemes for estimating stroke and bleeding risk. It also provides an update of the latest research concerning natural and pharmaceutical antithrombotics and includes a separate chapter covering the pros and cons of the new oral anticoagulants. Finally, it adds a chapter discussing stroke prevention based on occluding (closing off) the left atrial appendage where the vast majority of cardioembolic clots are generated.

This book would not have been possible without the whole-hearted support of my wife Judi who was instrumental in seeing it come to fruition. Without her word processing skills, editing advice, and encouragement I couldn't have accomplished it. Jackie Burgess, Patrick Chambers, MD, Norman Fisher, MD, Sadja Greenwood, MD, Martin Klughaupt, MD, FACC, and Frank McCabe also deserve my special, heartfelt thanks for taking the time to thoroughly review and comment on the first edition of *Thrombosis and Stroke Prevention*.

Hans R. Larsen
Victoria, BC, Canada
UPDATED (Third Edition) April 2018

Chapter 1

Mechanism of Thrombosis and Stroke

Atrial fibrillation without underlying structural heart disease (LAF) is not a life-threatening disorder and is not associated with fatal arrhythmias such as ventricular fibrillation. Several major clinical trials and epidemiologic studies have, however, concluded that atrial fibrillation is associated with an increased risk of ischemic stroke.

There are two types of ischemic stroke – thrombotic and embolic. Both involve the obstruction and subsequent stoppage of the blood supply to an area of the brain (infarction). However, the mechanism by which the obstruction occurs differs.

A thrombotic stroke involves the formation of atherosclerotic plaque and subsequent narrowing and clot (thrombus) formation at the point of obstruction. In an embolic stroke, on the other hand, the obstruction is caused by the lodging of an embolus (blood clot or atherosclerotic plaque) formed in the heart or in an artery outside the brain. Cardiogenic emboli (blood clots originating in the heart) can form on heart valves, particularly prosthetic ones, or as a result of mitral stenosis. Cardiogenic emboli can also originate from the walls of the heart as a result of a heart attack (myocardial infarction), atrial fibrillation or congestive heart failure or from a benign atrial tumour (myxoma).

The increased stroke risk associated with atrial fibrillation is clearly linked with embolic rather than thrombotic stroke and, more specifically, with embolic stroke caused by thrombi originating in the heart (cardio embolism). The risk of an atrial fibrillation associated stroke is markedly increased in the presence of certain well-defined risk factors:

- Hypertension
- Diabetes
- Heart failure
- Left ventricular ejection fraction below 0.35
- Coronary artery disease (heart disease)
- Rheumatic heart disease
- Presence of prosthetic heart valves
- Thyrotoxicosis (hyperthyroidism)
- A prior stroke (cerebrovascular event)
- A prior heart attack (myocardial infarction)
- A prior transient ischemic attack or TIA (mini-stroke)

It is still somewhat controversial as to whether advancing age increases stroke risk. Some studies point to an increased risk above the age of 75 years, but others consider the age-related risk increase to be minimal, if present at all [1,2].

To further complicate matters, there is emerging evidence that it may not be the presence of afib as such that increases the stroke risk, but rather the combination of atrial fibrillation with one or more of the above risk factors (comorbid conditions) which, in themselves, are known to be associated with a significantly increased stroke risk [3,4].

Nevertheless, whether or not one suffers from atrial fibrillation, having a stroke is a serious matter. Embolic stroke is actually a close cousin of pulmonary embolism except that in pulmonary embolism, the blood clot forms in the veins and travels to the lungs rather than forming in the heart or arteries and travelling to the brain. In a similar fashion, thrombotic stroke is a close cousin to heart attack except that the thrombus forms in the coronary arteries rather than in the brain. All three conditions can be fatal or severely disabling and are, unfortunately, very common. It is estimated that about 500,000 new strokes and 200,000 repeat strokes occurred in the United States in 2002 [5]. Of these, about 80% were ischemic strokes while the remaining 20% were hemorrhagic strokes, i.e. strokes caused by a burst blood vessel in the brain. Pulmonary embolism clocks in at about 650,000 cases per year and heart attacks occur at the rate of about 1.5 million per year in the United States [6,7].

It is clear that embolism or, more correctly, thromboembolism is a major health concern and a concerted effort should be made to prevent it whether or not one has atrial fibrillation. Thrombi can form in either the arterial system (the supply side involving the left side of the heart and the arteries) or in the venous system (the return side involving the veins, the right side of the heart and the lungs). The formation of a thrombus involves platelet activation, platelet aggregation, and blood coagulation. The body has a built-in mechanism for dealing with thrombi that no longer serve their purpose of preventing bleeding. This process is called fibrinolysis. Thrombi formed in the arteries tend to contain predominantly platelets (white thrombi) while those formed in the veins tend to be rich in fibrin and red blood cells (red thrombi).

The formation of a thrombus is a complicated process, but one that must be understood if approaches to preventing it is to be considered in a rational manner. Blood clotting is an integral part of the body's overall defense system. Its primary purpose is to stop bleeding from an injured blood vessel. Once the bleeding is stopped, the clot is gradually eliminated through fibrinolysis and healing of the injury proceeds. The blood, at all times, carries all the components necessary to initiate the platelet aggregation and coagulation process. The process can be activated when the blood is exposed to an injured or narrowed blood vessel, inflamed tissue, or a foreign object. The clotting process can also be initiated if the blood flow stagnates and the concentration of coagulation factors becomes excessive or the level of enzymes involved in fibrinolysis becomes deficient. Thrombus formation in the deep veins of the legs and in the left atrial appendage are examples of thrombus formation initiated by blood stagnation.

It is known that atrial fibrillation is associated with inflammation and fibrosis of the atria [8]. This can lead to exposure of sub-endothelial tissue (the layer below the outer lining) and subsequent initiation of thrombus formation. The thrombus formation initiated by sub-endothelial tissue exposure involves platelet aggregation to a much greater extent than does stagnation (stasis) induced coagulation, so it is likely that aspirin would be significantly more effective in preventing the former than the latter.

As mentioned above, thrombus formation and elimination involves three separate steps [9-12]:

- Platelet activation and aggregation
- Blood coagulation
- Fibrinolysis

Coagulation can follow one of two pathways:

- The intrinsic pathway, which is activated by contact with exposed sub-endothelial tissue, prosthetic implants or exposed cartilage, or by exposure to elevated blood levels of homocysteine, uric acid or certain long-chain saturated fatty acids.

- The extrinsic pathway, which is activated by the presence of tissue factor (factor III, thromboplastin) as a result of injury to tissue or blood vessel walls.

Both pathways ultimately coalesce into the common pathway, which results in the formation of insoluble (stabilized) fibrin from fibrinogen.

It is clear that thrombus formation can be retarded by reducing the concentration of the raw materials involved in its generation, ie. platelets and fibrinogen. Thrombus formation can also be inhibited by reducing the concentration of the enzymes and other factors involved in the thrombus-forming process or by inhibiting the conversion from their inactive to their active form. Finally, thrombus formation can be inhibited by promoting the fibrinolysis process. There are indeed many avenues for preventing thrombus formation and the resulting embolism and stroke. Aspirin and warfarin therapy are clearly only two of many possible approaches. To uncover other potentially beneficial approaches, it is necessary to take a closer look at each step of the overall thrombus formation process.

PLATELET ACTIVATION AND AGGREGATION

Platelets, like red and white blood cells, are an integral part of normal blood. In spite of their small size they contain an amazing variety of enzymes that interact with other plasma components crucial to the formation of blood clots. Among the more significant of these components are thromboxane A2, ADP (adenosine diphosphate) and von Willebrand factor.

The first step in the platelet aggregation process involves the adherence of platelets to sub-endothelial tissue or a foreign object. Von Willebrand factor is the main "glue" involved in platelet sticking to each other and to the vessel wall. Once the platelets begin to adhere, they change shape and develop small protrusions that facilitate subsequent aggregation and thrombus formation. Thromboxane A2 provides a further stimulus for platelet activation and aggregation and its release can be activated by arachidonic acid present in the blood stream. Thromboxane A2 is quite short-lived and is converted into inert thromboxane B2. Calcium ions are also involved in platelet activation.

Once platelets are activated, they begin sticking together and this process is associated with the release of ADP, thrombin, and additional thromboxane A2 as well as various platelet factors and possibly coagulation factors. Calcium ions are also involved in platelet aggregation and the process is inhibited by nitric oxide (NO) and prostacyclin released from neighbouring cells. The process of platelet aggregation exposes binding sites for fibrinogen, which can then be converted to fibrin (the main component of thrombi) through the action of thrombin. Fibrinogen binding sites on the platelet surface can also be exposed by contact with epinephrine (adrenaline), arachidonic acid, serotonin, zinc, collagen, thrombin and certain prostaglandins [9-11].

The total process of platelet activation and aggregation is, of course, considerably more complex than described here. However, from the above description, it is possible to suggest several approaches to inhibiting the process.

- Reduce overall level of von Willebrand factor or inhibit its release.
- Reduce overall level of thromboxane A2 or inhibit its release.
- Reduce level of prothrombin (the precursor of thrombin) or inhibit its release.
- Reduce fibrinogen level or inhibit its conversion to fibrin.
- Increase nitric oxide and prostacyclin availability.
- Maintain appropriately low blood levels of epinephrine, serotonin, arachidonic acid, zinc, and detrimental prostaglandins.

Each of the above approaches can, at least partially, help inhibit platelet activation and aggregation and thus lessen the risk of inappropriate thrombus formation. Aspirin and several naturally occurring compounds do indeed use one or more of the above options to achieve their preventive effect.

BLOOD COAGULATION

Intrinsic pathway

The initiation of the intrinsic pathway involves the activation of blood coagulation factor XII (Hageman factor). This activation requires the presence of prekallikrein, high molecular weight kinonokin, and an appropriate contact surface such as an activated platelet or exposed sub-endothelial tissue. Factor XII may also be activated by kallikrein in the absence of a contact surface.

Activated factor XII, in turn, activates factor XI which activates factor IX which, in turn, actives factor VIII. Factor VIII activation is the last step in the intrinsic pathway (factor VIII is lacking in hemophilia). Factor VIII is primarily found in a complex bound to von Willebrand factor. Activation of factor VIII by thrombin leads to the formation of factor X, the first step in the common pathway. It is interesting that the level of factor VIII increases with age in both men and women and, to a greater extent, in persons with blood types A, B and AB than in those with blood type O [11].

Extrinsic pathway
The initiation of the extrinsic pathway involves an interaction between tissue factor (thromboplastin) and coagulation factor VII which, when activated, results in the formation of factor X. The extrinsic pathway is the one involved in venous thrombosis and, most likely, in left atrial appendage thrombus formation as well [12].

Common pathway
An interaction between activated factor X, factor V, calcium ions, and platelet factor 3 leads to the activation of prothrombin which, in turn, is converted into thrombin through an intermediate step involving prothrombin fragment 1 and 2. Thrombin acts on fibrinogen to produce fibrin monomers and dimers (D-dimer), which then polymerize and are stabilized (cross-linked) into the final blood clot through the action of activated coagulation factor XIII. Fibrinogen levels are the same in men and women and increase slightly with age. Inflammation and stress are associated with an increased fibrinogen level [11].

The body also produces natural coagulation inhibitors such as antithrombin III and protein-C and its cofactor protein-S in order to keep the process from running away. About 5% of people of Western European origin have a mutation in coagulation Factor V (Factor V Leiden), which prevents protein-C from doing its job of controlling the coagulation reaction. The presence of Factor V Leiden causes a condition known as activated protein-C resistance (APC). APC has been linked to a significantly increased risk of venous thromboembolism, but evidence that it also increases the risk of arterial thrombosis is less convincing [13]. A recent study found no significant association between the presence of Factor V Leiden and stroke risk in a large sample of atrial fibrillation patients [14]. Nevertheless, since some afib-related strokes may be associated with stasis in the left atrial appendage, it is possible that the presence of Factor V Leiden could indeed increase the risk of ischemic stroke in a subset of afibbers, particularly if other cardiovascular risk factors are also present. More research is clearly required to establish this.

Despite the complexities in the blood coagulation process, several possible approaches to keeping it under control come to mind.

- Reduce overall level of one or more coagulation factors or inhibit their activation.
- Reduce the level of von Willebrand factor or inhibit its release.
- Reduce level of prothrombin or inhibit its conversion to thrombin.

- Reduce fibrinogen level or inhibit its conversion to fibrin.
- Promote the synthesis of natural coagulation inhibitors protein-C and its cofactors and antithrombin III.

Each of the above approaches can help control coagulation and thus lessen the risk of inappropriate thrombus formation. Aspirin, warfarin, heparin, ximelagatran, and several naturally occurring compounds indeed use one or more of the above methods to achieve their protective effect.

FIBRINOLYSIS

Fibrinolysis is the process by which the body rids itself of no longer needed or unwanted blood clots. The process involves the activation of plasminogen to plasmin, a proteolytic enzyme that dissolves the polymerized fibrin clot. Plasminogen is always present in blood plasma and is actually incorporated into blood clots where it is bound directly to fibrin. Plasminogen is converted into plasmin by plasminogen activators. Tissue type plasminogen activator (tPA) is found in the lining of small blood vessels and can also be secreted by macrophages (scavenger cells). Urokinase is present in the blood stream in trace amounts and assists the fibrinolysis process by activating fibrin-bound plasminogen [11].

To complicate matters further, there are also blood, platelet and tissue components that inhibit plasminogen activators; among them are plasminogen activator inhibitor 1 (PAI-1) and at least 5 plasma proteins that neutralize free plasmin, but not fibrin-bound plasmin. The release of endothelial plasminogen activators is enhanced by exercise, electric shock, and other forms of stress, as well as by activated factor X and certain substances released from platelets [12].

There is some evidence that fibrinolytic activity in the veins of the legs is subnormal; this may be a major underlying cause of deep vein thrombosis [12].

It is clear that fibrinolysis, like coagulation, is a very complex process indeed. However, it is also clear that there are several possible approaches to enhancing fibrinolysis.

- Inject or ingest compounds that activate plasminogen.
- Increase availability or activity of tPA and/or urokinase.
- Curtail the activity of plasminogen activator inhibitors.

CONCLUSION

It is clear that there are numerous ways of blocking the platelet aggregation and coagulation processes and also several approaches to enhancing the fibrinolysis process. It would seem logical to select an approach that targets factors that exhibit abnormal levels in afibbers. There is now emerging evidence that atrial fibrillation patients tend to have higher than normal levels of the following factors [15-22]:

- Fibrinogen
- Fibrin monomer
- Fibrin D-dimer
- Factor VIII c (functional part of factor VIII)
- von Willebrand factor
- Prothrombin fragments F1 and F2
- Thrombin-antithrombin complex (TAT)
- Tissue-type plasminogen activator

It has been observed that patients with non-valvular afib have lower levels of prekallikrein, perhaps indicating heightened kallikrein activity [17]. It is also of interest that British researchers have found that permanent afibbers have higher plasma levels of fibrinogen and fibrin D-dimer than do paroxysmal afibbers who, again, have higher levels than non-afibbers [16].

It is of interest to note that, of the factors elevated in afibbers, only prothrombin (vitamin K dependent) and fibrinogen conversion would be affected by warfarin therapy. Fortunately, as we shall discuss later, there are other substances, mostly natural, that do substantially reduce the level of the other afib-specific factors.

REFERENCES

1. ACC/AHA/ESC guidelines for the management of patients with atrial fibrillation: executive summary. Circulation, Vol. 104, October 23, 2001, pp. 2118-50
2. van Walraven, Carl, et al. A clinical prediction rule to identify patients with atrial fibrillation and a low risk for stroke while taking aspirin. Archives of Internal Medicine, Vol. 163, April 28, 2003, pp. 936-43
3. Wang, Thomas J, et al. A risk score for predicting stroke or death in individuals with new-onset atrial fibrillation in the community. JAMA, Vol. 290, August 27, 2003, pp. 1049-56
4. Waldo, Albert L. Stroke prevention in atrial fibrillation. JAMA, Vol. 290, August 27, 2003, pp. 1093-95
5. Broderick, JP. Stroke therapy in the year 2025: burden, breakthroughs, and barriers to progress. Stroke, December 11, 2003
6. Feied, Craig. Pulmonary embolism. www.emedicine.com/emerg/topic490.htm
7. www.emedicine.com/emerg/byname/myocardial-infarction.htm
8. Frustaci, A, et al. Histological substrate of atrial biopsies in patients with lone atrial fibrillation. Circulation, Vol. 96, August 19, 1997, pp. 1180-84
9. Wintrobe's Clinical Hematology, 9th edition, 1993, Lea & Febiger, Philadelphia, pp. 511-39
10. ibid pp. 540-65
11. ibid pp. 566-615
12. ibid pp. 1515-51

13. Wintrobe's Clinical Hematology, 10th edition, 1999, Lippincott, Williams & Wilkins, Philadelphia, pp. 1789-90

14. Go, AS, et al. Factor V Leiden and risk of ischemic stroke in nonvalvular atrial fibrillation. J Thromb Thrombolysis. Vol. 15, No. 1, February 2003, pp. 41-46

15. Topcuoglu, MA, et al. Plasma levels of coagulation and fibrinolysis markers in acute ischemic stroke patients with lone atrial fibrillation. Neurol Sci, Vol. 21, 2000, pp. 235-240

16. Lip, GYH, et al. Fibrinogen and fibrin D-dimer levels in paroxysmal atrial fibrillation: evidence for intermediate elevated levels of intravascular thrombogenesis. American Heart Journal, Vol. 131, April 1996, pp. 724-30

17. Gustafsson, C, et al. Coagulation factors and the increased risk of stroke in nonvalvular atrial fibrillation. Stroke, Vol. 21, January 1990, pp. 47-51

18. Kahn, SR, et al. Nonvalvular atrial fibrillation: evidence for a prothrombotic state. Canadian Medical Association Journal, Vol. 157, September 15, 1997, pp. 673-81

19. Perez, LA, et al. Hypercoagulability in atrial fibrillation and its relationship with risk factors for systemic embolism. Rev Med Chile, Vol. 130, October 2002, pp. 1087-94 [article in Spanish]

20. Foo Leong Li-Saw-Hee, et al. Effect of degree of blood pressure on the hypercoagulable state in chronic atrial fibrillation. American Journal of Cardiology, Vol. 86, October 1, 2000, pp. 795-97

21. Falk, Rodney H and Podrid, PJ, editors. Atrial Fibrillation: Mechanisms and Management. 2nd edition, 1997, Lippincott-Raven Publishers, Philadelphia, p. 291

22. Conway, DS, et al. Atrial fibrillation and the prothrombotic state in the elderly: the Rotterdam Study. Stroke, Vol. 34, February 2003, pp. 413-17

Chapter 2

Underlying Causes of Thrombosis

MEASURING COAGULATION TIME

Before discussing the underlying causes of thrombosis and embolism, it is informative to briefly review the methods for determining the tendency of blood to clot. It is indeed unfortunate that the test in general use today, the prothrombin time (INR), is not an absolute measure of the blood's tendency to form a clot (thrombus), but rather a measure of the blood level of those coagulation factors that depend on vitamin K for their synthesis and the factors they, in turn, activate. In other words, the universal test today is primarily designed to measure blood level of warfarin. You can take aspirin, nattokinase, vitamin E, fish oils, garlic or whatever, to your heart's content, and it will make absolutely no difference to your INR – and yet these substances all have proven preventive effects against thrombus formation.

The problem is that the INR test only measures blood coagulation time in the extrinsic and common pathways. Retardation of the coagulation sequence by anti-platelet aggregation medications (aspirin, clopidogrel, ticlopidine), for example, will not affect INR because the sequence is halted in the intrinsic pathway before vitamin K-dependent coagulation factors become involved. Similarly, if the coagulation process is initiated via the intrinsic pathway and prekallikrein, factor VIII or von Willebrand factor are blocked then the thrombus formation sequence will not proceed either, but the INR test, because it bypasses the intrinsic pathway, will not show that you are protected even though you clearly are.

There are tests that will measure blood coagulation tendency in other than INR terms. The problem is that they are generally only used if a coagulation disorder (thrombocytopenia, von Willebrand's disease, hemophilia, platelet dysfunction, etc.) is suspected. The most important tests for measuring the blood's tendency to aggregate and clot are [1]:

Platelet count   Partial thromboplastin time
Fibrinogen assay   Plasma thrombin time
Factor VIII assay   Plasma Prothrombin time
Homocysteine assay

PLATELET COUNT

The intrinsic pathway of coagulation involves platelet activation and aggregation so having an inordinate amount of platelets in the blood is not a desirable state for afibbers. The number of platelets is counted using a microscope or automated assay technique and the common range is 130,000 to 400,000 per microliter [2]. There are also various tests for measuring platelet adhesion and aggregation.

Fibrinogen assay
Fibrinogen is the raw material for the fibrin that forms the clot. Thus having a low fibrinogen level is clearly desirable. As a matter of fact, there is now evidence that fibrinogen levels above 400 mg/dL significantly increase the risk of a cardiovascular event (heart attack, stroke or sudden death) independent of the presence of other risk factors [3]. There are several laboratory tests for fibrinogen level and the normal range is 200-400 mg/dL [2].

Factor VIII assay
The level of factor VIII is somewhat difficult to measure, but the partial thromboplastin time (PTT) can provide some idea for screening purposes.

Homocysteine assay
Although homocysteine is not directly involved in platelet aggregation or the coagulation cascade, it does have an indirect effect. There is a strong association between the formation of tears in blood vessel walls and a high homocysteine level. Since tears in the vessel wall are a prime initiator of thrombus formation, it is clearly desirable to have a low blood level of this sulfur-containing amino acid.

Partial thromboplastin time (PTT)
The PTT measures the blood's tendency to coagulate via the intrinsic and common pathways. It thus provides an indication of the concentration and activity of prekallikrein, HMW kinogen, intrinsic factors XII, XI, IX and VIII, and common pathway factors X, V, prothrombin, and fibrinogen. The test involves measuring the coagulation time after adding a platelet substitute to the blood. The test does not measure the level of factor VII as it completely bypasses the extrinsic pathway. PTT is particularly sensitive to factor VIII [1].

Plasma thrombin time
This test involves adding preformed thrombin to the blood and essentially measures the rate at which fibrin is formed from fibrinogen [1].

Plasma prothrombin time
The prothrombin time (PT) specifically measures the level of factors VII, V, X, prothrombin and fibrinogen in the blood. In other words, it evaluates the rate of blood coagulation via the extrinsic and common pathways; it is especially sensitive to factor VII. The test is carried out by collecting a sample of venous blood in a test tube containing sodium citrate (to prevent premature clotting). The plasma is separated and a standardized preparation of thromboplastin (usually from rabbit brain) is added to convert prothrombin to thrombin. The mixture is kept at 37 degrees C for 1-2 minutes before calcium chloride is added to counteract the effect of sodium citrate and allow the clotting to proceed. The PT is the time it takes for the blood plasma to clot after addition of the calcium chloride. The normal prothrombin time is 11-15 seconds and can vary depending on the source of the thromboplastin [1].

The International Normalized Ratio (INR) was developed in order to make it possible to compare coagulation results obtained using thromboplastin from different sources. The normal value is 1.0 corresponding to a clotting time of 11-15 seconds. An INR of 2.0 means that the clotting time has doubled, a value of 3.0 means it has tripled, etc. The desired INR for stroke prevention using warfarin in afibbers is usually between 2.0 and 3.0 [4].

Conclusion
There are several different tests for determining coagulation time. In stroke prevention, the only widely used one is the prothrombin time, which is specifically designed to measure vitamin K-dependent coagulation factors; in other words, the factors inactivated by warfarin. The effectiveness of other stroke prevention protocols such as the use of aspirin and natural supplements is not reflected in the results of the standard prothrombin time (INR) test.

CAUSES OF THROMBOSIS

Blocking platelet aggregation and coagulation and enhancing fibrinolysis are obvious ways of reducing thrombosis and stroke risk. This reduction can be achieved through the use of antiplatelet agents (aspirin), anticoagulants (warfarin) or natural substances. It is indeed tempting to just use one or more of these agents to reduce stroke risk and leave it at that. However, to do so clearly falls into the trap of dealing with symptoms rather than causes. Thrombi do not just appear "out of the blue", there is a reason for their appearance. In otherwise healthy people without prosthetic heart valves, thrombus formation is aided and abetted by one or more of the following conditions:

- Dysfunctional artery walls
- Blood stasis (stagnation)
- Inflammation and fibrosis on the walls of the atria

Dealing directly with these causes is likely to prove far more rewarding than dealing with the thrombi once they are formed or are in the process of being formed. As a matter of fact, recent guidelines for stroke prevention issued by the American Heart Association estimates that women can reduce their risk of having a stroke by an astounding 84% by maintaining a desirable body weight, exercising regularly, not smoking, eating a healthy diet, and consuming only moderate amounts of alcohol [5]. There is no reason to believe that a similar risk reduction could not be obtained by men following the same guidelines. So yes, addressing the causes of thrombus formation can indeed be most rewarding!

DYSFUNCTIONAL ARTERY WALLS

Arterial vessel walls that are stressed, damaged or otherwise dysfunctional are prime breeding grounds not only for blood clots, but also for atherosclerotic plaque. Both blood clots (thrombi) and dislodged plaque fragments can cause an embolic stroke. The main causes of dysfunctional artery walls are:

- **Endothelial dysfunction** – involves an abnormality in the endothelium (inner lining of the blood vessel) that results in increased platelet adhesiveness, inflammation, impaired synthesis and release of NO (nitric oxide), a reduction in the ability of blood vessels to dilate in response to increased blood flow, and an increased risk of stroke and heart attack [6,7]. Endothelial dysfunction is the forerunner of essential hypertension and atherosclerosis and is also strongly implicated in diabetes [8,9].

- **Essential hypertension** – is associated with endothelial dysfunction; however, its main cause involves abnormalities in kidney function [10]. It is of interest to note that patients with hypertension have been found to have lower NO levels and high levels of D-dimer, an important coagulation promoter [11]. Recent research has also linked hypertension to elevated homocysteine levels [12]. The high blood pressure involved in hypertension contributes to arterial wall dysfunctionality by putting constant stress on the walls, thus making them more prone to tears and subsequent clot and plaque formation.

- **Smoking** – not only causes endothelial dysfunction but also increases fibrinogen and homocysteine levels as well as the level of C-reactive protein – a potent marker of inflammation. Smoking is a really bad actor when it comes to thrombosis formation and stroke. It is estimated that smokers have at least double the risk of having a stroke as compared to non-smokers, so by quitting smokers can reduce their stroke risk by 50%. It should be noted that exposure to second-hand smoke also causes endothelial dysfunction [13].

- **High homocysteine levels** – are strongly associated with an increased formation of tears in blood vessel walls. A team of American researchers found that men and women with a homocysteine level above 14.2 micromol/L had an 82% higher risk of having a stroke than did those with a level of 9.25 micromol/L or less [14]. Israeli researchers recently confirmed the association between high homocysteine levels and stroke risk [15].

- **Hyperlipidemia** – or elevated levels of triglycerides and cholesterol, especially low-density lipoprotein (LDL) cholesterol, is a recognized risk factor for ischemic stroke. LDL cholesterol and triglycerides are particularly detrimental due to their propensity to oxidation and subsequent formation of atherosclerotic plaque.

- **Oxidative stress** – occurs when the body's natural defenses against attack by free radicals are overwhelmed. It is a significant factor in reperfusion injury often following in the aftermath of an ischemic stroke. Oxidative stress is closely associated with inflammation, endothelial dysfunction, and atherosclerosis [16].

- **Low levels of nitric oxide** – NO is produced in the walls of healthy blood vessels and helps to relax them so as to facilitate the flow of blood. NO also helps inhibit platelet aggregation and the adherence of blood cells to vessel walls – two important functions in the prevention of thrombosis [17,18]. A shortage of NO in the left atrium has been found to increase the level of plasminogen activator inhibitor 1 (PAI-1). Such an increase would slow down fibrinolysis and thus contribute to thrombosis [18].

There are, no doubt, other causes of dysfunctional artery walls, but the ones discussed here are the major ones and ones that can, to a large extent, be controlled through diet and lifestyle changes combined with judicious supplementation. This will be discussed later in greater detail.

BLOOD STASIS

Stagnation of blood flow in the atrium, more specifically in the left atrial appendage (a small pouch connected to the left atrium), is an important factor in the formation of cardiogenic emboli and subsequent stroke. Japanese researchers checked 50 patients with permanent non-valvular atrial fibrillation and 12 patients with atrial flutter for the presence of thrombi in the left atrial appendage (LAA) using transesophageal echocardiography (TEE). They found no thrombi in patients with atrial flutter nor in those with lone atrial fibrillation; however, they did observe thrombi in 17% of afibbers whose AF did not fall in the category of "lone" [19]. Another group of Japanese researchers investigated 50 permanent afibbers with a history of prior cardioembolic stroke and found that 38% had thrombi in the LAA [20].

The developers of the PLAATO system for sealing off the LAA evaluated 15 permanent afibbers with severe cardiovascular disease and a high risk for stroke. They found LAA thrombi in 90% of the patients [21].

Researchers at the University of Louisville in the USA carried out a large study to determine the association between having a thrombus in the LAA and suffering a subsequent transient ischemic attack (TIA, mini-stroke). Their study involved 261 men and women who had been in atrial fibrillation for at least 4 days. About 70% had hypertension. Using transesophageal echocardiography (TEE) the researchers found that 18% of the participants had a thrombus in the LAA. The patients with thrombi were far more likely to have congestive heart failure (67% versus 30%), permanent afib (91% versus 67%) or to have suffered a prior cardiovascular event to TIA (52% versus 27%) than were patient without a discernible thrombus.

Clearly, the presence of thrombi in the LAA is related to the severity of the afib (permanent versus paroxysmal), the presence of heart failure, and a prior history of cardiovascular events. However, even among these quite sick people, thrombi were only found in 18% and the TIA rate among them was 9.2% per year as compared to 1.9% per year in the group without thrombi. The researchers noted that 75% of the participants with thrombi were on warfarin, but still had a total embolic event rate of 13.8% per year. They conclude that warfarin is not very effective in preventing or eliminating LAA thrombi in AF patients [22,23].

Other researchers have, however, found that prolonged anticoagulation with warfarin eventually resolves up to 90% of atrial thrombi [24].

It is clear that estimates of the incidence of thrombi in the LAA of permanent afibbers varies widely from 0-90% depending on prior stroke history and severity of underlying heart disease. However, it would seem that the incidence of LAA thrombi in otherwise healthy afibbers is negligible, particularly in the case of paroxysmal afibbers.

A landmark study, by cardiologists at the Medical College of Virginia, found that blood flow through the appendage was quite adequate (average ejection fraction of 46%) during normal sinus rhythm, but declined significantly (average ejection fraction of 26%) during an afib episode thus resulting in blood stagnation. Blood stagnation can promote thrombus formation because the concentration of coagulation factors tends to increase when blood flow is reduced and the blood is not regularly "cleaned up" by passing through the liver. The Virginia researchers also observed a very strong inverse correlation between heart rate during atrial fibrillation and LAA ejection fraction. They reason that a slower heart rates gives the left ventricle a better chance to fill up before it ejects its contents into the arteries. The wall of the left ventricle abuts the LAA so a more distended ventricle would tend to compress the LAA and then let it expand again when the ventricle empties. This would increase the blood flow in and out of the LAA and thus prevent stagnation [25]. These findings underscore the importance of keeping the heart rate under control, i.e. below 100 or, better still, below 90 bpm in order to avoid thrombus formation in the LAA. They also explain why emboli in the LAA are more common among afibbers with severe heart disease and reduced left ventricular ejection fraction [21].

Italian researchers have confirmed that the blood flow through the LAA is significantly lower during afib than during sinus rhythm and that thrombus formation in the LAA is associated with an exceptionally low rate of flow through the LAA [26]. American researchers have found that blood flow through the LAA is lower in older patients with heart disease-related atrial fibrillation than in younger patients [27]. Japanese researchers have found that blood flow through the LAA decreases with age in people with normal sinus rhythm [28]. Fortunately, a recent study also carried out by Japanese researchers concludes that lone afibbers (afibbers without underlying heart disease) and people with atrial flutter are at very low risk for thrombus formation in the LAA [19]. Of particular interest is the finding that thrombosis in the LAA may be related to elevated levels of von Willebrand factor [29,30].

INFLAMMATION AND FIBROSIS ON ATRIAL WALLS

Biopsies of atria in LAF patients have clearly shown the presence of inflammation and fibrosis and there is ample evidence that inflammation and infection are potent risk factors for ischemic stroke [31,32]. These abnormalities in the endothelial lining of the atria would have an effect similar to endothelial dysfunction as far as the activation and aggregation of platelets is concerned. It is also likely that the inflammation-induced platelet aggregation could lead to subsequent blood coagulation via the intrinsic pathway. Thus it would seem reasonable to assume that protocols aimed at reducing the risk of thrombi related to endothelial dysfunction would also be effective in reducing the risk of thrombi related to inflammation and fibrosis of atrial walls.

CONCLUSION

For younger lone afibbers with no atherosclerosis or hypertension, I would speculate that the left atrium walls would be the most likely source of thrombi; however, if hypertension, atherosclerosis or diabetes is present, then endothelial dysfunction in the arteries may increase in importance. I personally have a bit of a problem blaming atrial fibrillation for a stroke occurring in a patient with hypertension, diabetes or atherosclerosis. All of these conditions are, themselves, associated with an elevated risk of stroke and it is not at all clear how having afib as a comorbid condition would increase this already existing risk. Unless, of course, the rapid, irregular heart beat would facilitate the dislodging of an unstable plaque or blood clot in the arteries feeding the brain. I have seen no evidence that this actually happens.

Considering the Japanese and American findings, it is unlikely that thrombi originating in the left atrial appendage are a significant source of emboli in otherwise healthy afibbers. However, it is likely that blood stagnation in the LAA could become important with age, declining left ventricular ejection fraction, and a prior history of TIA or stroke [19,22, 23].

REFERENCES

1. Wintrobe's Clinical Hematology, 9th edition, 1993, Lea & Febiger, Philadelphia, pp. 1301-24
2. Harrison's Principles of Internal Medicine, 12th edition, 1991, McGraw-Hill, NY, p. A5
3. Palmieri, V, et al. Relation of fibrinogen to cardiovascular events is independent of preclinical cardiovascular disease: the Strong Heart Study. American Heart Journal, Vol. 145, March 2003, pp. 467-74
4. Wintrobe's Clinical Hematology, 9th edition, 1993, Lea & Febiger, Philadelphia, pp. 1515-51
5. Pearson, TA, et al. AHA guidelines for primary prevention of cardiovascular disease and stroke: 2002 update. Circulation, Vol. 106, July 16, 2002, pp. 388-91

6. Egashira, K. Clinical importance of endothelial function in arteriosclerosis and ischemic heart disease. Circulation Journal, Vol. 66, June 2002, pp. 529-33

7. Targonski, PV, et al. Coronary endothelial dysfunction is associated with an increased risk of cerebrovascular events. Circulation, Vol. 107, June 10, 2003, pp. 2805-09, 2766-68

8. Ercan, E, et al. Left ventricular hypertrophy and endothelial functions in patients with essential hypertension. Coron Artery Dis, Vol. 14, December 2003, pp. 541-44

9. Caballero, AE. Endothelial dysfunction in obesity and insulin resistance: a road to diabetes and heart disease. Obes Res, Vol. 11, November 2003, pp. 1278-89

10. Ritz, E, et al. Kidney and hypertension: causes. Herz, Vol. 28, No. 8, 2003, pp. 663-67

11. Zhang, WR, et al. Serum nitric oxide and D-dimer before and after administering antihypertensive drugs in essential hypertension. Hunan Yi Ke Da Xue Xue Boa, Vol. 28, August 2003, pp. 382-84 [article in Chinese] (abstract only)

12. Rodrigo, R, et al. Homocysteine and essential hypertension. J Clin Pharmacol, Vol. 43, December 2003, pp. 1299-1306

13. Tsiara, S, et al. Influence of smoking on predictors of vascular disease. Angiology, Vol. 54, September-October 2003, pp. 507-30

14. Bostom, AG, et al. Nonfasting plasma total homocysteine levels and stroke incidence in elderly persons. Annals of Internal Medicine, Vol. 131, September 7, 1999, pp. 352-55

15. Tanne, D and Sela, BA. Neurological implications of hyperhomocysteinemia in patients with atherothrombotic disease. Italian Heart Journal, Vol. 4, September 2003, pp. 577-79

16. Fenster, BE, et al. Endothelial dysfunction: clinical strategies for treating oxidant stress. American Hear Journal, Vol. 146, August 2003, pp. 218-26

17. Huang, PL. Endothelial nitric oxide synthase and endothelial dysfunction. Curr Hypertens Rep, Vol. 5, December 2003, pp. 473-80

18. Cai, H, et al. Down regulation of endocardial nitric oxide synthase expression and nitric oxide production in atrial fibrillation: potential mechanisms for atrial thrombosis and stroke. Circulation, Vol. 106, November 26, 2002, pp. 2764-66 and 2854-58

19. Narumiya, T, et al. Relationship between left atrial appendage function and left atrial thrombus in patients with nonvalvular chronic atrial fibrillation and atrial flutter. Circulation Journal, Vol. 67, January 2003, pp. 68-72

20. Ohyama, H, et al. Comparison of magnetic resonance imaging and transesophageal echocardiography in detection of thrombus in the left atrial appendage. Stroke, Vol. 34, October 2003, pp. 2436-39

21. Sievert, H, et al. Percutaneous left atrial appendage transcatheter occlusion to prevent stroke in high-risk patients with atrial fibrillation: early clinical experience. Circulation, Vol. 105, April 23, 2002, pp. 1887-89

22. Stoddard, MF, et al. Left atrial thrombus predicts transient ischemic attack in patients with atrial fibrillation. American Heart Journal, Vol. 145, April 2003, pp. 676-82

23. Sheahan, RG. Left atrial thrombus, transient ischemic attack, and atrial fibrillation: Does left atrial thrombus predict? Does absence protect? American Heart Journal, Vol. 145, April 2003, pp. 582-85

24. Collins, IJ, et al. Cardioversion of non-rheumatic atrial fibrillation: Reduced thromboembolic complications with 4 weeks of precardioversion anticoagulation are related to atrial thrombus resolution. Circulation, Vol. 92, 1995, pp. 160-63

25. Akosah, KO, et al.   Left atrial appendage contractile function in atrial fibrillation. Chest, Vol. 107, March 1995, pp. 690-96
26. Alessandri, N, et al. Thrombus formation in the left atrial appendage in the course of atrial fibrillation. Eur Rev Med Pharmacol Sci, Vol. 7, May-June 2003, pp. 65-73
27. Ilercil, A, et al. Influence of age on left atrial appendage function in patients with nonvalvular atrial fibrillation. Clin Cardiol, Vol. 24, January 2001, pp. 39-44
28. Tabata, T, et al. Influence of aging on left atrial appendage flow velocity patterns in normal subjects. J Am Soc Echocardiogr, Vol. 9, May-June 1996, pp. 274-80
29. Heppell, RM, et al.   Haemostatic and haemodynamics abnormalities associated with left atrial thrombosis in non-rheumatic atrial fibrillation. Heart, Vol. 77, 1997, pp. 407-11
30. Fukuchi, M, et al. Increased von Willebrand factor in the endocardium as a local predisposing factor for thrombogenesis in overloaded human atrial appendage. Journal of the American College of Cardiology, Vol. 37, 2001, pp. 1436-42
31. Frustaci, A., et al. Histological substrate of atrial biopsies in patients with lone atrial fibrillation. Circulation, Vol. 96, August 19, 1997, pp. 1180-84
32. Lindsberg, PJ and Grau, AJ. Inflammation and infections as risk factors for ischemic stroke. Stroke, Vol. 34, October 2003, pp. 2518-32

Chapter 3

Natural Approaches to Stroke Prevention

Effective prevention of thrombosis and stroke involves one or both of two approaches:

- Eliminate or reduce artery wall dysfunctionality, atrial inflammation and blood stasis.
- Use drugs or natural substances to prevent thrombosis.

Apart from regular exercise, it is not immediately obvious what can be done about reducing blood stasis in the left atrial appendage (LAA); so potential thrombus formation in the LAA is probably best prevented by the use of drugs or natural substances such as nattokinase.

While most pharmaceutical drugs are quite specific in their thrombosis-preventing action, several natural approaches not only inhibit specific promoters of platelet aggregation and coagulation, but also help to reduce inflammation and artery wall dysfunctionality.

VITAMIN B COCKTAIL

A daily vitamin B cocktail (vitamin B6, vitamin B12 and folic acid) is probably the most important supplement that an afibber, or anyone else for that matter, can take. The vitamin B cocktail effectively lowers the level of homocysteine in the blood. Homocysteine, a sulfur-containing amino acid, is certainly one of the arch villains when it comes to stroke, but is also involved in numerous other disease conditions:

- As mentioned in Chapter 2 of this book, a group of American researchers has found that a high blood level of homocysteine is associated with an increased risk of stroke even after adjusting for other known risk factors such as advanced age, hypertension, smoking, diabetes, heart disease, and atrial fibrillation. The researchers found that those of the 1947 study participants who had homocysteine levels greater than 14.2 micromol/L had an 82% greater incidence of stroke over the 10-year study period than did participants with an level of 9.25 micromol/L or less. It is interesting that the average annual stroke incidence among the study participants (average age of 70 years) was only 0.8% [1].

- Dutch researchers have found that high homocysteine levels are associated with a significantly higher risk of both stroke and heart attack. Their study involved 7983 elderly subjects who had their homocysteine level measured in July 1993. By December 1994, 120 of the participants had suffered a stroke and 104 had experienced a heart attack. The researchers found that stroke and heart attack risk increased linearly with an increase in homocysteine level so that a 1 micromol/L increase in homocysteine corresponded to a 6-7% increase in risk of stroke or heart attack. Study participants with the highest homocysteine level had a two times higher risk of stroke than did those with the lowest level after adjusting for age, sex, smoking, hypertension, cholesterol level, and diabetes. The increased stroke risk applied to both ischemic and hemorrhagic stroke and was further increased by the presence of hypertension. It is interesting to note that the annual incidence of stroke in the group was only 1.0% [2].

There are numerous other studies attesting to the association between high homocysteine levels and stroke risk. Many have found associations between high homocysteine levels and other disorders making homocysteine, without a doubt, one of the top villains on the health scene.

- Swiss researchers have observed a strong association between coronary artery disease and high homocysteine levels. They found that an increase of just 5 micromol/L corresponds to an increased risk of coronary artery disease of 60% in men and 80% in women. They also found that homocysteine levels increased in a linear fashion among 631 patients undergoing angiography from 9.2 micromol/L for patients with no coronary disease to 12.4 micromol/L in patients with three-vessel disease [3].

- Taiwanese researchers have found a strong link between high homocysteine levels and the presence of endothelial dysfunction and atherosclerosis. Perhaps not surprisingly, they also found that a high-protein meal will markedly elevate homocysteine levels. Fortunately, they also found that 5 weeks supplementation with the vitamin B cocktail reduces this protein-meal-induced homocysteine rise quite significantly [4].

- Researchers at the Boston University School of Medicine report that people with a homocysteine level above 14 micromol/L have nearly twice the risk of developing Alzheimer's disease as do people with lower levels. They also determined that a 5 micromol/L increase in homocysteine level corresponds to a 40% increased risk of Alzheimer's [5].

- Italian researchers have observed a strong correlation between elevated homocysteine levels and the incidence of deep vein thrombosis (DVT). They found that the incidence of DVT was twice as high among people with high homocysteine levels as among those with low levels [6]. This finding is particularly intriguing when considering that DVT is associated with blood stagnation in the veins of the legs. Blood stagnation is also a key factor in the formation of blood clots in the left atrial appendage (LAA). Thus it would seem likely that high homocysteine levels may be involved in thrombosis originating in the LAA and by inference, that measures that will prevent DVT and/or lower homocysteine levels will also have a salutary effect on LAA thrombosis.

- American researchers have established that the normal blood level of homocysteine is about 10-12 micromol/L. (NOTE: "normal" does not necessarily equate with "healthy"). Heart disease and stroke patients often have levels of 15 micromol/L or higher and elevated levels have also been observed among patients with intermittent claudication, hypothyroidism, lupus erythematosus, venous thrombosis, and psoriasis. High homocysteine levels are also common among patients taking medications such as methotrexate, levodopa, niacin, phenytoin (Dilantin), carbamazepine, and theophylline [7].

- Norwegian researchers have found that for every 5.0 micromol/L that the blood level of homocysteine exceeds 9.0 micromol/L, cardiovascular mortality increases by 50%, cancer mortality by 26%, and death from other causes (respiratory, gastrointestinal and central nervous system diseases) by 104%. They conclude that high homocysteine levels have a pervasive negative effect on longevity [8].

By now it should be abundantly clear that homocysteine is a very bad actor indeed and that maintaining low blood levels are of utmost importance. Taking steps to do so is particularly important for people eating a high-protein diet. Taiwanese researchers have found that consuming a high-protein meal rapidly increases homocysteine level to 20 micromol/L or more while at the same time constricting arterial blood flow [4].

Fortunately, it is easy, inexpensive, and safe to reduce homocysteine levels by regular supplementation with the vitamin B cocktail. "Regular" is a key term here. It takes about 4 to 5 weeks of supplementation to achieve maximum homocysteine reduction and much longer than that to reverse endothelial dysfunction. There is also evidence that homocysteine levels tend to rise again if daily supplementation is discontinued [9]. Numerous researchers have investigated just how much of the cocktail is required to achieve optimum results.

- Researchers at the Cleveland Clinic observed that a combination of 400 micrograms/day of folic acid plus 12.5 mg/day of vitamin B6 plus 500 micrograms/day of vitamin B12 reduced homocysteine levels in heart disease patients from an average of 13.8 micromol/L to 9.6 micromol/L over a 90-day period [10].

- Taiwanese researchers found that healthy women who supplemented with 5 mg/day of folic acid, 100 mg of vitamin B6, and 500 micrograms/day of vitamin B12 reduced their homocysteine level to 5.2 micromol/L after 5 weeks [4].

Other researchers have evaluated different protocols, but overall it would seem that 400-800 micrograms/day of folic acid plus 10-100 mg/day of vitamin B6 plus 500-1000 micrograms/day of vitamin B12 (a sublingual tablet is best) will do the trick. My own daily regimen is 400 micrograms of natural folate, 50 mg of vitamin B6, and a sublingual vitamin B12 tablet containing 1000 micrograms of methyl-cobalamin. Some very recent research has shown that the commonly used folic acid supplement (pteroylmonoglutamate) may not be converted to folate if doses above 400 micrograms are taken. It is not known what the long-term effects of an accumulation of unconverted pteroylmonoglutamate might be, so unless under a doctor's supervision, it would be prudent not to exceed a folic acid supplement intake of 400 micrograms/day or even better use natural 5-methyltetrahydrofolate as the folate source [11].

It is likely that the vitamin B cocktail works to prevent stroke not just by lowering homocysteine levels, but also by reducing the level of the thrombin-antithrombin III complex and by partial inhibition of thrombin generation [12].

In closing, high homocysteine levels are associated with inflammation. Inflammation is a key player in lone atrial fibrillation [13]. Is it possible that reducing homocysteine levels with the vitamin B cocktail would also reduce afib episode frequency? Time will tell.

VITAMIN B6 (PYRIDOXINE)

There is considerable evidence that low blood levels of vitamin B6 or, rather, its metabolite pyridoxal-5'-phosphate (PLP, P5P) are associated with an increased risk of stroke. This risk increase is independent of homocysteine level [14,15]. There is also evidence that low vitamin B6 levels increase the risk of deep vein thrombosis [6].

South African and Turkish researchers have found that vitamin B6 supplementation is effective in increasing bleeding time by about 65% and that the underlying mechanism involves a significant reduction in platelet aggregation through inhibition of both ADP (adenosine diphosphate)- and epinephrine-induced aggregation [16,17]. The Turkish researchers found that daily supplementation with about 350 mg (5 mg/kg) of vitamin B6 reduced ADP-induced aggregation by 48% and epinephrine-induced aggregation by 41% [17]. The South African researchers achieved similar results using 2 x 100 mg per day of vitamin B6 and also noted that B6 did not inhibit prostacyclin production [16].

Italian researchers have noted that people with low levels of vitamin B6 (less than 33.2 nanomol/L of PLP) have twice the risk of developing deep vein thrombosis than do people with levels above 46.5 nanomol/L [6]. The finding that high vitamin B6 levels may be protective against deep vein thrombosis is of particular interest to afibbers. It is highly likely that the mechanism (blood coagulation or inadequate fibrinolysis) involved in deep vein thrombosis is very similar to the mechanism involved in thrombus formation in the left atrial appendage. Thus, if vitamin B6 is protective against deep vein thrombosis, it may also be protective against thrombosis and stroke in atrial fibrillation.

Canadian researchers have found that supplementation with 100 mg/day of vitamin B6 for 10 weeks is associated with a 146% improvement in endothelial function in heart transplant patients [18]. More recently, researchers at the Harvard Medical School and the Massachusetts General Hospital discovered a strong association between stroke risk and blood level of PLP. This increased risk of stroke with low PLP levels was entirely independent of homocysteine levels confirming that vitamin B6, on its own, has significant stroke prevention properties. The researchers found that study participants with a plasma level of PLP of more than 80 nanomol/L had a 90% lower risk of stroke and transient ischemic attacks (TIAs) than did participants with a level below 20 nanomol/L. The risk decrease was independent of the presence of other risk factors such as hypertension, diabetes, and atrial fibrillation [15]. The researchers also noted a strong inverse correlation between C-reactive protein level and PLP level indicating that vitamin B6 may also have strong anti-inflammatory properties – an added plus for afibbers.

The 90% relative reduction in stroke risk among people with high PLP levels is very significant and compares extremely favourably with the oft-quoted relative risk reduction afforded by warfarin (64%) and aspirin (25%). Clearly, ensuring adequate blood levels of PLP is a must for all afibbers. Vitamin B6 is converted to its active metabolite PLP in the liver and there is some evidence that the liver can only handle about 50 mg of vitamin B6 at a time. Experiments have shown that the plasma concentration of PLP does not increase further if 100 mg rather than 50 mg of pyridoxine is ingested at any one time. So it is assumed that the conversion to PLP is limited by the liver's conversion capacity [19]. Other experiments have shown that supplementing (orally) with 40 mg of vitamin B6 will increase average plasma concentration from about 23 nmol/L (range: 18-37 nmol/L) to about 230 nmol/L within 3 days of beginning supplementation. No further increases were observed with 40 mg/day supplementation for a 12-week period [20].

The 230 nmol/L concentration achieved is well above the 80 nmol/L concentration associated with the 90% reduction in stroke risk observed by the Harvard researchers [15]. So 40-50 mg/day would seem to be sufficient for stroke protection and is considered entirely safe [20].

Vitamin B6 itself is, however, water-soluble and any excess is totally eliminated in the urine within about 9 hours. To keep the vitamin B concentration up, it would be necessary to take two or three 50 mg doses per day. However, in the case of stroke protection, one 50 mg dose per day is likely to be quite adequate, as PLP concentration does not vary much during the day once steady state conditions are achieved. Adequate amounts of vitamin B2 and magnesium are required in order to convert vitamin B6 to PLP. NOTE: If taking the vitamin B cocktail, there is no need for additional vitamin B6 in order to reap the benefits of its stroke prevention properties.

VITAMIN C

Vitamin C is a powerful antioxidant and as such helps to prevent oxidative stress, a major underlying cause of thrombosis and reperfusion injury. A low intake of vitamin C has been linked to a doubling of the risk of dying from a stroke [21, 22]. Finnish researchers recently reported that low vitamin C levels are also associated with an increased risk of actually having a stroke whether ischemic (caused by a blood clot) or hemorrhagic (caused by a burst blood vessel). Their study involved 2419 randomly selected middle-aged men (42 to 60 years of age) with no history of stroke at the baseline examination. The men were followed for an average of 10.4 years during which time 96 ischemic and 24 hemorrhagic strokes were documented. This corresponds to a total stroke incidence of 0.5% per year.

After adjusting for age, month of examination (vitamin C levels tend to vary with the seasons), body mass index, systolic blood pressure, smoking, alcohol consumption, total cholesterol level, and presence of diabetes or exercise-induced angina, the researchers observed that men with a plasma vitamin C level below 28.4 micromol/L had twice the risk of having a stroke when compared to men with a level above 65 micromol/L. The association was particularly pronounced among hypertensive men where low vitamin C levels were associated with a 2.6 times higher risk and among overweight men where low levels were associated with a 2.7-fold risk increase. The researchers have also observed a significant association between low vitamin C levels and elevated blood pressure (hypertension). They conclude that a low vitamin C level is an independent risk factor for both ischemic and hemorrhagic stroke, especially among hypertensive and overweight men. They call for clinical trials to test the efficacy of vitamin C supplements in the prevention of stroke among hypertensive and overweight (BMI greater than 25 kg/sq m) and obese men [23].

It is likely that vitamin C's stroke protection properties are associated with its ability to

- reduce endothelial dysfunction;
- reduce the level of von Willebrand factor;
- reduce the level of plasminogen activation inhibitor-1 (PAI-1)

Greek researchers have observed that daily supplementation with 2000 mg of vitamin C plus 800 IU of vitamin E markedly reduces plasma levels of PAI-1 and von Willebrand factor in smokers [24]. High PAI-1 levels are associated with a reduction in fibrinolytic activity and high von Willebrand factor levels are associated with enhanced coagulation.

Another group of Greek researchers found that daily supplementation with 2000 mg of vitamin C for 4 weeks significantly reduced endothelial dysfunction and decreased the level of von Willebrand factor in a group of patients with diabetes and coronary artery disease. The level of tissue plasminogen activator tPA) was also decreased corresponding to a decrease in fibrinolytic activity in this group of patients [25].

Other researchers have found that daily supplementation with 2 x 1000 mg of vitamin C for 6 months increases serum ascorbic acid levels by about 96%, increases fibrinolytic activity by 45-63%, and decreases platelet adhesive index by 27% [26]. The recently completed Rotterdam study found clear evidence that a high dietary intake of vitamin C significantly reduces the risk of ischemic stroke, especially among smokers [27]. It is interesting to note that the average incidence of ischemic stroke among the 5,197 participants in the Rotterdam study was 0.7% per year.

The above findings, particularly the Finnish study, underscores the importance of including vitamin C supplementation in a comprehensive stroke prevention program. The 50% relative risk reduction associated with high vitamin C levels compares favourably to the relative reduction quoted for warfarin (64%) and aspirin (25%). Tissue saturation with vitamin C (about 70 micromol/L in plasma) can be obtained by supplementing with 300-500 mg of vitamin C three times a day.

VITAMIN E

Vitamin E is a powerful, fat-soluble antioxidant that, together with vitamin C, protects cells against oxidative stress, an important underlying cause of stroke and cardiovascular disease. There is considerable epidemiologic evidence that supplementing with 100 IU/day or more of vitamin E is effective in reducing the incidence of heart disease by about 40% and the incidence of ischemic stroke by about 30% [28,29]. Larger daily intakes of vitamin E (800 IU/day) have been associated with a 77% reduction in the incidence of non-fatal heart attacks [30]. Other studies have concluded that vitamin E supplementation with 100 IU or more is effective in slowing the progression of atherosclerosis [31].

While there is little doubt about the benefit of vitamin E in *preventing* cardiovascular disease, two recent clinical trials concluded that it is not effective in *reversing* existing disease [32,33]. This is not really surprising. The main effect of antioxidants is that they help prevent (delay) the initiation of disease. They are not effective, certainly not in the amounts used in the trials, in reversing or even slowing down the progression of disease once it has taken hold. This is very basic antioxidant theory, but a point that seems to be ignored by many medical researchers. There are numerous studies that have shown vitamin E and Vitamin C to be effective in preventing many different conditions, but very few that have shown a curative effect.

Vitamin E produces its beneficial effects through three separate mechanisms:

- Prevention of lipid peroxidation, especially of low-density lipoprotein (LDL) cholesterol
- Improvement of endothelial function

- Inhibition of platelet aggregation and coagulation.

Vitamin E has been found to prevent or reverse endothelial dysfunction, especially in patients with cardiovascular disease, diabetes or high cholesterol level. It preserves or enhances the ability of endothelial tissue to produce nitric oxide and reduces the tendency of monocytes to adhere to vessel walls [34].

Vitamin E (100 IU/day) has been found to reduce platelet aggregation by inhibiting the release of arachidonic acid and thromboxane A2 [35]. Researchers at the Boston University School of Medicine found that a specific enzyme, protein kinase C (PKC), found in platelets will induce platelet aggregation and adhesion when stimulated by certain compounds. The researchers also discovered that supplementation with vitamin E completely suppresses this negative effect of PKC. Their experiment involved 15 volunteers who were given 400, 800 or 1200 IU/day of vitamin E for a 14-day period. The vitamin E content of the volunteers' platelets increased from 38.9 pmol/100 million platelets to 81.2, 96.0 and 160.5 pmol/100 million platelets respectively. PKC stimulation was completely inhibited at all three levels of vitamin E supplementation. The researchers conclude that vitamin E's ability to inhibit PKC stimulation and subsequent platelet aggregation and adhesion is an additional, beneficial effect that is not related to its ability to protect LDL against oxidation [36].

Other researchers have found that vitamin E profoundly inhibits platelet aggregation without affecting clotting time as measured with the prothrombin time test [37]. Yet, others have observed that vitamin E increases prostacyclin production and decreases von Willebrand factor activity [38]. Supplementation with 600 mg/day of vitamin E has been found to markedly decrease (by 25%) the blood level of prothrombin fragments 1 and 2 [39]. This would indicate that vitamin E can affect the common pathway in the coagulation cascade to possibly lengthen bleeding time. There is no indication that vitamin E affects the level of vitamin K-dependent coagulation factors except in people with certain specific coagulation disorders. There is also no indication that vitamin E alters the coagulation pattern in normal, warfarin-treated patients, so there is no reason to shun vitamin E supplementation when taking warfarin [40].

It is clear that vitamin E has a profound inhibitory effect on platelet aggregation and possibly some minor effect on thrombin generation. These effects, as well as its proven ability to combat oxidative stress and prevent or reverse endothelial dysfunction, are undoubtedly what underlies vitamin E's observed ability to reduce the incidence of ischemic stroke by about 30%.

It is interesting that combining vitamin E (300 mg/day) with vitamin C (600 mg/day), selenium (75 micrograms/day) and beta-carotene (27 mg/day) has an even more pronounced effect on platelet aggregation than does vitamin E alone. Finnish researchers found that supplementing with the above "cocktail" for 5 months reduced serum lipid peroxides by 20%, ADP-induced platelet aggregation by 24%, ATP release during aggregation by 42%, and produced an astounding 51% reduction in platelet-produced thromboxane B2[41].

The bottom line is that vitamin E is effective in preventing thrombosis related to platelet aggregation, is safe, does not cause bleeding, and does not interact with warfarin except possibly in some patients with specific coagulation disorders. An appropriate daily dose for stroke prevention is 400-600 IU/day. Vitamin E should always be taken in its natural form (d-alpha tocopherol) and in combination with vitamin C (3 x 300-500 mg/day).

NIACIN (VITAMIN B3)

Patients with peripheral arterial disease (PAD) have a high risk of stroke so are usually treated with warfarin. A recent clinical trial involving PAD patients found that warfarin therapy (INR 1.5-2.0) resulted in a significant drop in coagulation factor VIIc (18% drop as compared to placebo group) and in the level of prothrombin fragments 1 and 2 (48% drop as compared to placebo group). No significant decreases in fibrinogen or von Willebrand factor were observed.

As part of the trial a separate group of PAD patients were given 2 x 1500 mg of niacin (vitamin B3) daily. After one year, there was a significant 14% decrease in fibrinogen and a remarkable 60% decrease in prothrombin fragments 1 and 2. There was no effect on the level of von Willebrand factor. The researchers involved in the trial conclude that high-dose niacin has a potentially beneficial effect on coagulation parameters in patients with established PAD [42].

LYCOPENE

The carotenoid lycopene is a powerful antioxidant, particularly abundant in tomatoes. There is evidence that it helps prevent lung and prostate cancer [43,44]. Italian researchers have reported an inverse correlation between blood level of lycopene and the severity of atherosclerosis and peripheral vascular disease (intermittent claudication) [45]. Austrian researchers have reported that elderly people with microangiopathy-related cerebral damage have significantly higher blood levels of fibrinogen and significantly lower levels of lycopene and vitamin E [46].

Finnish researchers recently reported that middle-aged men with low lycopene levels have a 3.3-fold higher risk of suffering a heart attack or stroke than do men with normal levels. They also found that the intima-media thickness of the common carotid artery wall (a measurement of atherosclerosis) was 18% higher in men with a low lycopene level. They conclude that low levels of lycopene may play a role in the early stages of atherogenesis (endothelial dysfunction) [47].

It is not clear exactly how lycopene exerts its protective effects in cancer, heart disease and stroke; however, it is known that it is the most effective neutralizer of singlet oxygen, a powerful free radical [48]. Lycopene can be obtained from tomatoes or, even better, from processed tomato products such as tomato paste and juice. Supplements are also effective in increasing blood levels of lycopene [49].

MAGNESIUM

Not only is magnesium effective in reducing ectopic beats and perhaps atrial fibrillation episodes as well, there is now also emerging evidence that it may help protect against ischemic stroke. Austrian researchers recently investigated the association between serum magnesium levels and the risk of having an ischemic stroke or needing carotid revascularization (removal of the inner wall of the carotid artery or the placement of a stent to restore blood flow through the carotid artery). Their study involved 323 patients with advanced atherosclerosis (symptomatic peripheral artery disease and intermittent claudication). The patients (197 men and 126 women with an average age of 68 years) had their serum magnesium level measured and were then followed for 20 months. At the end of the study period, 35 patients had suffered an ischemic stroke or had needed revascularization or both. The researchers found that patients with a serum magnesium level below 0.76 mmol/L had a three times higher risk of experiencing a neurological event (stroke or revascularization) than did patients with a magnesium level of more than 0.84 mmol/L. Although these results, obtained in patients with advanced atherosclerosis, may not be directly applicable to lone afibbers they certainly do indicate that magnesium could play an important role in stroke prevention [50].

American researchers have reported that magnesium supplementation helps prevent the formation of blood clots in patients with coronary artery disease [51]. There is also evidence that magnesium injections given within 6 hours of suffering an ischemic stroke can markedly reduce stroke damage [52]. It is possible that magnesium may also, in a more indirect way, help to protect against stroke by preventing hypertension, a recognized risk factor for stroke.

Researchers at Harvard Medical School have reported that men whose daily magnesium intake is less than 250 mg/day have a 50% greater risk of developing hypertension than do men whose daily intake exceeds 400 mg [53]. Dutch researchers have found that magnesium supplementation is effective in lowering both systolic and diastolic blood pressure in women with moderate hypertension [54]. There is also evidence that magnesium supplementation is effective in reversing endothelial dysfunction, a recognized risk factor for stroke [55].

POTASSIUM

Several studies have observed that low potassium levels are associated with a greater mortality from stroke. American researchers have found that the risk of having a stroke also increases with low potassium levels. Their study involved 5600 men and women over the age of 65 years who were free of stroke at enrollment in 1990-93. All participants underwent a thorough medical examination at baseline, completed a food frequency questionnaire, and had blood serum potassium level determined. After 4 to 8 years of follow-up, a total of 473 strokes (404 ischemic) had occurred in the group. The researchers found that participants on diuretics had a 2.5 times increased risk of stroke if their serum level of potassium was below 4.1 mEq/L. Participants who were not taking diuretics were found to have a 50% increased risk of stroke if their dietary potassium intake was less than 2340 mg/day [56,57].

Researchers at Harvard Medical School studied 43,738 male health professionals. During 8 years of follow-up, 328 strokes (210 ischemic, 70 hemorrhagic, 48 unspecified) were observed. They found that men whose daily intake of potassium (as obtained from a food frequency questionnaire) averaged 4.3 grams/day had a 38% lower risk of experiencing a stroke than did men whose average daily intake was below 2.4 grams/day. Men who supplemented with potassium also had a substantially reduced risk of stroke, particularly if they were also taking diuretics (non-potassium-sparing) [58]. Harvard researchers have also found a substantially lower stroke risk among women with a high intake of calcium, magnesium, and potassium [59].

As in the case of magnesium, it is also possible that potassium acts indirectly to protect against stroke through its pronounced effect on blood pressure. Researchers at the Johns Hopkins University School of Medicine have come out in favour of using supplementation with potassium in the treatment and prevention of hypertension (high blood pressure). A group of seven medical researchers reviewed 33 randomized, controlled supplementation trials involving over 2600 participants. They conclude that potassium supplementation is effective in lowering both systolic and diastolic blood pressure. The average observed decrease in hypertensive patients was 4.4 mm Hg and 2.5 mm Hg for systolic and diastolic pressure respectively. In people with normal blood pressure, the observed decreases were 1.8 mm and 1.0 mm.

The amount of elemental potassium used in the studies varied from 60 mmol (2.5 grams) to 120 mmol (5.0 grams) daily. Sixty mmol of potassium is equivalent to 4.5 grams of potassium chloride, 6 grams of potassium bicarbonate or 20 grams of potassium citrate. Oral potassium supplementation appeared to be well tolerated in all the studies examined. The researchers conclude that potassium supplementation "should be considered as part of recommendations for prevention and treatment of hypertension." Potassium supplementation is particularly important in people who are unable to reduce their intake of sodium [60].

Medical researchers at Erasmus University Medical School in the Netherlands have discovered a natural mineral salt, which significantly lowers blood pressure in people suffering from mild to moderate hypertension. The salt, SagaSalt (Akzo Nobel), occurs naturally in Iceland and contains 41% sodium chloride, 41% potassium chloride, 17% magnesium salts, and 1% trace minerals. The researchers tested the salt in a randomized, double-blind, placebo-controlled trial involving 100 men and women aged 55 to 75 years. Half the group used the mineral salt in food preparation and at the table while the other half used common table salt (sodium chloride). After 8 weeks, the average blood pressure in the mineral salt group had fallen significantly. The systolic blood pressure (mean of measurement at weeks 8, 16 and 24) fell by 7.6 mm Hg and the diastolic pressure by 3.3 mm Hg in the mineral salt group as compared with the control group. The researchers conclude that replacing common table salt with a low sodium, high potassium, high magnesium mineral salt is an effective way of lowering blood pressure in older people suffering from mild to moderate hypertension [61].

Italian researchers have found that excessively high potassium levels increase stroke risk significantly [62]. Thus it is important to maintain potassium levels within a fairly narrow range. This should not be a problem if the kidneys are functioning normally. However, if kidney disease is present or potassium-sparing diuretics (spironolactone, triamterene) are used, then medical advice and extreme caution are advised if potassium supplementation or a switch to a high-potassium diet is contemplated.

FISH OILS

Studies carried out in 1994 by South African researchers concluded that fish oil (6 grams/day) reduces the level of coagulation factors V and VII in healthy men and women and also reduces factor X and fibrinogen levels in women [63]. Researchers at University of Oslo have found that fish oil supplementation is effective in reducing fibrinogen levels in men. Their study involved 64 healthy men between the ages of 35 and 45 years. The men were randomized to receive olive oil capsules or fish oil capsules daily for 6 weeks. The fish oil capsules supplied a daily intake of EPA (eicosapentaenoic acid) of 3.6 grams and a daily intake of DHA (docosahexaenoic acid) of 2.9 grams. At the end of the study period, the average fibrinogen levels had dropped by 13% (from 2.73 g/L to 2.37 g/L). The researchers conclude that the antithrombotic (blood clot preventing) effect of fish oils may be due to their ability to lower fibrinogen levels [64].

In January 2001, researchers at Harvard Medical School reported that women who consumed fish even just once a week reduced their stroke risk substantially. Their study involved 79,839 female nurses who were between the ages of 34 and 59 years at the start of the study in 1980. After 14 years of follow-up, a total of 574 strokes had occurred in the group. Most of the strokes (303) were ischemic, i.e. caused by a blood clot. There were also 181 hemorrhagic strokes, i.e. caused by a ruptured artery and 90 strokes of undetermined origin. After adjusting for age, smoking and other cardiovascular risk factors, the researchers concluded that women who ate fish once a week lowered their risk of having a stroke of any kind by 22% and those who consumed fish 5 or more times a week reduced their risk by 52%.

They ascribe the protective effect of fish consumption to the commensurate intake of fish oils. They estimate that women whose intake is 0.5 gram/day or more have a 30% lower risk of suffering a stroke than do women whose intake is below about 0.1 gram/day. There was no evidence that women with a high fish or fish oil consumption have an increased risk of hemorrhagic stroke. The researchers believe that the protective effects of fish oils are due to their ability to inhibit platelet aggregation, lower blood viscosity, suppress the formation of leukotrienes, reduce fibrinogen levels, and reduce blood pressure levels and insulin resistance. They also note that the beneficial effects of fish consumption were substantially more pronounced among women who did not take aspirin on a regular basis [65].

Shortly after the release of the Harvard study, researchers at Harvard School of Public Health released the results of another study involving male health professionals. Over 43,000 male health professionals aged 40 to 75 years were enrolled in the study in 1986. During a 12-year follow-up period, 608 strokes occurred (377 ischemic, 106 hemorrhagic, and 125 strokes of unknown origin). The participants completed food frequency questionnaires in 1986, 1990 and 1994.

Men who consumed fish at least once a month had a 44% lower risk of having an ischemic stroke than did men who consumed fish less than once per month. No significant association were found between fish or long chain omega-3 PUFA (polyunsaturated fatty acid) intake and the risk of hemorrhagic stroke, but a possible association could not be ruled out due to the relatively small number of hemorrhagic strokes that occurred in the group. The optimum protection was achieved at fish consumption once per week and more frequent fish consumption (5 or more times a week) did not reduce stroke risk further. The protective effect of fish consumption was not significantly affected by the use of aspirin or vitamin E supplements (about 25% of participants used aspirin for stroke protection and about 20% supplemented with vitamin E). The researchers calculated the intake of PUFAs (EPA and DHA) from fish and found that significant protection against ischemic stroke was achieved at a daily fish oil intake of between 50 mg and 200 mg. The level of daily intake of alpha-linolenic acid did not affect stroke risk. Additional fish oil supplementation did not reduce risk of ischemic stroke any further [66].

It is likely that some strokes, particularly in afibbers with hypertension or heart disease, may be caused by the dislodgement of fragments of atherosclerotic plaque from the walls of the arteries. Researchers at University of Southampton have just completed a clinical trial to see if fish oil supplementation would improve plaque stability and thus help prevent heart attack and thrombotic stroke. Their study involved 162 patients who were awaiting carotid endarterectomy (an operation involving the removal of atherosclerotic deposits from the carotid artery feeding the brain). The patients were randomly allocated to receive a placebo, fish oil or sunflower oil daily from the time they entered the study until the endarterectomy during which atherosclerotic plaque was removed for analysis. The placebo capsules contained an 80:20 blend of palm and soybean oils (a composition which closely matches that of the average UK diet); the sunflower oil capsules contained 1 gram of sunflower oil plus 1 mg of vitamin E (alpha-tocopherol); the fish oil capsules contained 1 gram of fish oil and 1 mg of vitamin E. The participants took 6 capsules daily providing a total to 3.6 grams linoleic acid (in the sunflower oil capsules) or 850 mg of EPA + 500 mg of DHA in the fish oil capsules.

The duration of supplementation varied between 7 and 189 days with the median being 42 days. Upon analysis of the removed plaque the researchers found that the supplemented fish oil (EPA and DHA) had been readily incorporated into the plaques and had resulted in favourable changes. Plaque from fish oil-treated patients tended to have thick fibrous caps and no signs of inflammation indicating more stability. Plaques from the control and sunflower oil groups, on the other hand, tended to have thin fibrous caps and signs of inflammation indicating less stability. The number of macrophages (large scavenger cells) in the plaque of fish oil-treated patients was also significantly less than the number observed in the control and sunflower oil groups. The researchers conclude that the increased plaque stability observed in the fish oil-treated patients could explain the reduction in fatal and non-fatal heart attacks and strokes associated with an increased intake of fish oils [67].

Italian researchers have concluded that fish oils are highly effective in preventing sudden cardiac death and point out that supplementation with fish oils shows its beneficial effect within a few weeks. They also emphasize that it is unlikely that the biological effects of fish oils would vary depending on source (oily fish or fish oil supplement) [68].

Some doctors and cardiologists caution against supplementing with fish oils if also taking warfarin or a daily aspirin. This concern would seem to be unwarranted. Norwegian medical researchers have found that fish oil supplementation does not increase the bleeding tendency in heart disease patients receiving aspirin or warfarin. Their study involved 511 patients who had undergone coronary artery bypass surgery. On the second day after the operation, half the patients were assigned in a random fashion to receive either a placebo or 4 grams of fish oil per day (providing 2 g/day of EPA, 1.3 g/day of DHA, and 14.8 mg/day of vitamin E). At the same time, the patients were also randomized to receive 300 mg of aspirin per day or warfarin aimed at achieving an INR of 2.5 to 4.2. The patients were evaluated every 3 months and questioned about bleeding episodes for the duration of the 9-month study period. The researchers concluded that fish oil supplementation did not result in a statistically significant increase in bleeding episodes in either the aspirin group or in the warfarin group [69].

It is clear that oily fish and fish oils are effective in stroke prevention with a relative risk reduction of 40-50% as compared to the 64% and 25% observed for warfarin and aspirin respectively. Other research has shown that fish and fish oils are highly protective against heart attacks, sudden cardiac death, and cardiovascular disease in general. However, there is, unfortunately, a flip side to this. Some fish can have mercury levels exceeding the current US standard of 1.0 ppm. Many more species of fish exceed the Canadian and New Zealand limit of 0.5 ppm.

To be on the safe side, it is best to eat fish and shellfish with an average mercury content of less than 0.10 ppm. Unfortunately, there are not too many species left that fulfill this requirement. King crab, scallops, catfish, salmon (fresh, frozen and canned), oysters, shrimp clams, flounder, and sole are all good choices. Salmon is my favourite because of its combination of a low mercury content with a high level of beneficial EPA and DHA. The following species should be avoided – tilefish, swordfish, king mackerel, shark, grouper, tuna, American lobster, halibut, pollock, sablefish, and Dungeness and blue crab. Limited sampling of the following also indicated high mercury levels – red snapper, marlin, orange roughy, and saltwater bass. Atlantic cod, haddock, mahi mahi, and ocean perch have mercury levels around 0.18 ppm, so should be eaten in moderation.

As more and more fish species join the "polluted list", it clearly becomes increasingly advantageous to use fish oil supplements rather than eating fish on a regular basis. However, caution is definitely in order here. All fish oil preparations are not created equal. Some contain impurities like mercury, dioxin or PCBs and others are rancid or become rancid if stored for any length of time. If you use fish oil supplements in gel capsules, you can check for rancidity be cutting open the capsule and smelling the contents. If there is any smell associated with the oil at all, then it is rancid and should not be used.

I have checked many fish oil preparations and have now taken Coromega (Coromega, Carlsbad, CA) for several years. A Norwegian company supplies the raw fish oil from which Coromega produces its product. The fish oil used by Coromega, in turn, is produced from the raw fish oil through a 3-stage process of purification and concentration that complies with European standards of Good Manufacturing Practice. This process yields oils that are highly refined and therefore represent a pharmaceutical preparation in which potential impurities, such as PCBs, mercury, other heavy metals, and dioxins, are effectively removed, as are pesticide residues, unwanted fatty acids, and oxidation products.

Coromega is emulsified to improve absorption and is packaged in individual foil pouches to prevent oxidation. Each pouch contains 350 mg of EPA and 230 mg of DHA as well as 3 IU of vitamin E serving as an antioxidant. James Donadio, MD of the Mayo Clinic, has evaluated Coromega extensively and highly recommends it. One pouch a day provides the recommended daily intake of EPA and DHA and is adequate for general health maintenance. However, Dr. Donadio recommends 2 pouches a day for heart disease and stroke prevention, 3 pouches a day for reduction of triglycerides, 5 pouches a day for alleviating symptoms of rheumatoid arthritis, and 5 pouches a day for patients with IgA nephropathy (a common kidney disorder) or end stage renal disease [70].

Additional information on Coromega fish oil can be found at
www.coromega.com

GARLIC

In the early 1990s, German researchers reported that daily supplementation with garlic tablets (800 mg/day) significantly reduced platelet aggregation (down by 56% after 4 weeks of supplementation) and diastolic blood pressure (down by 9.5%) [71,72]. These findings were later confirmed by American researchers who found that aged garlic extract (7.2 grams/day) inhibited platelet aggregation and platelet adherence to fibrinogen [73,74]. Other researchers have found that aged garlic extract helps prevent endothelial cell injury, inhibits lipid peroxidation and oxidative modification of LDL cholesterol, and reduces reperfusion damage after an ischemic stroke [75]. German researchers, after a 4-year clinical trial, concluded that garlic inhibits platelet aggregation, enhances fibrinolysis, decreases blood plasma viscosity, increases HDL cholesterol level by an average of 8% while lowering LDL level by 4%, and decreases blood pressure by an average of 7%. The researchers conclude that these benefits of garlic supplementation translate into a reduction of cardiovascular risk for stroke and heart attack of more than 50% [76].

Garlic, in many ways, acts similarly to aspirin. Garlic supplements should therefore, not be taken in combination with aspirin or warfarin [77,78].

GINKGO BILOBA

Animal experiments have shown that pre-treatment with ginkgo biloba extract substantially lessens the damaging effect of an ischemic stroke and that this beneficial effect persists even if the ginkgo biloba is given up to 2 hours after the stroke occurred [79]. It is believed that ginkgo biloba exerts its beneficial effects through its strong antioxidant properties, its ability to increase nitric oxide synthesis and vasodilatation, its beneficial effect on blood pressure, and its ability to increase cerebral blood flow [80,81].

A group of American researchers have reviewed the current state of the art in regard to ginkgo biloba and conclude that the herb shows promise in the treatment of Alzheimer's disease, traumatic brain injury, tinnitus, macular degeneration, and ischemic stroke. They recommend caution in giving ginkgo biloba to patients taking anticoagulants such as warfarin [82].

COENZYME Q10 (UBIQUINONE)

Animal experiments and a few small human studies have shown that coenzyme Q10 may help protect against ischemic stroke. There is also anecdotal evidence that taking 400 mg of coenzyme Q10 (with fat) immediately after suffering a stroke may markedly reduce the damage. About 100 mg a day (with fat or a fatty meal) is likely needed to provide meaningful protection against heart attack and ischemic stroke [83, 84].

L-ARGININE

Researchers at Stanford University School of Medicine have found that supplementation with the amino acid L-arginine is highly effective in reversing endothelial dysfunction. It has been established that L-arginine is the precursor for endothelium-derived nitric oxide (EDNO). EDNO, in turn, is a potent vasodilator and inhibits platelet aggregation and the adherence of circulating blood cells to blood vessel walls. L-arginine administration, either orally or intravenously, has been found useful in preventing and reversing atherosclerosis, in increasing coronary blood flow in heart disease patients, in alleviating intermittent claudication, and in improving functional status of heart failure patients. L-arginine infusions have been found to lower blood pressure and to inhibit restenosis (reclosing of arteries) after balloon angioplasty [85].

British researchers have found that intravenous administration of L-arginine to patients who have just undergone carotid endarterectomy (removal of the inner part of the artery wall including adhering clots and atherosclerotic plaque) markedly reduced post-operative formation of blood clots as measured by Doppler ultrasound. They ascribe this beneficial effect to the known ability of L-arginine to reduce platelet aggregation and adhesion [86].

The findings that L-arginine reduces platelet aggregation and adhesion, while at the same time increasing nitric oxide synthesis and reversing endothelial dysfunction, should make this common amino acid a good candidate for a highly effective, natural stroke prevention supplement. Unfortunately, I am not aware of any clinical trials that have evaluated its effectiveness.

The most commonly used dosage of L-arginine is between 6 and 30 grams per day.

RED WINE and RESVERATROL

Several studies have shown that moderate red wine consumption protects against heart attacks and stroke. The beneficial effect of wine consumption can be quite substantial. One study found that young women (aged 15 to 44 years) who consumed about 12 grams of alcohol per day (approximately 1 glass of wine) had a 45% lower risk of experiencing an ischemic stroke than did women who did not drink wine [87]. Red wine increases HDL cholesterol levels, helps prevent LDL cholesterol oxidation, and inhibits platelet aggregation [88-91]. There is also credible evidence from animal experiments that red wine effectively prevents homocysteine-induced endothelial dysfunction [92].

It is now clear that it is not the alcohol, but rather the polyphenol content of red wine that is responsible for its benefits. Polyphenols are exceptionally strong antioxidants. One component, resveratrol, has an antioxidant capacity 20 to 50 times greater than that of vitamins C and E and is now touted as a powerful cancer-preventing agent. Resveratrol also inhibits platelet aggregation and interferes with the release of inflammatory compounds. Red wine extract, as such, is also a potent initiator of NO (nitric oxide) production in endothelial tissue.

Afibbers have been found to have low levels of NO in their blood both during rest and exercise [93,94]. It has also been observed that NO levels are particularly low in the left atrium and left atrial appendage and some researchers believe that this could translate into a greater risk for stroke as NO has strong antithrombotic properties [95,96]. Red wine polyphenols have been found to increase NO production from endothelial cells [97].

Extensive research has shown that resveratrol is highly effective in preventing stroke damage and that both resveratrol and quercetin (a bioflavonoid found in red wine) significantly inhibit the synthesis of tissue factor, the component in the blood that initiates blood coagulation via the extrinsic pathway [98-100]. Inasmuch as thrombus formation in the left atrial appendage is probably initiated via the extrinsic pathway, it is likely that red wine, trans-resveratrol and quercetin would be highly effective in reducing stroke risk among afibbers.

TEA and FLAVONOIDS

Dutch researchers have observed that habitual tea drinking provides strong protection against stroke. Their study involved 552 men aged 50 to 69 years at baseline. During a 15-year follow-up, 42 of the participants suffered a stroke. An analysis of dietary data showed that men who consumed more than 4.7 cups of tea per day have a 69% lower risk of having a stroke than did men who drank 2.6 cups per day or less. The researchers believe that the protective effect of black tea is due to its high content of flavonoids (mainly quercetin). They calculate that men with a daily flavonoid intake of 28.6 mg or more have a 73% lower risk of suffering a stroke than do men with a lower intake (less than 18.3 mg/day). The Dutch researchers have previously reported that a high intake of flavonoids also protects elderly men against coronary heart disease [101].

Animal experiments have shown that pre-treatment with green tea extract can reduce stroke damage (infarct size) by as much as 60% [102]. Cell culture experiments have shown that quercetin is highly effective on its own in reducing stroke damage [103].

Drinking 5 cups of tea per day may not be everybody's "cup of tea"; however, it is highly likely that supplementing with 100-200 mg of quercetin before each meal would have a similar, beneficial effect.

NATTOKINASE

Nattokinase is a potent enzyme that is highly effective in dissolving blood clots (thrombi). It works both by dissolving the blood clot directly and by inactivating plasminogen activator inhibitor type 1 (PAI-1), a strong inhibitor of fibrinolysis [104]. Nattokinase is a highly purified extract from natto, a traditional fermented cheese-like food that has been used in Japan for centuries. Dr. Hiroyuki Sumi discovered nattokinase in 1980 and established that it was highly effective in dissolving blood clots [105].

Animal experiments have shown that nattokinase is about four times as effective as the body's endogenous "blood clot dissolver" plasmin [106]. Other research has clearly shown that nattokinase prevents the formation of blood clots on injured artery walls [107,108]. Some researchers believe it is superior to conventional clot-dissolving drugs such as urokinase. Other researchers have found that it contains ACE inhibitors and, in large doses, is effective in lowering blood pressure in hypertensive individuals [109]. The beneficial effects of nattokinase persist for 18 hours or more and positive effects have been observed with as little as 50 mg [110]. Martin Milner, ND, professor of cardiovascular and pulmonary medicine at the National College of Naturopathic Medicine and Bastyr University, has this to say about Nattokinase: *"In all my years of research as a professor of cardiovascular and pulmonary medicine, natto and nattokinase represents the most exciting new development in the prevention and treatment of cardiovascular related diseases. We have finally found a potent natural agent that can thin and dissolve clots effectively, with relative safety and without side effects."* [111]

PINOKINASE

Pinokinase is a recently developed proprietary blend of nattokinase and pycnogenol specifically aimed at preventing edema and venous thrombosis during long-haul flights. Pycnogenol is a water extract from the bark of French maritime pine and had been found effective in controlling edema. It is a strong antioxidant, has significant anti-inflammatory effects, and increases capillary wall resistance. Flite Tabs, the brand name pinokinase preparation, contains 150 mg of a proprietary mixture of nattokinase and pycnogenol and is manufactured by Aidan in Tempe, Arizona.

A group of British and Italian researchers recently reported that pinokinase (Flite Tabs) is indeed effective in preventing edema and venous thrombosis. Their clinical trial involved 204 airline passengers at high risk for venous thrombosis traveling between London and New York (a 7-8 hour flight). Half the passengers were randomized to receive 2 capsules of Flite Tabs two hours before the flight with 250 ml of water. The other half of the experimental group received placebo capsules in a similar fashion. The presence of blood clots in the veins of the leg was determined with ultrasound scanning within 90 minutes of the beginning and completion of the flight. The degree of edema experienced during the flight was determined through a combined edema score including ankle circumference, discomfort, subjective swelling, and a standard edema test.

The researchers observed no thrombotic events in the Flite Tabs group, but discovered 5 cases of deep vein thrombosis and 2 cases of superficial thrombosis in the control group. Thus the total incidence of venous thrombosis was 7.6% in the control group versus 0% in the Flite Tabs group. The average edema score increased by 12% in the control group after the flight, but decreased by 15% in the Flite Tabs group. The researchers conclude that Flite Tabs are effective in controlling edema and reducing thrombotic events during long-haul flights [112].

These findings add to the evidence of nattokinase's effectiveness in preventing thrombosis. Deep vein thrombosis is caused by blood stagnation in the veins, particularly in the legs. There is evidence that a significant source of blood clots in permanent afibbers with cardiovascular disease is the left atrial appendage where blood tends to stagnate during atrial fibrillation. It would seem likely that nattokinase might also be very effective in preventing thrombosis in the left atrial appendage.

EXERCISE

The body's coagulation system is constantly on the alert ready to spring into action at the first sign of bleeding. Coagulation factors are always present in the blood and, if not under strict control, can initiate inappropriate thrombosis. One of the most effective control mechanisms is the clearance and inactivation of activated coagulation factors by circulating the blood through the liver. Swiftly flowing blood is highly effective in dispersing activated factors not yet incorporated into the platelet aggregate and growing clot. The protective effect of flowing blood is clear when considering the increased risk of thrombosis associated with blood stagnation (stasis).

Exercise and physical activity, in general, is highly effective in increasing blood flow and the associated removal of activated coagulation factors in the liver. Thus, it is not surprising that a high level of physical fitness and regular physical activity have been associated with a substantially decreased risk of ischemic stroke. Doctors at a UK hospital have concluded that lifelong exercise provides a very significant protection against stroke. People who had been involved in vigorous exercise (running, swimming, cycling, playing tennis or squash) between the ages of 15 and 40 years were found to have a five times lower risk of suffering a stroke than had people who had never done any vigorous exercise. Being engaged in vigorous exercise between the ages of 15 and 25 years was found to be particularly beneficial but even people who began exercising in their forties or early fifties derived significant benefit. Interestingly enough, people who had just recently taken up walking for exercise were also found to be three times less likely to suffer from a stroke than were sedentary people [113].

American researchers involved in the Framingham Study have concluded that older men who maintain a medium level of physical activity reduce their risk of having a stroke by almost 60% [114]. Researchers at the Cooper Institute and West Texas A & M University followed over 16,000 men (aged 40 to 87 years at baseline) over a 10-year period and found that highly fit men (as determined via a treadmill test) had a 68% lower risk of dying from stroke than did men in the least fit group (bottom 20%). Moderately fit men had a 63% lower risk than did the least fit men. These risk reductions were not changed even after correcting for other known risk factors such as smoking, alcohol consumption, hypertension, diabetes, body mass index, and parental history of coronary heart disease [115].

Icelandic researchers have found that men who continued to engage in leisure-time physical activity after the age of 40 years reduced their risk of ischemic stroke by 38% [116]. Finnish researchers have observed that unfit men (maximum oxygen consumption during exercise (VO(2)max less than 25.2 mL/kg per minute) have a 3.5 times greater risk of suffering an ischemic stroke than do fit men (VO(2)max greater than 35.3 mL/kg per minute). They conclude that low cardiorespiratory fitness is in the same league as high blood pressure, obesity, smoking, and excessive alcohol consumption as a risk factor for stroke [117].

Physical activity is also protective against ischemic stroke (and other forms of stroke) in women. Researchers at the Harvard School of Public Health followed over 72,000 female nurses for 8 years and found that those who were highly physically active on a regular basis reduced their risk of ischemic stroke by 50% as compared to nurses who were generally physically inactive. This reduction was observed after adjusting for other known risk factors for stroke including age, obesity, and hypertension. Moderate intensity activities such as walking were also found to be effective with regular, brisk walking associated with a 40% reduction in the risk of ischemic stroke [118].

It is clear that there is much evidence that regular, moderate to vigorous physical activity is highly protective against ischemic stroke with an independent risk reduction somewhere between 40 and 70% even when corrected for other known risk factors for stroke. Some very recent research has, however, found that vigorous exercise when actually in afib, including when in persistent or permanent afib, may not be a good idea. It seems that platelet activation, an important step in the coagulation process, is enhanced during heavy physical activity when in afib. No increase in platelet activation was observed during moderate exercise [144]. Vigorous exercise also increases cortisol level and vagal tone so moderation is also important in avoiding afib episodes, especially among vagal afibbers.

INFLAMMATION

There is considerable evidence that a systemic inflammation is directly involved in atherosclerosis, angina, peripheral arterial disease (intermittent claudication), diabetes, depression, and most common cancers [119-124]. Recent research has added stroke to the list of diseases involving inflammation [125]. It is probably not an overstatement to conclude that 90% of all that ails us is caused by an underlying inflammation.

So why are we so inflamed? There are several possible explanations:

- Our lifestyle often emphasizes factors that are known to initiate inflammation – mental, emotional and physical stress, vigorous exercise, alcohol consumption, mercury poisoning (mostly from dental amalgams), and oxidative stress. Inflammation can also be initiated by a bacterial, viral or fungal infection.

- Many common foods are inflammatory given the right conditions. The excessively high ratio of omega-6 polyunsaturated fatty acids to omega-3 fatty acids found in our modern diet favours the production of inflammatory prostaglandins, which certainly does not help matters [126].

- Childhood exposure to bacteria and viruses has been sharply curtailed through vaccinations and an excessive preoccupation with cleanliness. According to the "hygiene hypothesis", this has created an imbalance in the body's T-cells (key immune system defenders) so that the ones that promote inflammation have become dominant [127].

So how can inflammation be eliminated? Clearly, a two-pronged approach is required:

- The factors that initiate inflammation must be avoided.
- The immune system must be rebalanced to prevent an excessive inflammatory response.

There are several approaches to dealing with a persistent inflammation. One involves rebalancing the immune system itself. Lymphocytes, a specialized kind of white blood cells, are important components of the immune system. They can be subdivided into B-lymphocytes, which produce antibodies, and T-lymphocytes (helper T-cells), which help identify foreign cells and antigens so that killer cells can dispose of them. T-cells come in two varieties – TH1 cells and TH2 cells. TH1 cells produce lymphokines that enhance the ability of the immune system to kill viruses, bacteria, fungi, and parasites. TH2 cells are involved in allergic reactions and release interleukin-6 (IL-6), a powerful marker of inflammation. A healthy immune system has an optimum balance of TH1 and TH2 cells. The results of too many TH2 cells are autoimmune diseases, allergies, inflammation and pain, while not enough TH1 cells can lead to cancer and infectious diseases [128].

Extensive research carried out at the University of Stellenbosch in South Africa has shown that a proprietary mixture of plant sterols and sterolins (Moducare) is very effective in increasing TH1 cell production (the "good" T cells) and decreasing TH2 cell production (the "bad" T cells). Moducare also normalizes the ratio between DHEA and cortisol [125]. Moducare has strong anti-inflammatory effects and sharply reduces IL-6 production. It has been found useful in the treatment of chronic viral infections, tuberculosis, and HIV infection [129]. Also, it has been found to reduce the inflammatory response associated with excessive physical exertion [130]. The recommended dosage of Moducare is two capsules one hour before the main meals for the first month and then one capsule one hour before breakfast, lunch and dinner.

Adjusting the ratio between pro-inflammatory eicosanoids and anti-inflammatory eicosanoids is another important approach to combating inflammation. Fish oil or rather its main component, the omega-3 fatty acids, EPA and DHA, is very effective in shifting the balance. EPA and DHA compete with arachidonic acid (the main omega-6 fatty acid in the body) for the enzymes required in the synthesis of eicosanoids. Having a surplus of EPA and DHA favours the production of anti-inflammatory eicosanoids while having a surplus of arachidonic acid favours the production of inflammatory eicosanoids.

There are several other natural substances that may be beneficial in reducing inflammation.

- Boswellia (Boswellia serrata, Frankincense) - This resin obtained from the Boswellia serrata tree has been used as an anti-inflammatory in Ayurvedic medicine for centuries. Recent research has found it to be highly effective in the treatment of ulcerative colitis, Crohn's disease and asthma [131-133].

- Curcumin – The yellow pigment of turmeric is as effective as cortisone in combating acute inflammation [134,135]. The recommended dosage is 400 mg three times daily preferably on an empty stomach [134].

- Bromelain – A mixture of enzymes found in pineapple has been found effective in the treatment of the inflammatory disease, rheumatoid arthritis [134,136]. The recommended dosage is 250-750 mg/day [134].

- Ginger (Zingiber officinalis) – It is a strong antioxidant that inhibits the formation of inflammatory compounds. It has been found highly useful in the treatment of rheumatoid arthritis [134,137]. The recommended dosage (fresh ginger root) is 8-10 grams/day [134].

- Pancreatic enzymes – These have been found to be beneficial in the treatment of chronic inflammatory conditions such as rheumatoid arthritis [138]. They should be taken before meals.

- Probiotics – A recent review of the benefits of probiotics (Lactobacillus and Bifidobacterium) concluded that the modification of gut microflora by probiotic therapy might help alleviate inflammatory diseases such as arthritis and inflammatory bowel disease [139].

- Antioxidants – Last, but certainly not least, it is very important to ensure an adequate daily intake of the major antioxidants (vitamin C, vitamin E, selenium, beta-carotene, proanthocyanidins and alpha-lipoic acid). They all help to combat oxidative stress, a potent source of inflammation.

Prednisone is the main pharmaceutical drug used in treating an acute inflammation. It has the potential for serious adverse reactions and its use is generally not recommended for extended periods of time. An unfavourable benefit/risk ratio also applies to the use of aspirin and other NSAIDs to combat inflammation. They do not get at the root cause of the inflammation and can cause serious bleeding complications.

Cholesterol-lowering (statin) drugs have been found effective in decreasing the levels of markers of inflammation and in reducing endothelial dysfunction [140,141]. There is also emerging evidence the statin drugs can lengthen the period between afib episodes. This effect is thought to be due to their anti-inflammatory actions and perhaps due to their ability to modulate the fatty acid composition and physiochemical properties of cell membranes, with resultant alterations in transmembrane ion channel properties [142].

Unfortunately, statin drugs come with many potentially serious side effects including memory loss, liver dysfunction, myopathy, rhabdomyolysis, and possibly cancer. Statin drugs also reduce coenzyme Q10 levels possibly leading to impaired cardiac function and congestive heart failure [143].

CONCLUSION

It is clear then that there is an astounding array of highly effective natural approaches to stroke prevention with some of them offering protection equal to or surpassing that of conventional pharmaceutical drugs such as aspirin and warfarin. What is more, the natural approaches do not increase the risk of hemorrhagic stroke or major bleeding – serious side effects of antithrombotic pharmaceutical drugs.

REFERENCES

1. Bostom, AG, et al. Nonfasting plasma total homocysteine levels and stroke incidence in elderly persons. Annals of Internal Medicine, Vol. 131, September 7, 1999, pp. 352-55
2. Bots, ML, et al. Homocysteine and short-term risk of myocardial infarction and stroke in the elderly: the Rotterdam study. Archives of Internal Medicine, Vol. 159, January 11, 1999, pp. 38-44
3. Schnyder, G, et al. Association of plasma homocysteine with the number of major coronary arteries severely narrowed. American Journal of Cardiology, Vol. 88, November 1, 2001, pp. 1027-30
4. Chao, CL, et al. Effects of short-term vitamin (folic acid, vitamins B6 and B12) administration on endothelial dysfunction induced by post-methionine load hyperhomocysteinemia. American Journal of Cardiology, Vol. 84, December 1, 1999, pp. 1359-61
5. Seshadri, S, et al. Plasma homocysteine as a risk factor for dementia and Alzheimer's disease. New England Journal of Medicine, Vol. 346, February 14, 2002, pp. 476-83, pp. 466-68

6.   Cattaneo, M, et al. Low plasma levels of vitamin B6 are independently associated with a heightened risk of deep-vein thrombosis. Circulation, Vol. 104, November 13, 2001, pp. 2442-46

7.   Moustapha, A and Robinson, K. Homocysteine: an emerging age-related cardiovascular risk factor. Geriatrics, Vol. 54, April 1999, pp. 41-51

8.   Vollset, SE, et al. Plasma total homocysteine and cardiovascular and noncardiovascular mortality: the Hordaland Homocysteine Study. American Journal of Clinical Nutrition, Vol. 74, July 2001, pp. 130-36, p. 3

9.   Brouwer, IA, et al. Low-dose folic acid supplementation decreases plasma homocysteine concentrations. American Journal of Clinical Nutrition, Vol. 69, January 1999, pp. 99-104

10. Lobo, A, et al. Reduction of homocysteine levels in coronary artery disease by low-dose folic acid combined with vitamins B6 and B12. American Journal of Cardiology, Vol. 83, March 15, 1999, pp. 821-25

11. Lucock, M. Is folic acid the ultimate functional food component for disease prevention? British Medical Journal, Vol. 328, January 24, 2004, pp. 211-14

12. Undas, A, et al. Treatment of hyperhomocysteinemia with folic acid and vitamins B12 and B6 attenuates thrombin generation. Thromb Res, Vol. 95, September 15, 1999, pp. 281-88

13. Frustaci, A, et al. Histological substrate of atrial biopsies in patients with lone atrial fibrillation. Circulation, Vol. 96, August 19, 1997, pp. 1180-84

14. Robinson, K, et al. Low circulating folate and vitamin B6 concentrations: Risk factors for stroke, peripheral vascular disease, and coronary artery disease. Circulation, Vol. 97, 1998, pp. 437-43

15. Kelly, PJ, et al. Low vitamin B6 but not homocysteine is associated with increased risk of stroke and transient ischemic attack in the era of folic acid grain fortification. Stroke, Vol. 34, June 2003, pp. e51-e54

16. van Wyk, V, et al. The in vivo effect in humans of pyridoxal-5'-phosphate on platelet function and blood coagulation. Throm Res, Vol. 66, June 15, 1992, pp. 657-68

17. Sermet, A., et al. Effect of oral pyridoxine hydrochloride supplementation on in vitro platelet sensitivity to different agonists. Arzneimittelforschung, Vol. 45, January 1995, pp. 19-21

18. Miner, SE, et al. Pyridoxine improves endothelial function in cardiac transplant recipients. J Heart Lung Transplant, Vol. 20, September 2001, pp. 964-69

19. Khaw, KT and Woodhouse, P. Interrelation of vitamin C, infection, haemostatic factors, and cardiovascular disease. British Medical Journal, Vol. 310, June 17, 1995, pp. 1559-63

20. Zempleni, J. Pharmacokinetics of vitamin B6 supplements in humans. Journal of the American College of Nutrition, Vol. 14, 1995, pp. 579-86

21. Vakur, BM, et al. Plasma vitamin B6 vitamers before and after oral vitamin B6 treatment. Clinical Chemistry, Vol. 49, 2003, pp. 155-61

22. Gale, CR, et al. Vitamin C and risk of death from stroke and coronary heart disease in cohort of elderly people. British Medical Journal, Vol. 310, June 17, 1995, pp. 1563-66

23. Kurl, S, et al. Plasma vitamin C modifies the association between hypertension and risk of stroke. Stroke, Vol. 33, June 2002, pp. 1568-73

24. Antoniades, C., et al. Effects of antioxidant vitamins C and E on endothelial function and thrombosis/fibrinolysis system in smokers. Thromb Haemost, Vol. 89, June 2003, pp. 990-95

25. Tousoulis, D, et al. Vitamin C affects thrombosis/fibrinolysis system and reactive hyperemia in patients with type 2 diabetes and coronary artery disease. Diabetes Care, Vol. 26, October 2003, pp. 2749-53

26. Bordia, AK. The effect of vitamin C on blood lipids, fibrinolytic activity and platelet adhesiveness in patients with coronary artery disease. Atherosclerosis, Vol. 35, February 1980, pp. 181-87

27. Voko, Z, et al. Dietary antioxidants and the risk of ischemic stroke: the Rotterdam Study. Neurology, Vol. 61, No. 9, November 11, 2003, pp. 1273-75

28. Stampfer, MJ, et al. Vitamin E consumption and the risk of coronary disease in women and men. New England Journal of Medicine, Vol. 328, May 20, 1993, pp. 1444-56

29. Stampfer, MJ and Rimm, EB. Epidemiologic evidence for vitamin E in prevention of cardiovascular disease. American Journal of Clinical Nutrition, Vol. 62 (suppl), December 1995, pp. 1365S-69S

30. Stephens, NG, et al. Randomised controlled trial of vitamin E in patients with coronary disease: Cambridge Heart Antioxidant Study (CHAOS), The Lancet, Vol. 347, March 23, 1996, pp. 781-86

31. Azen, SP, et al. Effect of supplementary antioxidant vitamin intake on carotid arterial wall intima-media thickness in a controlled clinical trial of cholesterol lowering. Circulation, Vol. 94, November 15, 1996, pp. 2369-72

32. Yusuf, S, et al. Vitamin E supplementation and cardiovascular events in high-risk patients. New England Journal of Medicine, Vol. 342, January 20, 2000, pp. 154-60

33. MRC/BHF Heart Protection Study of antioxidant vitamin supplementation in 20,536 high-risk individuals: a randomised placebo-controlled trial. The Lancet, Vol. 360, July 6, 2002, pp. 23-33

34. Brown, AA and Hu, FB. Dietary modulation of endothelial function: implications for cardiovascular disease. American Journal of Clinical Nutrition, Vol. 73, 2001, pp. 673-86

35. Jain, SK, et al. Relationship of blood thromboxane-B_2 (TxB_2) with lipid peroxides and effect of vitamin E and placebo supplementation on TxB_2 and lipid peroxide levels in type 1 diabetic patients. Diabetes Care, Vol. 21, September 1998, pp. 1511-16

36. Freedman, JE, et al. Alpha-tocopherol inhibits aggregation of human platelets by a protein kinase C-dependent mechanism. Circulation, Vol. 94, November 15, 1996, pp. 2434-40

37. Bakaltcheva, I, et al. Effects of alpha-tocopherol on platelets and the coagulation system. Platelets, Vol.12, No. 7, November 2001, pp. 389-94

38. Huang, N, et al. Alpha-tocopherol, a potent modulator of endothelial cell function. Thromb Res, Vol. 50, No. 4, May 1988, pp. 547-57

39. De, CR, et al. Plasma protein oxidation is associated with an increase of pro-coagulant markers causing an imbalance between pro- and anticoagulant pathways in healthy subjects. Thromb Haemost, Vol. 87, January 2002, pp. 58-67

40. Kim, JM and White, RH. Effect of vitamin E on the anticoagulant response to warfarin. American Journal of Cardiology, Vol. 77, March 1, 1996, pp. 545-46

41. Salonen, JT, et al. Effects of antioxidant supplementation on platelet function. American Journal of Clinical Nutrition, Vol. 53, May 1991, pp. 1222-29

42. Chesney, CM, et al. Effect of niacin, warfarin, and antioxidant therapy on coagulation parameters in patients with peripheral arterial disease in the

Arterial Disease Multiple Intervention Trial (ADMIT). American Heart Journal, Vol. 140, October 2000, pp. 631-36

43. Kucuk, O, et al. Phase II randomized clinical trial of lycopene supplementation before radical prostatectomy. Cancer Epidemiology, Biomarkers & Prevention, Vol. 10, August 2001, pp. 861-68

44. Michaud, DS, et al. Intake of specific carotenoids and risk of lung cancer in 2 prospective US cohorts. American Journal of Clinical Nutrition, Vol. 72, October 2000, pp. 990-97, pp. 901-02

45. Gianetti, J, et al. Inverse association between carotid intima-media thickness and the antioxidant lycopene in atherosclerosis. American Heart Journal, Vol. 143, March 2002, pp. 467-74

46. Schmidt, R., et al. Risk factors for microangiopathy-related cerebral damage in the Austrian stroke prevention study. J Neurol Sci, Vol. 152, No. 1, November 6, 1997, pp. 15-21

47. Rissanen, T, et al. Lycopene, atherosclerosis, and coronary heart disease. Exp Biol Med (Maywood), Vol. 227, No. 10, November 2002, pp. 900-07

48. Mascio, P, et al. Lycopene as the most efficient biological carotenoid singlet oxygen quencher. Archives of Biochemistry and Biophysics, Vol. 274, No. 2, November 1, 1989, pp. 532-38

49. Paetau, I, et al. Chronic ingestion of lycopene-rich tomato juice or lycopene supplements significantly increases plasma concentrations of lycopene and related tomato carotenoids in humans. American Journal of Clinical Nutrition, Vol. 68, December 1998, pp. 1187-95

50. Amighi, J, et al. Low serum magnesium predicts neurological events in patients with advanced atherosclerosis. Stroke, Vol. 35, January 2004, pp. 22-27

51. Shechter, M, et al. Oral magnesium supplementation inhibits platelet-dependent thrombosis in patients with coronary artery disease. American Journal of Cardiology, Vol. 84, July 15, 1999, pp. 152-56

52. Muir, KW. Magnesium in stroke treatment. Postgraduate Med J, Vol. 78, November 2002, pp. 641-45

53. Ascherio, A, et al. A prospective study of nutritional factors and hypertension among US men. Circulation, Vol. 86, November 1992, pp. 1475-84

54. Witteman, JCM, et al. Reduction of blood pressure with oral magnesium supplementation in women with mild to moderate hypertension. American Journal of Clinical Nutrition, Vol. 60, July 1994, pp. 129-35

55. Shechter, M, et al. Oral magnesium therapy improves endothelial function in patients with coronary artery disease. Circulation, Vol. 102, November 7, 2000, pp. 2353-58

56. Green, DM, et al. Serum potassium level and dietary potassium intake as risk factors for stroke. Neurology, Vol. 59, August 2002, pp. 314-20

57. Levine, SR and Coull, BM. Potassium depletion as a risk factor for stroke. Neurology, Vol. 59, August 2002, pp. 302-03

58. Ascherio, A, et al. Intake of potassium, magnesium, calcium, and fiber and risk of stroke among US men. Circulation, Vol. 98, September 22, 1998, pp. 1198-1204

59. Iso, H, et al. Prospective study of calcium, potassium, and magnesium intake and risk of stroke in women. Stroke, Vol. 30, September 1999, pp. 1772-79

60. Whelton, PK, et al. Effects of oral potassium on blood pressure. JAMA, Vol. 277, May 28, 1997, pp. 1624-32

61. Geleijnse, JM, et al. Reduction in blood pressure with a low sodium, high potassium, high magnesium salt in older subjects with mild to moderate hypertension. British Medical Journal, Vol. 309, August 13, 1994, pp. 436-40

62. Mazza, A, et al. Predictors of stroke mortality in elderly people from the general population. European Journal of Epidemiology, Vol. 17, No. 12, 2001, pp. 1097-104

63. Oosthuizen, W., et al. Both fish oils and olive oil lowered plasma fibrinogen in women with high baseline fibrinogen levels. Thromb Haemost, Vol. 72, No. 4, October 1994, pp. 557-62

64. Flaten, H, et al. Fish-oil concentrate: effects of variables related to cardiovascular disease. American Journal of Clinical Nutrition, Vol. 52, 1990, pp. 300-06

65. Iso, H, et al. Intake of fish and omega-3 fatty acids and risk of stroke in women. JAMA, Vol. 285, January 17, 2001, pp. 304-12

66. He, K, et al. Fish consumption and risk of stroke in men. JAMA, Vol. 288, December 25, 2002, pp. 3130-36

67. Thies, F, et al. Association of n-3 polyunsaturated fatty acids with stability of atherosclerotic plaques. The Lancet, Vol. 361, February 8, 2003, pp. 477-85

68. De Caterina, R, et al. Antiarrhythmic effects of omega-3 fatty acids: from epidemiology to bedside. American Heart Journal, Vol. 146, September 2003, pp. 420-30

69. Eritsland, J, et al. Long-term effects of n-3 polyunsaturated fatty acids on haemostatic variables and bleeding episodes in patients with coronary artery disease. Blood Coagulation and Fibrinolysis, Vol. 6, 1995, pp. 17-22

70. Donadio, JV. Overview of the Potential Benefits of Omega-3 Fatty Acids with Suggested Doses of Coromega for Each Category of Disease. Newsletter, Mayo Nephrology Collaborative Group, Rochester, MN, November 2003

71. Kiesewetter, H, et al. Effect of garlic on platelet aggregation in patients with increased risk of juvenile ischaemic attack. European Journal of Clinical Pharmacology, Vol. 45, No. 4, 1993, pp. 333-36

72. Kiesewetter, H, et al. Effect of garlic on thrombocyte aggregation, microcirculation, and other risk factors. Int J Clin Pharmacol Ther Toxicol, Vol. 29 April 1991, pp. 151-55

73. Steiner, M and Li, W. Aged garlic extract, a modulator of cardiovascular risk factors: a dose-finding study on the effects of AGE on platelet functions. Journal of Nutrition, Vol. 131 (suppl), 2001, pp. 980S-84S

74. Steiner, M and Lin, RS. Changes in platelet function and susceptibility of lipoproteins to oxidation associated with administration of aged garlic extract. Journal of Cardiovascular Pharmacology, Vol. 31, June 1998, pp. 904-08

75. Borek, C. Antioxidant health effects of aged garlic extract. Journal of Nutrition, Vol. 131 (suppl), 2001, pp. 1010S-15S

76. Siegel, G, et al. Pleiotropic effects of garlic. Wien Med Wochenschr, Vol. 149, No. 8-10, 1999, pp. 217-24 [article in German]

77. Fugh-Herman, A. Herb-drug interactions. The Lancet, Vol. 355, January 8, 2000, pp. 134-38

78. Miller, LG. Herbal medicinals. Archives of Internal Medicine, Vol. 158, November 9, 1998, pp. 220-21

79. Lee, EJ, et al. Acute administration of Ginkgo biloba extract (EGb 761) affords neuroprotection against permanent and transient focal cerebral ischemia in Sprague-Dawley rats. J Neurosci Res, Vol. 68, No. 5, June 1, 2002, pp. 636-45

80. Sasaki, Y, et al. Effects of Ginkgo biloba extract (EGb 761) on cerebral thrombosis and blood pressure in stroke-prone spontaneously hypertensive rats. Clin Exp Pharmacol Physiol, Vol. 29, November 2002, pp. 963-67

81. Zhang, WR, et al. Protective effect of ginkgo extract on rat brain with transient middle cerebral artery occlusion. Neurol Res, Vol. 22, No. 5, July 2000, pp. 517-21

82. Diamond, BJ, et al. Ginkgo biloba extract: mechanisms and clinical indications. Arch Phys Med Rehabil, Vol. 81, May 2000, pp. 668-78

83. Ely, JTA, et al. Hemorrhagic stroke in human pretreated with coenzyme Q10: exceptional recovery as seen in animal models. Journal of Orthomolecular Medicine, Vol. 13, No. 2, 2ⁿᵈ Quarter 1998, pp. 105-09

84. Ely, JTA and Krone, CA. A brief update on ubiquinone (coenzyme Q10). Journal of Orthomolecular Medicine, Vol. 15, No. 2, 2ⁿᵈ Quarter 2000, pp. 63-68

85. Maxwell, AJ and Cooke, JP. Cardiovascular effects of L-arginine. Current Opinion in Nephrology & Hypertension, Vol. 7, January 1998, pp. 63-70

86. Kaposzta, Z, et al. L-arginine and S-nitrosoglutathione reduce embolization in humans. Circulation, Vol. 103, May 15, 2001, pp. 2371-75

87. Malarcher, AM, et al. Alcohol intake, type of beverage, and the risk of cerebral infarction in young women. Stroke, Vol. 32, January 2001, pp. 77-83

88. Miyagi, Y, et al. Inhibition of human low-density lipoprotein oxidation by flavonoids in red wine and grape juice. American Journal of Cardiology, Vol. 80, December 15, 1997, pp. 1627-31

89. Fuhrman, B, et al. Consumption of red wine with meals reduces the susceptibility of human plasma and low-density lipoprotein to lipid peroxidation. American Journal of Clinical Nutrition, Vol. 61, March 1995, pp. 549-54

90. Renaud, S and de Lorgeril, M. Wine, alcohol, platelets, and the French paradox for coronary heart disease. The Lancet, Vol. 339, June 20, 1992, pp. 1523-26

91. Mansvelt, EP, et al. The in vivo antithrombotic effect of wine consumption on human blood platelets and hemostatic factors. Annals of the New York Academy of Sciences, Vol. 957, May 2002, pp. 329-32

92. Fu, W, et al. Red wine prevents homocysteine-induced endothelial dysfunction in porcine coronary arteries. J Surg Res, Vol. 115, No. 1, November 2003, pp. 82-91

93. Takahashi, N, et al. Impaired exercise-induced vasodilatation in chronic atrial fibrillation – role of endothelium-derived nitric oxide. Circulation Journal, Vol. 66, June 2002, pp. 583-88

94. Minamino, T, et al. Plasma levels of nitrite/nitrate and platelet cGMP levels are decreased in patients with atrial fibrillation. Arteriosclerosis, Thrombosis, and Vascular Biology, Vol. 17, 1997, pp. 3191-95 http://atvb.ahajournals.org/cgi/content/full/17/11/3191

95. Cai, H, et al. Downregulation of endocardial nitric oxide synthase expression and nitric oxide production in atrial fibrillation. Circulation, Vol. 106, November 26, 2002, pp. 2854-58

96. Rubart, M and Zipes, DP. NO hope for patients with atrial fibrillation. Circulation, Vol. 106, November 26, 2002, pp. 2764-66

97. Leikert, JF, et al. Red wine polyphenols enhance endothelial nitric oxide synthase expression and subsequent nitric oxide release from endothelial cells. Circulation, Vol. 106, September 24, 2002, pp. 1614-17

98. Sinha, K, et al. Protective effect of resveratrol against oxidative stress in middle cerebral artery occlusion model of stroke in rats. Life Sciences, Vol. 71, No. 6, June 28, 2002, pp. 655-65

99. Di Santo, A, et al. Resveratrol and quercetin down-regulate tissue factor expression by human stimulated vascular cells. J Thromb Haemost, Vol. 1, May 2003, pp. 1089-95

100. Vidavalur R, et al. Significance of wine and resveratrol in cardiovascular disease: French paradox revisited. Exp. Clin Cardiology, Vol 11(3), Fall 2006, pp. 217-25

101. Keli, SO, et al. Dietary flavonoids, antioxidant vitamins, and incidence of stroke. Archives of Internal Medicine, Vol. 156, March 25, 1996, pp. 637-42

102. Hong, JT, et al. Protective effect of green tea extract on ischemia/reperfusion-induced brain injury in Mongolian gerbils. Brain Research, Vol. 888, January 5, 2001, pp. 11-18

103. Dajas, F, et al. Cell culture protection and in vivo neuroprotective capacity of flavonoids. Neurotox Res, Vol. 5, No. 6, 2003, pp. 425-32

104. Uranos, T, et al. The profibrinolytic enzyme subtilisin NAT purified from Baccillus subtilis cleaves and inactivates plasminogen activator inhibitor type 1. Journal of Biological Chemistry, Vol. 276, No.27, July 6, 2001, pp. 24690-96

105. Sumi, H, et al. A novel fibrinolytic enzyme (nattokinase) in the vegetable cheese Natto; a typical and popular soybean food in the Japanese diet. Experientia, Vol. 43, No. 10, October 15, 1987, pp. 1110-11

106. Fujita, M, et al. Thrombolytic effect of nattokinase on a chemically induced thrombosis model in rats. Biol Pharm Bull, Vol. 18, October 1995, pp. 1387-91

107. Suzuki, Y, et al. Dietary supplementation of fermented soybean, natto, suppresses intimal thickening and modulates the lysis of mural thrombi after endothelial injury in rat femoral artery. Life Sciences, Vol. 73, No. 10, July 25, 2003, pp. 1289-98

108. Suzuki, Y, et al. Dietary supplementation with fermented soybeans suppresses intimal thickening. Nutrition, Vol. 19, March 2003, pp. 261-64

109. Sumi, H, et al. Enhancement of the fibrinolytic activity in plasma by oral administration of nattokinase. Acta Haematol, Vol. 84, No. 3, 1990, pp. 139-43

110. Calvino, N. The enzyme of enzymes.
www.encognitive.com/files/The%20Enzyme%20of%20Enzymes.pdf

111. Better Health International. Nattokinase: potent fibrinolytic enzyme extract of traditional Japanese food.
http://www.betterhealthinternational.com/lib_Nattokinase.asp

112. Cesarone, MR, et al. Prevention of venous thrombosis in long-haul flights with Flite Tabs. Angiology, Vol. 54, No. 5, Sept-Oct, 2003, pp. 531-39

113. Shinton, R and Sagar, G. Lifelong exercise and stroke. British Medical Journal, Vol. 307, July 24, 1993, pp. 231-34

114. Kiely, DK, et al. Physical activity and stroke risk: the Framingham Study. American Journal of Epidemiology, Vol. 140, October 1, 1994, pp. 608-20

115. Lee, CD and Blair, SN. Cardiorespiratory fitness and stroke mortality in men. Medicine & Science in Sports & Exercise, Vol. 34, April 2002, pp. 592-95

116. Agnarsson, U, et al. Effects of leisure-time physical activity and ventilatory function on risk for stroke in men: the Reykjavik Study. Annals of Internal Medicine, Vol. 130, June 15, 1999, pp. 987-90

117. Kurl, S, et al. Cardiorespiratory fitness and the risk of stroke in men. Archives of Internal Medicine, Vol. 163, July 28, 2003, pp. 1682-88

118. Hu, FB, et al. Physical activity and risk of stroke in women. JAMA, Vol. 283, June 14, 2000, pp. 2961-67

119. Kiechl, Stefan, et al. Chronic infections and the risk of carotid atherosclerosis. Circulation, Vol. 103, February 27, 2001, pp. 1064-70

120. Biasucci, L.M., et al. Inflammation and acute coronary syndromes. Herz, Vol. 25, March 2000, pp. 108-12

121. Ridker, Paul M., et al. Novel risk factors for systemic atherosclerosis, JAMA, Vol. 285, May 16, 2001, pp. 2481-85

122. Pradhan, Aruna D., et al. C-reactive protein, interleukin 6, and risk of developing type 2 diabetes mellitus. JAMA, Vol. 286, July 18, 2001, pp. 327-34

123. Brown, Phyllida. A mind under siege. New Scientist, June 16, 2001, pp. 34-37

124. O'Byrne, K.J. and Dalgleish, A.G. Chronic immune activation and inflammation as the cause of malignancy. British Journal of Cancer, Vol. 85, No. 4, August 2001, pp. 473-83

125. Chamorro, A. Role of inflammation in stroke and atherothrombosis. Cerebrovascular Diseases, Vol. 17 (suppl 3), 2004, pp. 1-5

126. Simopoulos, Artemis P. Omega-3 fatty acids in health and disease and in growth and development. American Journal of Clinical Nutrition, Vol. 54, 1991, pp. 438-63

127. Helm, R.M. and Burks, A.W. Mechanisms of food allergy. Curr Opin Immunol, Vol. 12, No. 6, December 2000, pp. 647-53

128. Vanderhaeghe, Lorna R. And Bouic, Patrick J.D. The Immune System Cure, 1999, Prentice Hall Canada, Don Mills, ON

129. Bouic, P.J. and Lamprecht, L.H. Plant sterols and sterolins: a review of their immune-modulating properties. Alternative Medicine Review, Vol. 4, June 1999, pp. 170-77

130. Bouic, P.J., et al. The effects of B-sitosterol (BSS) and B-sitosterol glucoside (BSSG) mixture on selected immune parameters of marathon runners: inhibition of post marathon immune suppression and inflammation. International Journal of Sports Medicine, Vol. 20, May 1999, pp. 258-62

131. Gupta, I., et al. Effects of Boswellia serrata gum resin in patients with ulcerative colitis. European J Med Res, Vol. 2, January 1997, pp. 37-43

132. Gerhardt, H., et al. Therapy of active Crohn's disease with Boswellia serrata extract H 15. Z Gastroenterol, Vol. 39, January 2001, pp. 11-17 [article in German]

133. Gupta, I., et al. Effects of Boswellia serrata gum resin in patients with bronchial asthma: results of a double-blind, placebo-controlled, 6-week clinical study. European J Med Res, Vol. 3, November 17, 1998, pp. 511-14

134. Murray, Michael and Pizzorno, Joseph. Encyclopedia of Natural Medicine, revised 2nd edition, 1998, Prima Publishing, Rocklin, CA 95677, pp. 770-89

135. Srimal, R. and Dhawan, B. Pharmacology of diferuloyl methane (curcumin), a non-steroidal anti-inflammatory agent. J Pharm Pharmac, Vol. 25, 1973, pp. 447-52

136. Cohen, A. and Goldman, J. Bromelain therapy in rheumatoid arthritis. Pennsylvania Medical Journal, Vol. 67, 1964, pp. 27-30

137. Srivastava, K.C. and Mustafa, T. Ginger (Zingiber officinale) and rheumatic disorders. Medical Hypothesis, Vol. 29, 1989, pp. 25-28

138. Murray, Michael T. Encyclopedia of Nutritional Supplements, 1996, Prima Publishing, Rocklin, CA 95677, p. 397

139. Isolauri, Erika. Probiotics in human disease. American Journal of Clinical Nutrition, Vol. 73 (suppl), June 2001, pp. 1142S-46S

140. Kwak, Br, et al. Atherosclerosis: anti-inflammatory and immunomodulatory activities of statins. Autoimmun Rev, Vol. 2, No. 6, October 2003, pp. 332-38

141. Tiefenbacher, CP, et al.   ACE-inhibitors and statins acutely improve endothelial dysfunction of human coronary arterioles. Am J Physiol Heart Circ Physiol, November 26, 2003

142. Siu, CW, et al. Prevention of atrial fibrillation recurrence by statin therapy in patients with lone atrial fibrillation after successful cardioversion. American Journal of Cardiology, Vol. 92, December 1, 2003, pp. 1343-45

143. Compendium of Pharmaceuticals and Specialties, 35th edition, Canadian Pharmacists Association, 2000, pp. 1258-60

144. Goette, A. et al. Effect of physical exercise on platelet activity and the von Willebrand factor in patients with persistent lone atrial fibrillation. J. Interv Card Electrophysiol, Vol. 10, No. 2, April 2004, pp. 139-46

Chapter 4

Stroke Risk Estimates

Hypertension (high blood pressure) is a potent risk factor for both ischemic and hemorrhagic stroke. Having stage 1 hypertension (blood pressure 140-159/90-99 mm Hg) increases the risk of suffering an ischemic stroke by a factor of 2.8 when compared to the risk at a normal blood pressure of less than 140/90 mm Hg. The risk of having a hemorrhagic stroke if diagnosed as having stage 1 hypertension increases risk by a factor of 4.9 when compared to the risk at a normal blood pressure. A history of bleeding also markedly increases the risk of a hemorrhagic stroke [1].

Other important risk factors for ischemic stroke are:

- Congestive heart failure
- Coronary artery disease (heart disease)
- Peripheral arterial disease (Intermittent claudication)
- Valvular heart disease
- Diabetes
- Old age

Atrial fibrillation, if coexisting with one or more of the above risk factors, can significantly increase the risk of an ischemic stroke caused by a blood clot released from the left side of the heart (cardioembolic stroke) [2].

Two classification schemes have been developed and validated to help physicians judge the stroke risk for individual atrial fibrillation patients.

NATIONAL REGISTRY OF ATRIAL FIBRILLATION SCHEME
This classification scheme, also known as the **CHADS$_2$** Index, was created by consolidating the Atrial Fibrillation Investigators (AFI) classification scheme with that developed by the Stroke Prevention and Atrial Fibrillation (SPAF) investigators.

The creation of the CHADS$_2$ score involved following a cohort of 1733 men and women with documented non-valvular atrial fibrillation who had been admitted to hospital with an ischemic stroke during a 1.2 year period. The mean age of the group was 81 years (65-95 years) and 58% were women. The cohort definitely could not be classified as healthy with 56% having hypertension, 56% having congestive heart failure, 23% having diabetes and 25% having suffered a previous stroke or TIA. None of the patients were on warfarin at the time of their stroke.

The CHADS$_2$ scheme assigns a score of 0 to atrial fibrillation patients with no additional risk factors. One point is added for the presence of worsening congestive heart failure, hypertension, age 75 years or older, and diabetes (1 point for each) and 2 points for a history of stroke or TIA (transient ischemic attack).

CHADS2 Risk Score

75 years of age or older	1 point
Hypertension (1)	1 point
Diabetes (2)	1 point
Congestive heart failure (3)	1 point
Stroke or TIA (4)	2 points

(1) Treated hypertension or blood pressure above 140/90 mm Hg
(2) Diagnosis of diabetes or fasting glucose level above 126 mg/dL (7 mmol/L)
(3) Congestive heart failure that has worsened recently
(4) Ever experienced an ischemic stroke or transient ischemic attack (TIA)

During follow-up 94 study participants (5.4%) were admitted to hospital with an ischemic stroke. The risk of experiencing a stroke was closely related to a patient's CHADS2 score as shown in the table below.

Annual Stroke Risk

CHADS2 Score	Annual Stroke Rate
0	1.9%
1	2.8%
2	4.0%
3	5.9%
4	8.5%
5	12.5%
6	18.2%

The developers of the CHADS2 scheme emphasize that the 1,733 patients involved in validating the scheme were quite old (between 65 and 95 years of age) and sick and that it is likely that the stroke risks predicted from the score would have been lower if they had been derived from a younger and healthier population of afibbers. They also point out that the only study specifically addressing the stroke risk in elderly patients with lone atrial fibrillation and no additional risk factors found an annual stroke incidence of only 0.9%. Thus it is likely that the estimated stroke risk for scores of 0 and 1 is high [3].

Researchers at Kaiser Permanente in California have confirmed that the annual stroke risk assigned to individual CHADS2 scores by the developers of the

CHADS$_2$ index are indeed high. The Kaiser researchers compared CHADS$_2$ scores to actual event rates among 5,089 atrial fibrillation patients (non-valvular) not on warfarin. The actual event rates were as follows [4]:

Annual Stroke Risk (Kaiser)

CHADS2 Score	Annual Stroke Rate
0	0.49%
1	1.52%
2	2.50%
3	5.27%
4	6.02%
5	6.88%
6	6.88%

It is clear that the stroke rates observed by the Kaiser Permanente researchers are substantially lower than those predicted by the original CHADS$_2$ developers. However, it is likely that the Kaiser estimates are more realistic as they included three times as many patients with a much broader spectrum of age and underlying conditions and were based on data obtained in actual clinical practice rather than in clinical trials.

The original risk predictions can, of course, not be ignored, but a more realistic estimate of stroke risk versus CHADS$_2$ score may be had by combining the original estimate with the Kaiser estimate. Calculating the average of the results of the two trials (weighted by the number of patients in each trial) yields the following estimates:

Combined Annual Stroke Risk

CHADS2 Score	Annual Stroke Risk
0	0.8%
1	1.8%
2	2.9%
3	5.4%
4	6.6%
5	8.3%
6	9.8%

FRAMINGHAM HEART STUDY SCHEME

The Framingham Heart Study investigators followed 705 patients with new onset non-valvular atrial fibrillation (not on warfarin) for 4 years to determine their risk of ischemic stroke. The average age of the study participants was 75 years, 47% were women, 51% were being treated for hypertension, 35% had congestive heart failure or had suffered a heart attack, 15% had diabetes and 15% had suffered a prior stroke or TIA. NOTE: 22% of participants were on aspirin when their stroke occurred.

Based on the actual incidence of ischemic stroke in the group the investigators arrived at the risk scores and associated stroke risks shown below.

Framingham Risk Score

Risk Factor	Points
Age below 60 years	0
Age 60-62 years	1
Age 63-66 years	2
Age 67-71 years	3
Age 72-74 years	4
Age 75-77 years	5
Age 78-81 years	6
Age 82-85 years	7
Female gender	6
Systolic blood pressure 120-139 mm Hg	1
Systolic blood pressure 140-159 mm Hg	2
Systolic blood pressure 160-179 mm HG	3
Diabetes (1)	5
Previous ischemic stroke or TIA	6

(1) Diagnosed with diabetes or having a fasting glucose level above 126 mg/dL (7 mmol/L)

Annual Stroke Risk (Framingham)

Framingham Score	5-year Stroke Rate	Annual Stroke Rate
0 - 1	5%	1.0%
2 – 3	6%	1.2%
4	7%	1.4%
5	8%	1.6%
6 – 7	9%	1.8%
8	11%	2.2%
9	12%	2.4%
10	13%	2.6%
11	14%	2.8%
12	16%	3.2%

Annual Stroke Risk (Framingham) - continued

Framingham Score	5-year Stroke Rate	Annual Stroke Rate
13	18%	3.6%
14	19%	3.8%
15	21%	4.2%
16	24%	4.8%
17	26%	5.2%
18	28%	5.6%
19	31%	6.2%
20	34%	6.8%
21	37%	7.4%
22	41%	8.2%
23	44%	8.8%
24	48%	9.6%
25	51%	10.2%
26	55%	11.0%
27	59%	11.8%
28	63%	12.6%
29	67%	13.4%
30	71%	14.2%
31	75%	15.0%

The Framingham investigators point out that their prediction scheme is conservative. Thus the actual incidence of stroke in the group predicted to have a risk of 1.5% per year was only 1.1% per year and the incidence in the group predicted to have a risk of 2.0% per year was actually only 1.5% per year. They conclude that individuals with an annual stroke risk of 2% or less may not realize additional benefit from warfarin compared with aspirin and their risk of ischemic stroke may not exceed the risk of life-threatening bleeding with warfarin [5].

COMPARISON OF PREDICTION SCHEMES
The annual stroke risks predicted by using the original CHADS$_2$ validation, the Kaiser Permanente validation and the Framingham score and validation are significantly different as shown in the following tables.

Examples of Predicted Annual Stroke Risks for Men

Age	Risk Factor	CHADS$_2$ Original	Kaiser	Framingham
64	None	1.9%	0.5%	1.2%
64	Hypertension (1)	2.8%	1.5%	1.4%
64	Diabetes + Hypertension	4.0%	2.5%	2.4%
64	Prior Stroke (2)	4.0%	2.5%	2.2%

Examples of Predicted Annual Stroke Risks for Men

Age	Risk Factor	CHADS$_2$ Original	Kaiser	Framingham
76	None	2.8%	1.5%	1.6%
76	Hypertension (1)	4.0%	2.5%	1.8%
76	Diabetes + Hypertension	5.9%	5.3%	3.2%
76	Prior Stroke (2)	5.9%	5.3%	2.8%

Examples of Predicted Annual Stroke Risks for Women

Age	Risk Factor	CHADS$_2$ Original	Kaiser	Framingham
64	None	1.9%	0.5%	2.2%
64	Hypertension (1)	2.8%	1.5%	2.6%
64	Diabetes + Hypertension	4.0%	2.5%	4.2%
64	Prior Stroke (2)	4.0%	2.5%	3.8%

Examples of Predicted Annual Stroke Risks for Women

Age	Risk Factor	CHADS$_2$ Original	Kaiser	Framingham
76	None	2.8%	1.5%	2.8%
76	Hypertension (1)	4.0%	2.5%	3.6%
76	Diabetes + Hypertension	5.9%	5.3%	5.6%
76	Prior Stroke (2)	5.9%	5.3%	5.2%

1) Stage 1 hypertension (systolic blood pressure 140-159 mm Hg)
2) History of prior ischemic stroke or transient ischemic attack (TIA)

The Framingham formula for stroke risk prediction assumes that female afibbers have an inherently higher risk of ischemic stroke than do male afibbers. The Kaiser Permanente study and the original CHADS$_2$ score make no such assumption. I have been unable to determine if the presumed increased stroke risk for women is age-related. However, it would make sense that it could be. There is ample evidence that women are at greatly increased risk for heart attacks and the development of cardiovascular disease after menopause. It is likely that the risk of ischemic stroke would also increase after menopause.

It is clear that the stroke risk predicted by the original CHADS$_2$ validation is substantially higher than the Kaiser Permanente and Framingham estimates. However, both the Kaiser and Framingham studies confirm that male atrial fibrillation patients under the age of 65 years with no other risk factors for stroke (lone afibbers) have an annual stroke risk of ischemic stroke close to that found in the general population.

Although the prediction schemes do give an indication of the additional stroke risk associated with various disease conditions they do, by no means, tell the whole story. Smoking, high homocysteine levels and lack of exercise are all associated with an approximate doubling of stroke risk; in other words, they equal diabetes and hypertension in importance. Hopefully, future stroke prediction schemes will be expanded to include these and other modifiable risk factors.

REFERENCES

1) Song, YM, et al. Blood pressure, hemorrhagic stroke, and ischemic stroke: the Korean national prospective occupational cohort study. British Medical Journal, Vol. 328, February 7, 2004, pp.324-25
2) Hart, RG, et al. Lessons from the Stroke Prevention in Atrial Fibrillation trials. Annals of Internal Medicine, Vol. 138, May 20, 2003, pp. 831-38
3) Gage, BF, et al. Validation of clinical classification schemes for predicting stroke: Results from the National Registry of Atrial Fibrillation. JAMA, Vol. 285, June 13, 2001, pp. 2864-70
4) Go, AS, et al. Anticoagulation therapy for stroke prevention in atrial fibrillation: How well do randomized trials translate into clinical practice? JAMA, Vol. 290, November 26, 2003, pp. 2685-92
5) Wang, TJ, et al. A risk score for predicting stroke or death in individuals with new-onset atrial fibrillation in the community: The Framingham Heart Study. JAMA, Vol. 290, August 27, 2003, pp. 1049-56

Chapter 5

Pharmaceutical Drugs for Stroke Prevention

Pharmaceutical drugs prescribed for stroke prevention are aimed at inhibiting platelet aggregation or coagulation. They are also used to promote fibrinolysis of blood clots after a stroke has occurred. They do not address the underlying causes of thrombosis except in the case of aspirin, which has anti-inflammatory properties, and the statin drugs, which have anti-inflammatory and cholesterol-lowering properties.

Several clinical trials have found both aspirin and warfarin effective in preventing ischemic stroke in atrial fibrillation patients. The overall outcome of these trials was that daily aspirin therapy reduces relative stroke risk by 20-30% while warfarin therapy reduces it by about 65%. In other words, if afibbers with additional risk factors have an annual stroke rate of 3%, then taking aspirin would reduce this to about 2.3% while taking warfarin would reduce it to 1.0%. Both aspirin and warfarin significantly increase the risk of hemorrhagic stroke and major gastrointestinal bleeding, so the net benefit of prophylaxis with these two drugs is substantially less than quoted above.

Unfortunately, the original trials involving aspirin and warfarin had one very major shortcoming – they did not stratify the outcome of therapy according to the number and severity of other risk factors for stroke. Fortunately, there is now growing awareness that the overall benefit of aspirin and warfarin therapy varies enormously from patient to patient. Thus an afibber with no other risk factor for stroke may be worse off taking warfarin because of the risk of hemorrhagic stroke, while an afibber with hypertension and diabetes may derive substantial benefit from warfarin therapy. Says the Stroke Prevention in Atrial Fibrillation Investigators in a recent review article, *"It is no longer relevant to discuss the merits of antithrombotic prophylaxis in patients with atrial fibrillation without considering stroke risk subgroups."*[1]

Several researchers have recently gone back and reviewed the original clinical trial data and, where possible, stratified the benefits of aspirin and warfarin therapy by risk subgroups. These investigations provide a substantially different picture of the relative efficacy of aspirin and warfarin therapy. It has also long been clear that results obtained in strictly controlled trials may not be indicative of what happens in the "real world" where patients are selected with less care and INR measurements may be less frequent and less accurate than in clinical trials.

ANTIPLATELET AGENTS

Aspirin

Aspirin (acetylsalicylic acid) is the most widely used drug for the prevention of platelet aggregation – the first step in the intrinsic pathway of thrombosis. Aspirin was the first commercially successful, synthetic drug ever produced and celebrated its centenary in 1997. It is estimated that over 35 tons of the drug are consumed every day in the US alone and that millions of Americans now take a daily aspirin to ward off a heart attack or stroke [2-3]. Aspirin is an effective painkiller and has significant anti-inflammatory properties. It has also been found quite effective in preventing a second (secondary) heart attack, but not in preventing a first (primary) heart attack.

British doctors report that while daily aspirin usage may benefit some men, it may actually harm others. Their study involved 5499 men between the ages of 45 and 69 years who were at increased risk of coronary heart disease. The men were given either a placebo or 75 mg aspirin in a controlled-release formulation. The researchers found that the younger men with a relatively low systolic blood pressure (less than 130 mm Hg) benefited significantly from taking aspirin while the older men (over 65 years) and the men with higher systolic pressure (above 145 mm Hg) actually were worse off if taking aspirin. The researchers point out that a recent large-scale study in the UK found that men who take 75 mg of aspirin per day have a 2.3 times higher risk of developing bleeding ulcers than do men not taking aspirin. They conclude that, "it may be that four or five heart attacks would be avoided by treating 1000 men for a year, but the risk of serious non-cerebral bleeding would also need to be taken into account." They further conclude that, *"men with higher blood pressure derive no cardio-protective benefit from aspirin but risk possible serious bleeding."* [4]

Attempts have been made to reduce the bleeding risk by coating or buffering the aspirin tablet or by reducing the amount taken from the standard 325 mg to 75 mg or 81 mg per day. Several studies have concluded that these measures do not decrease bleeding risk and may, in fact, increase it [3,5,6].

Five clinical trials designed to determine the benefits of aspirin therapy in the prevention of a first heart attack were recently reviewed in a study funded by Bayer, the manufacturer of aspirin. Two of the trials, the Physicians Health Study and the British Doctors Trials, involved a total of 27,210 healthy men aged 40-84 years. The participants were followed for a mean of 5 and 6 years respectively. The rate of nonfatal heart attack was 0.28% per year in the aspirin group and 0.40% per year in the placebo group; that is, an absolute risk reduction of 0.12% or a relative risk reduction of 30%. Two other studies involving men and women at high risk for cardiovascular disease revealed an incidence rate of 0.53% per year for nonfatal heart attack in the aspirin group versus 0.76% in the placebo group; that is, an absolute risk reduction of 0.23% or a relative risk reduction of 31%. [7]

Considering that the risk of hemorrhagic stroke and fatal bleeding is about 0.2% per year, and that of major gastrointestinal bleeding is about 0.5% per year, it is imminently clear that long-term aspirin therapy for the prevention of a first heart attack or stroke (primary prevention) is not appropriate. This is fully recognized in the FDA's decision not to approve aspirin for long-term use in the primary prevention of stroke and heart attack [8].

Aspirin does, however, have a significant role to play in preventing death when a first heart attack is actually experienced. Several large-scale trials have shown that taking as aspirin as soon as possible after feeling the first symptoms of a heart attack can reduce the risk of dying by 23%. Medical doctors at the Texas Southwestern Medical School have found that the aspirin should be chewed rather than swallowed whole in order to minimize the time it takes for it to take effect. Aspirin works by blocking the synthesis of thromboxane, a metabolite of arachidonic acid, which is involved in the formation of blood clots. Aspirin enters the blood stream very quickly and swallowing a chewed tablet with water was found to inhibit thromboxane formation by 50% after 5 minutes and by 90% after 14 minutes [9].

Despite its lack of benefit in preventing a first heart attack, aspirin is still recommended for and widely used by afibbers to prevent a first ischemic stroke. A team of American, Canadian, Dutch and Danish medical researchers has concluded that a daily aspirin provides adequate stroke prevention in a large segment of afibbers irrespective of age. Individual patient data from 6 major clinical trials of the use of aspirin in stroke prevention was re-examined by the researchers. The trials involved 2501 patients with non-valvular AF who took 75 to 325 mg of aspirin daily. During 4689 person-years of follow-up 166 participants experienced a transient ischemic attack (TIA) or an ischemic (caused by a blood clot) or a hemorrhagic stroke (caused by a burst blood vessel). The overall event rate was 3.5/100 person-years (3.5% per year). This compares to the overall general population rate of 1.2/100 person-years observed in the large Framingham Heart Study. NOTE: Less than 2.8% of male participants and less than 2.2% of female Framingham Study participants had atrial fibrillation.

The researchers reasoned that afibbers without certain other risk factors for TIAs and stroke might have a significantly lower risk than would those with these risk factors. They determined the combined TIA and stroke incidence for a subgroup of 1661 afibbers who did not have hypertension (systolic blood pressure greater than 140 mm Hg), angina or diabetes and who had not suffered a previous heart attack, stroke or TIA. The overall TIA plus stroke incidence in this low-risk group was 1.0 event per 100 person-years. This compares to an event rate for a gender and age matched cohort in the Framingham Study of 1.2 events per 100 person-years. In other words, this low-risk group of afibbers using aspirin daily for prevention had a TIA plus stroke rate slightly less than that observed in a comparable group of afib-free individuals. Afibbers who did not satisfy the requirements for low risk, on the other hand, had an event rate of 4.2 events per 100 person-years – significantly higher than the expected rate of 1.3 events per 100 person-years. Of the 2501 study participants, 588 (23.5%) were classified as low risk. Their mean age was 67 years and 23.6% were female. It is interesting to note that of the 900 patients older than 75 years, 16% were classified as low risk. The prediction that low risk afibbers could safely use a daily aspirin for stroke prevention was validated in the remaining group of 840 study participants.

The researchers also looked at the effectiveness of oral anticoagulation (warfarin therapy) among participants in the 6 trials. The event rate in the low-risk group (as defined above) was 1.5 per 100 person-years (higher than in the aspirin group) and the rate in the remaining moderate- to high-risk group was 3.4 per 100 person-years (1 event per 100 person-years lower than in the high-risk aspirin group). The researchers conclude that irrespective of age, afibbers who satisfy the criteria for low risk can safely take aspirin for stroke prevention and would not benefit from oral anticoagulation. They estimate that about one quarter of all afibbers would fall in the low-risk group [10]. The conclusion of this study is good news for lone afibbers. I would estimate that around 80% of the over 300 afibbers who have participated in our surveys fall in the low-risk group.

Other researchers have concluded that afibbers with a predicted annual stroke risk of 2% or less may not realize additional benefit from warfarin compared with aspirin and their risk of stroke may not exceed the risk of life-threatening bleeding with warfarin. Thus anticoagulation therapy may not be justified in individuals with low predicted rates of stroke [11, 12].

The multinational team of researchers specifically point out that their study did not address whether patients, classified as low risk, would have as favourable an outcome with no therapy as with aspirin. They also express uncertainty whether the benefits of aspirin offset the increased bleeding risk in low risk afibbers [10].

In view of the fact that aspirin therapy does carry a significant risk of internal bleeding, it is clearly important to establish whether long-term aspirin therapy is beneficial or detrimental for afibbers at low to moderate risk for ischemic stroke.

A review of six clinical trials on the use of aspirin in stroke prevention concluded that long-term aspirin therapy reduces the risk of ischemic stroke by an average of 22%. The six trials included patients who had previously experienced a stroke or TIA and no attempt was made to stratify the benefit of aspirin therapy by risk factor status. It is thus highly likely that the relative benefit of aspirin therapy would be less than 22% in afibbers at low to moderate stroke risk. A 22% relative risk reduction means that a person whose annual stroke risk is 1.2% with no medication would have a stroke risk of 0.9% a year if treated long-term with aspirin [13].

The estimated excess bleeding risk associated with daily aspirin use varies between 0.5% and 1.0% per year. Pooled data from clinical trials comparing placebo and aspirin in the treatment of patients with atrial fibrillation show that aspirin therapy increases the risk of hemorrhagic stroke (intracranial bleeding) by 0.1% per year, that of fatal bleeding by 0.1% per year, and that of major bleeding requiring hospitalization and blood transfusion by 0.5% per year for a total risk of serious internal bleeding of 0.7% per year over and above the risk experienced by placebo users [14].

Researchers involved in the Framingham Heart Study have developed a system for predicting stroke risk in the presence of various common risk factors [11]. Combining their findings with the above mentioned estimates for bleeding risk yields the following estimates of the overall benefit of aspirin therapy in afibbers with low to moderate risk of ischemic stroke associated with blood pressure level:

Estimated Net Benefit of Aspirin Therapy
Risk of Ischemic Stroke and Bleeding, %/year

	Age	Systolic Blood Pressure	Stroke Risk Placebo	Stroke Risk Aspirin	Bleeding Risk	Net Benefit
Men	55-62	120-139	1.2	0.9	0.7	-0.4
	55-62	140-159	1.2	0.9	0.7	-0.4
	63-71	120-139	1.4	1.1	0.7	-0.4
	72-77	120-139	1.8	1.4	0.7*	-0.2
Women	55-62	120-139	2.2	1.7	0.7	-0.2
	55-62	140-159	2.4	1.9	0.7	-0.2
	63-71	120-139	2.6	2.0	0.7	-0.1
	72-77	120-139	3.2	2.5	0.7*	0

* Bleeding risk increases sharply over age 75 so it is likely that the 0.7% a year estimate would be much too low in this age group; thus making the long-term use of aspirin even more detrimental in this age group.

In conclusion, there is no convincing evidence that the ritual of the daily aspirin is beneficial for afibbers at low- to moderate-risk for ischemic stroke. As a matter of fact, the net benefit would appear to be negative, at least in individuals with an estimated annual risk for stroke of 3% or less. So is there any place for long-term aspirin therapy in atrial fibrillation patients? Probably not. At an annual risk of 3% or less, the net benefit of aspirin is in serious doubt; and, at a risk above 3%, anticoagulation (with warfarin) would be the officially recommended therapy.

Aspirin imparts its stroke prevention effect by preventing blood platelets from sticking together (aggregation). Vitamin E also works by inhibiting platelet aggregation and adhesion and two large studies carried out at the Harvard Medical School concluded that people who had taken 100 IU of vitamin E for 2 years or more had a 30% lower incidence of ischemic stroke – this is equal or better than the protection offered by aspirin. Fish oils, vitamin C, vitamin B6, and garlic also inhibit platelet aggregation and have been associated with relative risk reduction for ischemic stroke in the general population of 40-60%.

What all this adds up to is that a regimen of natural antiplatelet supplements may well be the best stroke prevention option for low risk lone afibbers and, of equal importance, this protection does not carry the risk of internal bleeding experienced with aspirin and warfarin use. Paroxysmal afibbers may benefit from supplementing with nattokinase at the onset and termination of episodes. This would also help protect against cardioembolic strokes whereas aspirin would not.

Clopidogrel

Clopidogrel (Plavix) inhibits ADP-induced platelet aggregation. It has been evaluated in patients at risk for ischemic events (stroke, heart attack, or sudden death). The study found that clopidogrel (75 mg/day) was slightly more effective than aspirin (325 mg/day) in preventing ischemic events – overall annual incidence was 2.8% with clopidogrel and 3.1% with aspirin. Clopidogrel was also found to be associated with a lower risk of intracranial bleeding (0.33 versus 0.47%) and major gastrointestinal bleeding (0.52 versus 0.72%). There were no atrial fibrillation patients included in the study [15].

A recent pilot study concluded that aspirin + clopidogrel are more effective than aspirin alone in preventing platelet aggregation in patients with congestive heart failure and heightened platelet activity [16]. A small study in patients with non-valvular atrial fibrillation found that a combination of aspirin (300 mg/day) and clopidogrel (75 mg/day) was superior to aspirin alone in inhibiting platelet function, but had no significant effect on the coagulation cascade itself [17].

A study (ACTIVE) is currently underway to compare the effect of aspirin + clopidogrel with that of aspirin or warfarin alone in patients with atrial fibrillation. Results are expected sometime in 2004 [18].

Ticlopidine

Ticlopidine (Ticlid) is a platelet aggregation inhibitor. It has been found effective in preventing recurrent stroke but carries a significant risk (0.85%) of severe neutropenia (a decrease in the number of white blood cells – neutrophils) [19]. Ticlopidine is usually only prescribed if aspirin or clopidogrel cannot be used. It is less effective than clopidogrel [20].

Dipyridamole

Dipyridamole (Persantine) is not terribly effective on its own, but does enhance the effect of aspirin. The 2nd European Stroke Prevention Study evaluated dipyridamole in combination with aspirin. Over 6000 patients with prior stroke or transient ischemic attack (TIA) were randomized to receive aspirin (25 mg twice a day), modified-release dipyridamole alone (400 mg/day), a combination of the two or a placebo. The combination reduced the relative risk of stroke by 37% as compared to a risk reduction of 18% with aspirin alone and 16% with dipyridamole alone. Bleeding complications were less common with dipyridamole than with aspirin, but headache was a common adverse event among dipyridamole users. Only 6.5% (429) of the patients had atrial fibrillation [21].

Indobufen

Indobufen (Ibustrin) inhibits platelet cyclooxygenase activity and has been found to be effective in preventing thromboembolic events in heart disease patients at risk for embolism. Italian researchers have evaluated it in comparison to warfarin in a group of 916 afibbers who had suffered a stroke or TIA. The participants were randomized to receive 100 or 200 mg of indobufen twice a day or warfarin to an INR of 2.0 to 3.5 for a 12-month period. The frequency of primary events (nonfatal stroke including intracranial bleeding, pulmonary or systemic embolism, nonfatal heart attack and vascular death) was similar in the warfarin and indobufen groups (9% versus 10.6%) as was the incidence of recurrent stroke (4% versus 5%). Bleeding complications were significantly more common in the warfarin group [22]. Indobufen is not currently available in the United States.

Glycoprotein GP11b/111a Inhibitors

Glycoprotein GP11b/111a inhibitors (abciximab, eptifibatide, tirofiban) inhibit the fibrinogen receptor sites on activated platelets. An intravenous form of these drugs has been used with some success in connection with angioplasty operations, but results of trials involving the use of oral preparations in ischemic heart disease have been disappointing [18]. No large scale trials have been performed to investigate their use in stroke prevention in atrial fibrillation patients.

CONCLUSION

Antiplatelet agents have been found reasonably effective in preventing a second (secondary) heart attack. They are not nearly as effective in preventing a first (primary) heart attack and the FDA recently refused to approve aspirin for this purpose. Antiplatelet agents are not very effective in preventing stroke in afibbers and there is considerable doubt that the benefits outweigh the risk (intracranial and gastrointestinal bleeding) - at least in afibbers with no other risk factors for stroke. Some afib-related strokes are likely caused by emboli originating in the left atrial appendage. Antiplatelet agents are not effective in preventing this type of thromboembolism as it does not involve platelet aggregation. Anticoagulants are the preferred drugs for preventing cardioembolic strokes originating in the LAA.

ANTICOAGULANTS

Warfarin

Warfarin was first isolated in the 1920s after farmers noted that their cows often bled to death after eating spoiled sweet clover. It was patented as a powerful rat poison in 1948. By the mid-fifties, it was beginning to be used as an anticoagulant in humans. The drug lost in popularity during the 1970s when it was realized that it probably caused as many deaths from bleeding as it prevented deaths from stroke. One of the major problems was the need to adjust the dosage for each individual patient. This, combined with the fairly unreliable test methods used at the time, resulted in a less-than-sterling experience with the drug. For the last 20 years, warfarin has experienced a resurgence, partly because of the development of an improved test for bleeding time (International Normalized Ratio) and partly because of a superb marketing campaign by the manufacturer of Coumadin. Warfarin works by inhibiting the activation of vitamin K-dependent coagulation factors V, VII and X in the extrinsic and common pathways of the coagulation cascade.

Several studies were carried out in the early 1990s to determine the effectiveness of warfarin in preventing stroke in atrial fibrillation patients. Unfortunately, these studies did not distinguish between AF with underlying heart disease and AF without heart disease (lone atrial fibrillation). One major trial (SPAF II) specifically excluded lone afibbers and all trials included a large proportion of patients not only with heart disease, but also with one or more risk factors for stroke (hypertension, diabetes, heart failure or a prior stroke or TIA). Thus the applicability of the trial data to lone afibbers, and in particular lone afibbers without risk factors, is very much in doubt. The average annual rates of ischemic stroke among all patients included in the five trials were as follows [23]:

Annual Incidence of Ischemic Stroke

Factors	Placebo	Warfarin	Relative Risk Reduction
Age less than 65 years			
No risk factors	1.0%	1.0%	0%
One or more risk factors	4.9%	1.7%	65%
Age 65 to 75 years			
No risk factors	4.3%	1.1%	74%
One or more risk factors	5.7%	1.7%	70%
Age over 75 years			
No risk factors	3.5%	1.7%	51%
One or more risk factors	8.1%	1.2%	85%

It is clear that there is no reason to prescribe warfarin for afibbers below the age of 65 years who have no additional risk factors for stroke and, indeed, this is fully recognized in the 2001 Guidelines for the Management of Atrial Fibrillation [24].

The data would, however, indicate that prescribing warfarin for afibbers over the age of 75 years having one or more risk factors might be prudent. The SPAF II trial found that the risk of an ischemic stroke in this age group was 3.6% when on warfarin and 4.8% when on aspirin. However, when looking at the combined total of fatal and disabling ischemic and hemorrhagic strokes there was little difference – 4.6% in the warfarin group and 4.3% in the aspirin group. So again, the wisdom of prescribing warfarin rather than aspirin for older afibbers is by no means clear-cut. It should also be kept in mind that the SPAF II trial was a clinical trial with frequent and accurate monitoring of INR levels. Even though close monitoring would presumably reduce the risk of major bleeding, the SPAF II study found the risk of major internal bleeding in patients over 75 years to be 4.2%, thus largely cancelling out the benefit of ischemic stroke protection [25].

More recently, a group of American researchers evaluated stroke risk among 700 elderly participants (mean age of 75 years) in the Framingham Heart Study and concluded that afibbers with a predicted annual stroke risk of 2% or less (irrespective of age) may not realize additional benefit from warfarin compared with aspirin and their risk of stroke may not exceed the risk of life-threatening bleeding with warfarin. Thus anticoagulation therapy may not be justified in individuals with low predicted rates of stroke [11,12].

A team of American, Canadian, Dutch, and Danish medical researchers looked at the effectiveness of warfarin therapy among participants in six major trials. The annual rate of stroke in the low-risk group (no hypertension, angina or diabetes and no history of stroke or TIA) was 1.5% on warfarin as compared to 1.0% with aspirin and 1.2% in an age and gender matched cohort without afib. The stroke risk in the remaining moderate- to high-risk group was 3.4% per year with warfarin, 4.2% with aspirin, and 1.3% in an age and gender matched cohort without afib or risk factors. The researchers conclude that, irrespective of age, afibbers who satisfy the criteria for low risk can safely take aspirin for stroke prevention and would not benefit from oral anticoagulation. They estimate that about one quarter of all afibbers would fall in the low-risk group [10].

Researchers at Kaiser Permanente in northern California recently concluded that results regarding warfarin efficacy obtained in tightly- controlled clinical trials may not necessarily be indicative of what is going on in the "real world". They followed 11,526 patients with nonvalvular atrial fibrillation for an average of 2.2 years (25,341 person years). About half the patients (6,320) were treated with warfarin while the remainder (5,089) took daily aspirin or used no drugs for stroke prevention. The average age of the patients was 71 years with about 40% being over the age of 74 years and about 24% being below the age of 65 years. Most of the participants had one or more risk factors for stroke (previous ischemic stroke [8%], heart failure [28.5%], hypertension [50.1%], diabetes [16.8%], and coronary heart disease [27.7%]). Almost half (43%) of patients were women. This survey population thus has little in common with a representative group of lone afibbers.

During the follow-up period, the researchers observed 141 ischemic strokes, 59 hemorrhagic strokes (intracranial bleeding), and 118 major gastrointestinal bleeds in the warfarin group and 231 ischemic strokes, 29 hemorrhagic strokes, and 119 major gastrointestinal bleeds in the aspirin/no drug therapy group. Results are detailed below in the following tables. [26]

Annual Incidence of Stroke and Bleeding, %
Patients on Warfarin

Condition	Ischemic Stroke	Hemorrhagic Stroke*	Major Bleed*	Total A	Total B
No risk factors	0.21	0.46	0.91	0.67	1.58
Prior stroke	3.24	0.46	0.91	2.78	3.69
Diabetes	2.06	0.46	0.91	2.52	3.43
Hypertension	1.59	0.46	0.91	2.05	2.96
Heart failure	1.22	0.46	0.91	1.68	2.59
Heart disease	1.57	0.46	0.91	2.03	2.94
Age over 75	1.43	0.46	0.91	1.89	2.80
Total population	1.11	0.46	0.91	1.57	2.48

Annual Incidence of Stroke and Bleeding, %
Patients on Aspirin or no Drug Therapy

Condition	Ischemic Stroke	Hemorrhagic Stroke*	Major Bleed*	Total A	Total B
No risk factors	0.43	0.23	0.96	0.66	1.62
Prior stroke	7.40	0.23	0.96	7.63	8.59
Diabetes	3.56	0.23	0.96	3.79	4.75
Hypertension	2.55	0.23	0.96	2.78	3.74
Heart failure	3.54	0.23	0.96	3.77	4.73
Heart disease	2.94	0.23	0.96	3.17	4.13
Age over 75	3.22	0.23	0.96	3.45	4.41
Total population	1.88	0.23	0.96	2.11	3.07

* Assuming these rates are independent of ischemic stroke risk factors
A = Incidents of ischemic stroke + hemorrhagic stroke (intracranial bleeding)
B = Incidents of ischemic stroke + hemorrhagic stroke + major bleeding

74

Difference in Annual Incident Rate
Warfarin vs. No Warfarin
Net Benefit, %/year

Condition	Ischemic	Ischemic+Hemorrh	Ischemic+Hemorrh +Major Bleed
No risk factors	0.22%	-0.01%	0.04%
Prior stroke	4.16%	4.85%	4.90%
Diabetes	1.50%	1.27%	1.32%
Hypertension	0.96%	0.73%	0.78%
Heart failure	2.32%	2.09%	2.14%
Heart disease	1.37%	1.14%	1.19%
Age over 75 years	1.79%	1.56%	1.61%
Total Population	0.77%	0.53%	0.59%

In reviewing these results, it should be kept in mind that a hemorrhagic stroke is usually more devastating than an ischemic stroke, so what really matters to the patient is the combined incidence of the two. The incidence of major gastrointestinal hemorrhage (defined as death or hospitalization requiring blood transfusion) was similar in the two groups at about 1% per year. This is likely due to the fact that the non-warfarin group included patients taking aspirin. Regular aspirin usage has been associated with a 0.7-1.0% per year excess bleeding risk in other studies [3, 14].

It is clear that warfarin does indeed have a moderate overall beneficial effect on the combined incidence of stroke (ischemic plus hemorrhagic) in patients with non-valvular atrial fibrillation. For every 1000 patients treated with warfarin for a year, 5 strokes are avoided. This corresponds to a relative risk reduction of 25% when compared to patients taking aspirin or using no drug therapy. It also means that for every 1000 patients treated with warfarin for a year 995 receive no benefit.

The benefit of warfarin therapy is substantial for patients having suffered a prior ischemic stroke. In this group, 49 strokes would be avoided for every 1000 patients treated for a year (a 63% relative benefit). There would be no benefit for afibbers with no risk factors for stroke (zero strokes per year avoided or a 0% benefit). This finding, of course, is in line with numerous previous studies. The benefit of warfarin therapy for afibbers with hypertension is 7 strokes avoided for every 1000 patients treated for a year for a relative benefit of 26%. This is significant, but not impressive.

Overall, it is apparent that 1,000 patients need to be treated with warfarin for a year in order to prevent 5.3 strokes. Treating one patient for a year would cost an estimated $830 (8 lab tests @ $50/test + 4 doctor's visits per year @ $75/visit + drug cost @ $130). Thus treating 1,000 patients would cost $830,000 or $157,000 per annual stroke avoided. The cost per annual stroke avoided in patients with a prior stroke would be $20,000 and that for patients with hypertension - $86,000 per stroke per year. The cost would, of course, be astronomical for patients with no risk factors.

The Kaiser Permanente researchers conclude that, *"Warfarin is very effective in preventing ischemic stroke in patients with atrial fibrillation in clinical practice while the absolute increase in the risk of intracranial hemorrhage is small"*.

I find this conclusion hard to reconcile with the actual data presented in the report. I would conclude that warfarin therapy is contraindicated for afibbers without risk factors, is quite effective for patients with heart failure and for those who have suffered an ischemic stroke previously, and is marginally effective for afibbers with hypertension. However, the cost of warfarin therapy to the healthcare system is considerable with an estimated annual cost of about $86,000 per stroke avoided among afibbers with hypertension.

A group of 7500 California Medicaid recipients with afib and one or more of the following conditions – hypertension (58%), congestive heart failure (48%), diabetes (34%), prior stroke (17%) or prior heart attack (14%) participated in a recent study to evaluate the effectiveness of warfarin therapy. During follow-up, stroke occurred in 514 patients with a rate of 3.4 per 100 person-years in patients treated with warfarin and a rate of 4.1 per 100 person-years for those not on warfarin. This corresponds to an overall absolute risk reduction of 0.7% per year. Bleeding occurred in 302 patients with a rate of 3.0 per 100 person-years in patients treated with warfarin and a rate of 2.2 per 100 person-years for those not on warfarin. This corresponds to an absolute increase in bleeding risk of 0.8% per year. The researchers conclude that, "Warfarin therapy, in clinical practice, has a relatively modest benefit in terms of reducing stroke rates, with the greatest benefit occurring among patients with moderate stroke risk. However, this benefit is somewhat offset by the increased risk of bleeding events" [27].

Unfortunately, quite apart from its limited efficacy, warfarin also has other significant shortcomings:

- Several studies have shown that 14-44% of patients with atrial fibrillation have at least one contraindication to its use [24]. Thus prescribing warfarin to an afibber without thoroughly checking for contraindications is not advisable.

- Reliably maintaining an INR within the customary range of 2.0 to 3.0 is still a very dicey proposition. Two recent, tightly-controlled clinical trials found that only 57% and 66% respectively of participants were consistently within the desired range during the trial [28, 29]. The number of patients within the range in a much less controlled, actual daily practice would be considerably lower. Having an INR above 3.0 increases the risk of internal bleeding while having an INR below 2.0 significantly increases the risk of thrombus formation.

- Appropriate monitoring of INR levels requires frequent visits to a testing laboratory and results in considerable inconvenience to the patient plus a significant financial burden on the health care system.

- INR levels are strongly affected by many foods and herbs adding further to the difficulty of maintaining the desired ratio.

- Warfarin interacts with at least 60 common drugs. Some of the interactions, particularly with relatively high doses of acetaminophen (Tylenol, Paracetemol), can be fatal as a combination of warfarin and acetaminophen can raise INR to 6.0 or higher [30-32].

- Warfarin can cause hemorrhagic stroke, gastrointestinal bleeding, osteoporosis and bone fractures (with long-term use), skin necrosis in some cases involving amputation of breast or penis, and, no doubt, a host of other less common complications [30,33].

The many shortcomings of warfarin and the relative under-utilization of anticoagulation for prevention of thrombosis and embolism have led to a concerted effort to find an effective replacement. First off the mark in the search for a warfarin replacement is the new oral anticoagulant ximelagatran.

Ximelagatran

Ximelagatran (Exanta) was developed by the Swedish arm of AstraZeneca and, by now, is probably one of the most carefully tested of all pharmaceutical drugs. Ximelagatran or rather its metabolite, melagatran, prevents blood coagulation by directly inhibiting the final step in the coagulation process – namely, the conversion of fibrinogen to insoluble fibrin by thrombin. Warfarin, on the other hand, works less directly by reducing the blood level of vitamin K-dependent coagulation factors. Early clinical trials of ximelagatran concluded that it has many advantages over warfarin.

- One size fits all. Two 36 mg tablets of ximelagatran taken daily provide anticoagulation equivalent to or better than that afforded by warfarin. There is no need for periodic monitoring of clotting time.

- Ximelagatran is not metabolized by the cytochrome P450 enzyme system in the liver so its effect is not altered by foods, herbs or supplements. There is no need to be concerned about what foods or supplements are safe to take when on ximelagatran.

- There are no known interactions between ximelagatran and other pharmaceutical drugs.

- Ximelagatran does increase bleeding risk, but the increase in risk is no greater than what is experienced with warfarin in the 2.0-3.0 INR range.

- Ximelagatran has no known major adverse effects in the short-term (about 18 months); however, it is not known whether it may have adverse effects in the long-term. A significant elevation in liver enzymes has been noticed in about 5% of patients, but this increase usually disappears with continued use or can be reversed by discontinuing the drug.

It is clear that ximelagatran has many advantages over warfarin, but is it equally effective?

Clinical trials of ximelagatran

Several clinical trials have evaluated the effectiveness of ximelagatran as compared to warfarin. For ethical reasons, ximelagatran has not been evaluated against placebo. One trial involved heart attack patients, two trials involved patients with venous thromboembolism while the five SPORTIF (Stroke Prevention Using Oral Thrombin Inhibitor in Atrial Fibrillation) trials involved patients with atrial fibrillation.

Ximelagatran in heart disease patients

This trial (ESTEEM) involved 1833 patients who had suffered a heart attack. The patients were randomized to placebo or 24 mg, 36 mg, 48 mg or 60 mg of ximelagatran twice daily. All participants also received 160 mg of aspirin daily. During the 6-month duration of the trial, 16.3% of the placebo group members suffered another non-fatal heart attack, died or developed severe recurrent ischemia. The corresponding number for the combined ximelagatran groups was 12.7% indicating that adding ximelagatran to a daily aspirin can reduce risk by an absolute 3.6% or a relative reduction of 22% over and above the protection provided by aspirin alone.

The incidence of major bleeding was 1.8% in the combined ximelagatran group and 0.9% in the aspirin only (placebo) group. The concentration of the liver enzyme, alanine transaminase, was more than 3 times the upper normal limit in 4% of the participants receiving 24 mg of ximelagatran twice daily as compared to 1% in the placebo group. The underlying mechanism for this increase is under investigation. No major adverse effects were observed during the 6-month trial. The researchers conclude that aspirin plus 24 mg of ximelagatran twice daily provides an absolute additional risk reduction of 4% over aspirin alone, has an acceptable risk of major bleeding, and a manageable rise in liver enzymes. It is of interest to note that the total incidence of internal bleeding (minor and major) was 22% in the combined ximelagatran group versus 13% in the aspirin only group [34].

Ximelagatran in prevention of venous thromboembolism

This Swedish trial involved 1233 patients from 18 countries with confirmed venous thromboembolism who had been treated for 6 months with anticoagulant therapy without reoccurrence of thromboembolism. The participants were randomized to receive placebo or 24 mg of ximelagatran twice daily for an 18-month period after discontinuing warfarin therapy. No coagulation tests were carried out during the trial period. At the end of the period, 12 patients (2%) in the ximelagatran group had experienced a new thromboembolism versus 71 patients (12%) in the placebo group – a 10% absolute and an 84% relative risk reduction. The risk of minor or major internal bleeding was 22% and 18% in the ximelagatran and placebo groups respectively. Major hemorrhage accounted for about 1% in each group. The cumulative incidence of elevation of alanine aminotransferase to more than 3 times upper normal level was 6.4% in the ximelagatran group and 1.2% in the placebo group. The researchers conclude that oral ximelagatran is effective in extended prevention of venous thromboembolism [35].

Ximelagatran after knee replacement

Venous thromboembolism occurs in 40 to 84% of patients undergoing total knee replacement if they do not receive anticoagulation therapy. About 7% of patients experience a pulmonary embolism and, in about 0.2 to 0.7% of cases, the embolus is fatal. Anticoagulation with warfarin reduces the overall incidence of venous thromboembolism to about 47%.

A group of researchers from Brazil, Canada, Israel, Mexico and the United States carried out a study to determine the relative efficacy of warfarin and ximelagatran in the prevention of venous thromboembolism after total knee replacement. The 1851 study participants were randomized to receive warfarin (INR = 2.0-3.0) or 24 mg or 36 mg of oral ximelagatran twice daily for 7-12 days following surgery. At the end of the trial, 128 patients in the 36 mg ximelagatran group (20%) had either died or developed venous thromboembolism while 168 patients in the warfarin group (28%) had done likewise. Minor or major bleeding occurred in 5.3% of the patients in the 36 mg ximelagatran group and in 4.5% of those in the warfarin group. (NOTE: This after only 7-12 days of therapy). Levels of alanine aminotransferase were not noticeably elevated in either group after this short treatment. The researchers conclude that 36 mg of ximelagatran administered twice daily is superior to warfarin in preventing venous thromboembolism following total knee replacement [36].

Ximelagatran in atrial fibrillation

Following a small preliminary trial (SPORTIF II) to investigate optimal dosing and alleviate safety concern, two major trials were undertaken to evaluate the efficacy of ximelagatran in stroke prevention among patients with non-valvular atrial fibrillation. SPORTIF III involved 3407 patients from 23 countries and SPORTIF V involved 3922 patients from 409 locales in North America. All study participants had one or more risk factors for stroke (about 40% had coronary artery disease and about 75% had hypertension) and 89% of participants had persistent rather than paroxysmal afib. Thus results are not directly applicable to paroxysmal afibbers with no risk factors for stroke. The 7300 high-risk patients were randomized to receive either 36 mg of ximelagatran twice daily or warfarin adjusted to an INR of 2.0-3.0. After an average follow-up of about 18 months, 91 patients (1.6%) in the combined ximelagatran groups (SPORTIF III and V) had suffered an ischemic or hemorrhagic stroke or had experienced a systemic thromboembolic event. The corresponding figure for the combined warfarin groups was 93 patients (1.6%).

Minor and major bleeding events were significantly lower in the ximelagatran groups at 37% versus 47% in the warfarin groups (NOTE: A rate of 37% or 47% of patients experiencing internal bleeding during an 18-month period is still, or ought to be, a major cause for concern). If deaths, strokes and major bleeding events were combined the incidence was 5.2% in the ximelagatran groups compared to 6.2% with warfarin - a significant relative risk reduction of 16%. Elevated liver enzyme levels (alanine aminotransferase) were noted in about 6% of ximelagatran users and in about 1% of warfarin users. The investigators conclude that fixed-dose ximelagatran is at least as effective as well-controlled warfarin in preventing stroke and systemic embolism in high-risk patients with atrial fibrillation [29, 37, 38].

Conclusion

Trials involving close to 10,000 patients have shown that ximelagatran is equivalent or superior to warfarin in preventing ischemic stroke and systemic embolism. Bleeding rates are similar although, in my opinion, unacceptably high if applied to patients at low risk for stroke. Significant elevation of liver enzymes occurs in about 5% of patients on ximelagatran, but appears to be reversible. No other major adverse effects have been observed in trials lasting up to 20 months, but longer-term effects are unknown. It is also not yet clear how excessive bleeding will be stopped in the case of accidents and other trauma.

Ximelagatran is superior to warfarin in ease of administration and control. The dosage is fixed at 24 or 36 mg twice daily and no monitoring of coagulation parameters is required. It also has the great advantage of not being affected by different foods, herbs and supplements and not interacting with other commonly used drugs. However, liver enzymes do need to be checked monthly for the first 6 months of therapy.

Ximelagatran has successfully passed phase III trials and has been approved for short term use in Europe, but has so far not obtained approval in Canada and the USA.

While ximelagatran would likely be advantageous for afibbers with one or more risk factors for stroke, I do not believe it would be any more appropriate for afibbers with no risk factors than is warfarin.

Heparin

Heparin is a natural anticoagulant that is produced in the mast cells of most animals. It is particularly abundant in the liver, lungs, and intestines and commercial preparations are extracted from porcine and bovine intestines or from the lungs of cows. Heparin works by promoting the activity of antithrombin III, the primary inhibitor of coagulation factor activation. It also neutralizes factor X and prevents the conversion of prothrombin to thrombin. The main complication of heparin therapy is hemorrhage [39]. Heparin is primarily used to prevent blood clotting during and immediately after surgical procedures. It is administered intravenously or by subcutaneous injection as the oral formulation is poorly absorbed. Heparin may also be administered subcutaneously for a short period of time before permanent warfarin therapy is begun. Because it cannot be given orally, heparin is of little interest for continuous stroke prevention therapy and has not been evaluated in afibbers for this purpose.

Low molecular weight heparin (LMWH)

Low molecular weight heparin is produced by fractionating or depolymerising heparin. It is less likely to cause bleeding than is heparin as such because it is less efficient in promoting antithrombin III activity, the main factor involved in heparin-induced bleeding. It does inhibit factor X and is just as effective as heparin in clinical practice [39]. The most popular LMWH preparations are enoxaparin (Lovenox) and nadroparin (Fraxiparine).

LMWH has been evaluated in two small trials involving patients with atrial fibrillation. Results were inconclusive [18]. Again, it is not likely that LMWH will become popular as an anticoagulant among afibbers since it cannot be taken orally.

OTHER MEDICATIONS FOR STROKE PREVENTION

Statin Drugs

There is evidence that statin drugs (lovastatin, atorvastatin, pravastatin, simvastatin, etc.) reduce the relative risk of heart attack or an ischemic stroke in patients who have already suffered a cardiovascular event (secondary prevention) by about 30% [40]. However, there is much less, if any, evidence that statin therapy does anything to prevent a first heart attack or stroke [41, 42].

The main effect of statin therapy is cholesterol reduction. A recent review found that statin therapy can be expected to reduce total cholesterol by 22%, LDL cholesterol by 29%, triglycerides by 12%, and increase HDL cholesterol by 6% [41]. There is emerging evidence that the protective effects of statin drugs may not be due to their cholesterol-reducing effects alone. Research has shown that statins help reverse endothelial dysfunction, increase NO availability, decrease vascular inflammation and enhance plaque stability [42-44].

Although used by millions of people and generally considered safe by the medical profession, statin drugs do, unfortunately, have several potentially serious adverse effects. Several cases of rhabdomyolysis (an often fatal muscle disease) associated with statin therapy have been reported and one statin drug, cerivastatin (Baycol), was withdrawn from the market after having caused the death of over 100 users[45, 46]. There is also evidence that statin therapy can cause memory loss and seriously depletes coenzyme Q10 levels potentially increasing the risk of congestive heart failure [47, 48].

Thus, considering there is little evidence that statin drugs are effective in primary stroke prevention and that no clinical trials have found them effective in preventing stroke in afibbers, there would seem to be little reason to take them unless natural remedies have failed to reduce high cholesterol levels. The other desirable properties of statin drugs (increase in NO availability, reversal of endothelial dysfunction, enhanced plaque stability, and reduced inflammation) can all be obtained in a much safer and more effective way by supplementing with fish oils.

ACE Inhibitors

ACE (angiotensin converting enzyme) inhibitors are used extensively in the treatment of hypertension. The benefits of using ACE inhibitors in secondary stroke prevention are still not clear. Two trials have found them beneficial while one has found them detrimental [49-51]. In any case, all the research done in this field have involved patients who had already suffered a heart attack or stroke or had cardiovascular disease or diabetes as well as other risk factors. The HOPE study involved 267 hospitals in 19 countries and lasted 4.5 years. A total of 9296 patients with vascular disease or diabetes plus an additional risk factor were randomized to receive either 10 mg of ramipril (Altace) or placebo daily. At the end of the study, 156 patients (3.4%) in the ramipril group had suffered a stroke as compared to 226 patients (4.9%) in the placebo group, i.e. a 32% relative reduction in risk.

The risk reduction was even greater in the case of fatal strokes. Seventeen patients (0.4%) in the ramipril group suffered a fatal stroke as compared to 44 patients (1.0%) in the placebo group, i.e. a 61% relative risk reduction. The researchers conclude that patients at high risk for stroke should be treated with ramipril [49]. This approach, unfortunately, may not benefit afibbers as one of the more common side effects of ramipril is irregular heartbeat. Moreover, serious questions have been raised about the conduct of the study. Several medical doctors have pointed out that the benefits of ramipril treatment may have been significantly overstated. One doctor points out that the absolute risk reduction with ramipril is only 0.33% per year for fatal stroke and 0.2% per year for non-fatal stroke. Another doctor points out that the cost of preventing a single stroke by treatment with ramipril over 4.5 years is somewhere in the range of US$ 64,000 – 160,000. So the jury is very definitely still out in regard to the benefits of ramipril in stroke prevention [52].

The PROGRESS study involved 6105 patients with a prior history of cardiovascular events. Participants were randomized to receive 4 mg/day of perindopril (Aceon) or placebo. After an average follow-up period of 3.9 years, 10% of the patients in the placebo group had suffered an ischemic stroke as compared to 8% in the perindopril group – a relative risk reduction of 24% in this group of high risk patients [50].

The CAPPP study involved 10,985 patients enrolled at 536 health centers in Sweden and Finland. All participants had high blood pressure (diastolic pressure above 100 mm Hg). Patients were randomized to treatment with captopril (Capoten) or conventional antihypertensive treatment (diuretics, beta-blockers). During follow-up 189 patients (3.4%) in the captopril group suffered a stroke as compared to 148 patients (2.7%) in the conventionally treated group. Thus, there is no indication that captopril is effective in preventing stroke in patients with hypertension and some indication that it may be detrimental [51].

No clinical trials have been done involving afibbers without risk factors for stroke, so there is no evidence that ACE inhibitors may help prevent stroke in otherwise healthy afibbers.

THROMBOLYTIC AGENTS

Thrombolytic agents are used after the fact, that is, to dissolve an already formed blood clot. They are not employed in the prevention of thrombosis, ischemic stroke or heart attack. Thrombolytic agents work by activating plasminogen which, in turn, activates plasmin, the proteolytic enzyme that dissolves the polymerized fibrin clot. Plasminogen is always present in blood plasma and is actually incorporated into blood clots where it is bound directly to fibrin. The body has its own natural plasminogen activators, tissue type plasminogen activator (tPA), which is found in the lining of small blood vessels, and urokinase which is present in the blood stream in trace amounts [53].

Both tPA and urokinase (Abbokinase) have been synthesized and are used to dissolve blood clots involved in a heart attack or venous thrombosis. They are also used to a more limited extent to dissolve blood clots in the brain (ischemic stroke). The main problem with their use is their very major tendency to cause internal bleeding. One study found that patients infused with high doses of tPA developed bleeding complications in 47% of cases and suffered a hemorrhagic stroke (intracranial bleeding) in 1.6% of cases [53]. The "window of opportunity" for the successful use of thrombolytic agents is very narrow. Blood clots tend to become more and more difficult to dissolve with time, so if the plasminogen activator is injected more than 3 hours after the cardiovascular event, it is not very effective at all, but its capacity to cause bleeding remains undiminished. For this reason, thrombolytic agents are not approved for use beyond 3 hours after the event.

Considering today's waiting times in emergency wards, the need to get the appropriate stroke specialist involved and the need to ensure, via a CAT scan, that the stroke was not caused by intracranial bleeding, it is clear that very few ischemic stroke victims actually benefit from the use of thrombolytic agents. The use of these agents is, of course, contraindicated in patients taking anticoagulants such as warfarin or ximelagatran and cannot be used in cases of trauma or where the blood clot occurs in connection with surgery.

The importance of timing in the use of thrombolytic agents was demonstrated by Australian researchers using streptokinase. Streptokinase (Streptase) is the least expensive of the agents and is an extract of streptococci bacteria. The Australian researches determined survival after 3 months in 340 ischemic stroke patients who received an infusion of streptokinase (1.5 million units) or placebo over a 1-hour period. Seventy of the patients received the infusion within 3 hours of the event while the remaining 270 patients received it between 3 and 4 hours after the event. The mortality in the group receiving the streptokinase infusion beyond the 3-hour window was twice as high as that experienced among those infused with placebo. Those that received the infusion within the 3-hour window had equivalent death rates whether they received streptokinase or placebo. Only 3% of the placebo-treated patients developed a haematoma as compared to 13.2% in the group infused with streptokinase. The researchers conclude that, *"while treatment within 3 hours of stroke was safer and associated with significantly better outcomes than later treatment, it showed no significant benefit over placebo."*[54]

Interventional radiologists and neurologists use imaging procedures to diagnose stroke type (ischemic or hemorrhagic) and to guide a small catheter to the tiny arteries in the brain so as to be able to inject the thrombolytic agent directly into the clot or break it up mechanically. The use of this treatment extends the safe period for injection to 6 hours, but requires highly sophisticated equipment and the presence of a team of highly-skilled specialists unlikely to be available on short notice in the average emergency ward.

The bottom line is that the use of thrombolytic agents is unlikely to be of benefit to the great majority of stroke victims. It is likely to be of more benefit for heart attack patients where the need to ensure the absence of intracranial bleeding does not enter into the picture.

SURGICAL APPROACHES

Eliminating atrial fibrillation by surgical intervention (Maze procedure) or catheter ablation (pulmonary vein isolation) would be expected to reduce the risk of ischemic stroke to that of the general population. The Maze procedure includes the surgical removal or obliteration of both atrial appendages, thus eliminating the danger of clot formation in the left atrial appendage. A 12-year follow-up study concluded that, *"the Maze procedure essentially abolishes the risk of stroke associated with atrial fibrillation"* [55]. Because of the relative newness of the PVI procedure, no studies concerning long-term stroke risk in successfully ablated patients have been reported so far. However, it would seem highly likely that a successful PVI would also reduce stroke risk to that of the general population.

A team of cardiologists from Germany, Italy and the United States have reported that blocking the opening of the left atrial appendage (LAA) can effectively seal it off and eliminate the danger of clot formation. Their clinical trial involved 15 patients with permanent atrial fibrillation who, for one reason or another, could not tolerate warfarin therapy. All patients had a self-expanding nitinol cage coated with expanded polytetrafluoroethylene plastic inserted so as to completely seal off the opening to the LAA. The cage was delivered to the LAA (in collapsed form) via a catheter threaded through a vein in a procedure similar to that used in radiofrequency ablation. The expanded cage ranged in diameter from 18 to 32 mm with the average being 26 mm. The cage was successfully placed in all 15 patients with only one experiencing excessive bleeding. The entire procedure took about 90 minutes. The researchers have since performed an additional 16 procedures and conclude that the implantation of a mechanical device to close off the LAA can be done safely and with relative ease. They call for further trials to evaluate the long-term safety and effectiveness of the device (PLAATO system) in reducing stroke incidence in AF patients [56].

Other researchers contend that the PLAATO system should be deemed as treatment of last resort and one that must be considered only for AF patients at high-risk of a thromboembolism with contraindication to anticoagulation and in whom no other form of curative treatment appears likely [18].

The idea of closing off the LAA with a suture or staples during open heart surgery is also under investigation in the LAAOS Study. A total of 2500 patients with AF or at elevated risk for ischemic stroke will participate in the 5-year study [57].

CONCLUSION

Aspirin, warfarin (Coumadin) and eventually ximelagatran (Exanta) are the mainstay pharmaceutical drugs used in the prevention of thrombosis, embolism, and ischemic stroke. They all carry a significant risk of intracranial bleeding (hemorrhagic stroke) and gastrointestinal bleeding. Their risks probably outweigh their benefits in afibbers with no underlying heart disease or other risk factors for stroke. However, they are likely to be of benefit to afibbers who have already suffered a stroke or TIA or have congestive heart failure.

REFERENCES

1. Hart, RG, et al. Lessons from the Stroke Prevention in Atrial Fibrillation trials. Annals of Internal Medicine, Vol. 138, May 20, 2003, pp. 831-38
2. Jack, DB. One hundred years of aspirin. The Lancet, Vol. 350, August 9, 1997, pp. 437-39
3. Derry, S and Loke, YK. Risk of gastrointestinal haemorrhage with long term use of aspirin: meta-analysis. British Medical Journal, Vol. 321, November 11, 2000, pp. 1183-87
4. Meade, TW, et al. Determination of who may derive most benefit from aspirin in primary prevention: subgroup results from a randomised -controlled trial. British Medical Journal, Vol. 321, July 1, 2000, pp. 13-17
5. Sorensen, HT, et al. Risk of upper gastrointestinal bleeding associated with use of low-dose aspirin. American Journal of Gastroenterology, Vol. 95, September 2000, pp. 2218-24
6. Kelly, JP, et al. Risk of aspirin-associated major upper-gastrointestinal bleeding with enteric-coated or buffered product. The Lancet, Vol. 348, November 23, 1996, pp. 1413-16
7. Eidelman, RS, et al. An update on aspirin in the primary prevention of cardiovascular disease. Archives of Internal Medicine, Vol. 163, September 22, 2003, pp. 2006-10

8. U.S. Food & Drug Administration. Use of Aspirin for Primary Prevention of Heart Attack and Stroke.
https://www.fda.gov/drugs/resourcesforyou/consumers/ucm390574.htm

9. Feldman, M and Cryer, B. Aspirin absorption rates and platelet inhibition times with 325-mg buffered aspirin tablets (chewed or swallowed intact) and with buffered aspirin solution. American Journal of Cardiology, Vol. 84, August 15, 1999, pp. 404-09

10. van Walraven, C, et al. A clinical prediction rule to identify patients with atrial fibrillation and a low risk for stroke while taking aspirin. Archives of Internal Medicine, Vol. 163, April 28, 2003, pp. 936-43

11. Wang, TJ, et al. A risk score for predicting stroke or death in individuals with new-onset atrial fibrillation in the community. Journal of the American Medical Association, Vol. 290, August 27, 2003, pp. 1049-56

12. Waldo, AL. Stroke prevention in atrial fibrillation. Journal of the American Medical Association, Vol. 290, August 27, 2003, pp. 1093-95 (editorial)

13. Hart, RG, et al. Antithrombotic therapy to prevent stroke in patients with atrial fibrillation. Annals of Internal Medicine, Vol. 131, October 5, 1999, pp. 492-501

14. Artang, R and Vidaillet, H. Alternatives to warfarin for thromboembolism prophylaxis in nonrheumatic atrial fibrillation. Journal of Interventional Cardiac Electrophysiology, Vol. 10, February 2004, pp. 33-44

15. CAPRIE Steering Committee. A randomized, blinded, trial of clopidogrel versus aspirin in patients at risk of ischemic events. The Lancet, Vol. 348, November 16, 1996, pp. 1329-39

16. Serebruany, VL, et al. Effects of clopidogrel and aspirin combination versus aspirin alone on platelet aggregation and major receptor expression in patients with hear failure. American Heart Journal, Vol. 146, No. 4, October 2003, pp. 713-20

17. Muller, I, et al. Effects of aspirin and clopidogrel versus oral anticoagulation on platelet function and on coagulation in patients with nonvalvular atrial fibrillation. Pathophysiol Haemost Thromb, Vol. 32, Jan-Feb 2002, pp. 16-24

18. Artang, R and Vidaillet, H. Alternatives to warfarin for thromboembolism prophylaxis in nonrheumatic atrial fibrillation. Journal of Interventional Cardiac Electrophysiology, Vol. 10, February 2004, pp. 33-44

19. Noble, S and Goa, KL. Ticlopidine: A review of its pharmacology, clinical efficacy and tolerability in the prevention of cerebral ischaemica and stroke. Drugs and Aging, Vol. 8, March 1996, pp. 214-32

20. Casella, G, et al. Safety and efficacy evaluation of clopidogrel compared to ticlopidine after stent implantation. Italian Heart Journal, Vol. 4, October 2003, pp. 677-84

21. Diener, HC, et al. European Stroke Prevention Study: dipyridamole and acetylsalicylic acid in the secondary prevention of stroke. J Neurol Sci, Vol. 143, November 1996, pp. 1-13

22. Morocutti, C, et al. Indobufen versus warfarin in the secondary prevention of major vascular events in nonrheumatic atrial fibrillation. Stroke, Vol. 28, No. 5, 1997, pp. 1015-21

23. Falk, Rodney H and Podrid, PJ, editors. Atrial Fibrillation: Mechanisms and Management. 2ⁿᵈ edition, 1997, Lippincott-Raven Publishers, Philadelphia, p. 282

24. ACC/AHA/ESC guidelines for the management of patients with atrial fibrillation: executive summary. Circulation, Vol. 104, October 23, 2001, pp. 2118-50

25. Warfarin versus aspirin for prevention of thromboembolism in atrial fibrillation: Stoke Prevention in Atrial Fibrillation II Study. The Lancet, Vol. 343, March 19, 1994, pp. 687-91

26. Go, AS, et al. Anticoagulation therapy for stroke prevention in atrial fibrillation. JAMA, Vol. 290, November 26, 2003, pp. 2685-92

27. Warfarin of only modest benefit. Circulation, Vol. 108, No. 17, October 28, 2003, p. IV-757, abstract #3419

28. Petersen, Palle, et al. Ximelagatran versus warfarin for stroke prevention in patients with nonvalvular atrial fibrillation. Journal of the American College of Cardiology. Vol. 41, May 7, 2003, pp. 1445-51

29. Stroke prevention with the oral direct thrombin inhibitor ximelagatran compared with warfarin in patients with non-valvular atrial fibrillation (SPORTIF III). The Lancet, Vol. 362, November 22, 2003, pp. 1691-98

30. Wintrobe's Clinical Hematology, 9th edition, Lea & Febiger, 1993, p. 1530-31

31. Wells, PS, et al. Interactions of warfarin with drugs and food. Annals of Internal Medicine, Vol. 121, November 1, 1994, pp. 676-83

32. Hylek, EM, et al. Acetaminophen and other risk factors for excessive warfarin anticoagulation. JAMA, Vol. 279, March 4, 1998, pp. 657-62, 702-03

33. Carabballo, PJ, et al. Long-term use of oral anticoagulation and the risk of fracture. Archives of Internal Medicine, Vol. 159, August 9/23, 1999, pp. 1750-56

34. Wallentin, Lars, et al. Oral ximelagatran for secondary prophylaxis after myocardial infarction: The ESTEEM randomised controlled trial. The Lancet, Vol. 362, September 6, 2003, pp. 789-97

35. Schulman, Sam, et al. Secondary prevention of venous thromboembolism with the oral direct thrombin inhibitor ximelagatran. New England Journal of Medicine, Vol. 349, October 30, 2003, pp. 1713-21

36. Francis, Charles W., et al. Comparison of ximelagatran with warfarin for the prevention of venous thromboembolism after total knee replacement. New England Journal of Medicine, Vol. 349, October 30, 2003, pp. 1703-12

37. Halperin, JL, et al. Ximelagatran compared with warfarin for prevention of thromboembolism in patients with nonvalvular atrial fibrillation: rationale, objectives, and design of a pair of clinical studies and baseline patient characteristics (SPORTIF III and V). American Heart Journal, Vol. 146, September 2003, pp. 431-38

38. Halperin, JL. SPORTIF V: Stroke prevention using oral thrombin inhibitor in atrial fibrillation. www.medscape.com/viewarticle/464545

39. Spivak, JL and Eichner, ER, eds. The Fundamentals of Clinical Hematology, 3rd edition, 1993, Johns Hopkins University Press, pp. 387-98

40. Hennekens, CH, et al. Additive benefits of pravastatin and aspirin to decrease risk of cardiovascular disease. Archives of Internal Medicine, Vol. 164, January 12, 2004, pp. 40-44

41. Vrecer, M, et al. Use of statins in primary and secondary prevention of coronary heart disease and ischemic stroke. Int J Clin Pharmacol Ther, Vol. 41, December 2003, pp. 567-77

42. Vaughan, CJ. Prevention of stroke and dementia with statins: effects beyond lipid lowering. American Journal of Cardiology, Vol. 91, No. 4A, February 20, 2003, pp. 23B-29B

43. Pierre-Paul, D and Gahtan, V. Noncholesterol-lowering effects of statins. Vasc Endovascular Surg, Vol. 37, No. 5, Sep-Oct 2003, pp. 301-13

44. Liao, JK. Beyond lipid lowering: the role of statins in vascular protection. International Journal of Cardiology, Vol. 86, No. 1, November 2002, pp. 5-18

45. Jamil, S and Iqbal, P. Rhabdomyolysis induced by a single dose of a statin. Heart, Vol. 90, January 2004, p. e3

46. How a statin might destroy a drug company. The Lancet, Vol. 361, March 8, 2003, p. 793

47. Pagan, S. You're my wife? New Scientist, December 6, 2003, p. 14

48. Langsjoen, PH and Langsjoen, AM. The clinical use of HMG CoA-reductase inhibitors and the associated depletion of coenzyme Q10. Biofactors, Vol. 18, No. 1-4, 2003, pp. 101-11

49. Bosch. J, et al. Use of ramipril in preventing stroke. British Medical Journal, Vol. 324, March 23, 2002, pp. 699-702

50. Chapman, N, et al. Effects of a perindopril-based blood pressure-lowering regimen on the risk of recurrent stroke according to stroke subtype and medical history. Stroke, Vol. 35, January 2004, pp. 116-21

51. Hansson, L, et al. Effect of angiotensin-converting-enzyme inhibition compared with conventional therapy on cardiovascular morbidity and mortality in hypertension. The Lancet, Vol. 353, February 20, 1999, pp. 611-16

52. Preventing stroke with ramipril. British Medical Journal, Vol. 325, August 24, 2002, pp. 439-41

53. Wintrobe's Clinical Hematology, 9th edition, Lea & Febiger, 1993, p. 1515-51

54. Donnan, GA, et al. Streptokinase for acute ischemic stroke with relationship to time of administration. JAMA, Vol. 276, September 25, 1996, pp. 961-66

55. Cox, JL, et al. Impact of the maze procedure on the stroke rate in patients with atrial fibrillation. J Thorac Cardiovasc Surg, Vol. 118, 1999, pp. 833-40

56. Sievert, H, et al. Percutaneous left atrial appendage transcatheter occlusion to prevent stroke in high-risk patients with atrial fibrillation. Circulation, Vol. 105, April 23, 2002, pp. 1887-89

57. Crystal, E, et al. Left Atrial Appendage Occlusion Study (LAAOS). American Heart Journal, Vol. 145, 2003, pp. 174-78

Chapter 6

Effectiveness of Antithrombotic Agents

The effectiveness of an antithrombotic agent, whether natural or synthetic, depends on four aspects:

1. How well does the agent inhibit or eliminate the underlying causes of thrombosis?
2. How effective is the agent in inhibiting the various factors promoting platelet aggregation?
3. How effective is the agent in inhibiting the various factors promoting coagulation?
4. How effective is the agent in enhancing the various factors promoting fibrinolysis?

1. Inhibiting Effects on Underlying Causes

Table 1 summarizes the inhibitory effects on the underlying causes of thrombosis of the various antithrombotic agents discussed in chapters 3 and 5.

It is clear that natural antithrombotic agents are far more effective than pharmaceutical antithrombotic agents when it comes to inhibiting or eliminating the underlying causes of thrombosis. It is likely that most natural antithrombotics owe their effectiveness as much to their ability to deal with underlying causes as to their ability to interfere with the platelet aggregation, coagulation or fibrinolysis processes themselves. It is also clear that a supplementation program can easily be designed to provide effective protection against all the most common underlying causes of thrombosis.

Aspirin, statin drugs and ACE inhibitors also have significant inhibitory effects on some underlying causes of thrombosis, but warfarin and ximelagatran do not.

2. Inhibiting Effects on Platelet Aggregation

The most important components involved in platelet aggregation are:

- Thromboxane A2
- ADP (adenosine diphosphate)
- Von Willebrand factor
- Prothrombin
- Fibrinogen
- Nitric oxide (inhibits platelet aggregation)

- Prostacyclin (inhibits platelet aggregation)

Table 2 summarizes the known effects on platelet aggregation of the various antithrombotic agents discussed in chapters 3 and 5.

TABLE 1
Beneficial Effects on Underlying Causes of Thrombosis

Agent	Dysf	BP	Hcy	Lipids	Oxi	NO	Inflam
Vitamin B cocktail	X		X				X
Vitamin B6	X		X				X
Vitamin C	X	X			X		
Vitamin E	X				X		
Niacin (vitamin B3)				X			
Lycopene	X				X	X	
Magnesium	X	X			X		
Potassium		X					
Fish oils	X	X		X			X
Garlic	X	X		X	X		
Ginkgo biloba		X			X	X	
L-arginine	X					X	
Red wine	X			X	X	X	X
Resveratrol	X			X	X	X	X
Tea/flavonoids					X		
Nattokinase		X					
Exercise		X		X			
Aspirin							X
Clopidogrel						X	
Warfarin							
Ximelagatran							
Statin drugs	X			X		X	X
ACE inhibitors		X					

Dys = Endothelial dysfunction
BP = Hypertension
Hcy = Homocysteine level
Lipids = Hyperlipidemia (high cholesterol levels)
Oxi = Oxidative stress
NO = Nitric oxide deficiency
Inflam = Inflammation

TABLE 2
Beneficial Effects on Platelet Aggregation

Agent	PLA	A2	ADP	vonW	Proth	Fib	NO	Prostcy
Vitamin B cocktail	X				X			
Vitamin B6	X		X					
Vitamin C	X			X				
Vitamin E	X	X		X	X		X	X
Niacin	X				X	X		
Fish oils	X					X		
Garlic	X							
Ginkgo biloba	X						X	
L-arginine	X						X	
Red wine	X					X		
Resveratrol	X					X		
Nattokinase								
Aspirin	X	X	X					
Clopidogrel	X		X					
Warfarin								
Ximelagatran								
Statin drugs	?						X	
ACE inhibitors	?							

PLA = Overall inhibition of platelet aggregation
A2= Thromboxane A2 (inhibition is beneficial)
ADP = Adenosine diphosphate (inhibition is beneficial)
vonW = von Willebrand factor (inhibition is beneficial)
Proth = Prothrombin (inhibition is beneficial)
Fib = Fibrinogen (reduced level is beneficial)
NO = Nitric oxide (increased level is beneficial)
Prostcy = Prostacyclin (increased level is beneficial)

It is clear that a judicious combination of natural antiplatelet agents can effectively inhibit or enhance, as the case may be, all the major factors involved in platelet aggregation. Aspirin, on the other hand, only inhibits the production of thromboxane A2 and ADP-induced platelet aggregation. Clopidogrel only inhibits ADP-induced platelet aggregation. Warfarin, ximelagatran and ACE inhibitors have no effect on platelet aggregation, but statin drugs may inhibit it somewhat due to their ability to increase NO production.

The antiplatelet effects of natural supplements are by no means negligible. Vitamin B6 reduces ADP-induced platelet aggregation by 48% and epinephrine-induced aggregation by 41%. Vitamin E reduces the level of prothrombin (fragments 1 and 2) by 25%; high-dose niacin reduces it by 60% and, in addition, reduces fibrinogen level by 14%. Fish oil supplementation reduces fibrinogen levels by about 13% [1-4].

It is indeed unfortunate that there have been no clinical trials comparing aspirin with natural supplements in the prevention of platelet aggregation. Were such trials ever to be under taken, I would suspect that natural antiplatelet agents would come out the winner and, what's more, they carry none of the serious, inherent bleeding risks of aspirin.

3. Inhibiting Effects on Coagulation Process

The most important parameters involved in blood coagulation are:

- Intrinsic pathway factors XII, XI, IX and VIII
- Extrinsic pathway factor VII
- Common pathway factors X and V
- von Willebrand factor
- Tissue factor (thromboplastin)
- Prothrombin, thrombin and fibrin dimers (D-dimer)
- Fibrinogen
- Antithrombin III and protein-C and -S

Table 3 summarizes the known effect on coagulation parameters of the various antithrombotic agents discussed in chapters 3 and 5.

It is clear that the effect of natural antithrombotic agents is less pronounced when it comes to inhibiting the coagulation process than when it comes to inhibiting platelet aggregation. Vitamin C and vitamin E do inhibit the intrinsic pathway through their ability to lower von Willebrand factor and vitamin E and the vitamin B cocktail also play a role in reducing the conversion of prothrombin to thrombin as does niacin. Niacin and fish oils reduce fibrinogen levels and red wine and resveratrol reduce the level of tissue factor (thromboplastin), which initiates the extrinsic pathway.

Aspirin, clopidogrel and the remaining natural substances do not directly influence the coagulation process unless it is initiated by platelet activation.

Warfarin interrupts the coagulation cascade by inhibiting the activation of vitamin K dependent coagulation factors V, VII and X in the extrinsic and common pathways.

TABLE 3
Beneficial Effects on Coagulation

Agent	PLA	Int	Ext	Com	vonW	TisF	Proth	Fib
Vitamin B cocktail	X			X			X	
Vitamin B6	X							
Vitamin C	X	X			X			
Vitamin E	X	X		X	X		X	
Niacin	X			X			X	X
Fish oils	X			X				X
Garlic	X							
Ginkgo biloba	X							
L-arginine	X							
Red wine	X		X			X		
Resveratrol	X		X			X		
Nattokinase								
Aspirin	X							
Clopidogrel	X							
Warfarin			X	X				
Ximelagatran							X	
Statin drugs	?							
ACE inhibitors	?							

PLA = Overall inhibition of platelet aggregation
Int = Inhibiting intrinsic pathway factors VIII, IX, XI and XII
Ext =Inhibiting extrinsic pathway factor VII
Com = Inhibiting common pathway factors V and X
vonW = Reducing concentration of von Willebrand factor
TisF = Reducing level of tissue factor (thromboplastin)
Proth = Inhibiting conversion of prothrombin to thrombin
Fib = Reducing level of fibrinogen or inhibiting conversion to fibrin

Ximelagatran inhibits the final step in the coagulation process; namely, the conversion of fibrinogen to insoluble fibrin by thrombin.

There is very little information on the magnitude of the effect of natural supplements on the coagulation cascade although South African and Turkish researchers have reported that vitamin B6 increases bleeding time by about 65% [1,5].

4. Effects on Fibrinolysis

The most important factors involved in fibrinolysis are:
- Plasminogen
- Plasminogen activators (tPA and urokinase)
- Plasminogen activator inhibitor 1 (PAI-1)

Table 4 summarizes the known effects on fibrinolysis of the various antithrombotic agents discussed in chapters 3 and 4.

TABLE 4
Effects on Fibrinolysis

Agent	Fibrinolytic Activity	Plas	tPA	PAI-1	Direct
Vitamin C	X			X	
Nattokinase	X			X	X
Aspirin					
Warfarin					
Ximelagatran					
Statin drugs					
ACE inhibitors					

Plas = Plasminogen (increase is beneficial)
tPA = Plasminogen activators (increase is beneficial)
PAI-1 = Plasminogen activator inhibitor PAI-1 (reduction is beneficial)
Direct = Direct clot dissolving effect

The fibrinolysis process is obviously difficult to influence through the use of drugs or supplements. There are drugs that can be used to dissolve existing blood clots. However, these drugs must be injected and their effect is hard to control, so they are only used for treatment once a stroke or heart attack has actually occurred; they are not used for prevention.

This leaves vitamin C and nattokinase as the only viable alternatives for increasing fibrinolytic activity as a stroke prevention measure. Both of these supplements work by reducing the level of plasminogen activator inhibitor 1 (PAI-1), a compound that prevents the conversion of plasminogen to plasmin, the body's endogenous clot dissolver. Nattokinase also works by dissolving blood clots directly and is about four times as effective as plasmin in doing so. Other research has shown that nattokinase prevents the formation of blood clots on injured artery walls [6-8]. A recent clinical trial found nattokinase to be 100% effective in preventing deep vein thrombosis in air travellers at high risk for developing thrombi in the veins [9]. Vitamin C supplementation has been found to increase fibrinolytic activity by 45-63% [10].

EFFECTIVENESS IN STROKE PREVENTION

While antithrombotic drugs like aspirin, warfarin and ximelagatran have been exhaustively evaluated to determine their effectiveness in stroke prevention, very few clinical trials have been performed to evaluate the effectiveness of natural compounds. Nevertheless, it is possible to get a reasonable idea of the relative benefits of natural antithrombotic agents by considering data from large-scale epidemiologic studies.

In doing so, it should be kept in mind that most ischemic strokes suffered by atrial fibrillation patients have the same underlying causes and the same mechanism of thrombosis as do ischemic strokes occurring in the general population except, perhaps, in the case of permanent afibbers with heart failure where blood stasis may play a greater role. Thus the effectiveness of stroke prevention measures observed in the general population should be a direct indication of the effectiveness that could be expected among low-risk atrial fibrillation patients.

Table 5 summarizes the effects and effectiveness of natural and pharmaceutical stroke prevention agents.

It is clear that there is a vast array of natural antithrombotic agents that can provide very meaningful protection against ischemic stroke in afibbers with no other risk factors for stroke. It is also evident that these agents are far superior to aspirin and warfarin when <u>net benefit</u> is considered, ie. when reduction in ischemic stroke risk is adjusted for increased risk of major bleeding and hemorrhagic stroke. There is no evidence that any of the natural agents increase the risk of major bleeding or hemorrhagic stroke.

There is, unfortunately, no data in the medical literature regarding the effectiveness of natural antithrombotics in stroke prevention among afibbers with one or more risk factors for stroke. This makes the design of a rational stroke prevention program a whole lot more challenging.

TABLE 5
Effect and Effectiveness of Antithrombotics

Agent	Beneficial Effect on				Risk Reduc, %		Ref #
	Causes	Aggr	Coag	Fibrin	Stroke	Net	
Vitamin B cocktail	X	X	X		80	80	11
Vitamin B6	X	X			90	90	12
Vitamin C	X	X	X	X	50	50	13
Vitamin E	X	X	X		30	30	14,15
Niacin (B3)	X	X	X		?	?	
Lycopene	X				?	?	
Magnesium	X				?	?	

TABLE 5 [continued]
Effect and Effectiveness of Antithrombotics

Agent	Beneficial Effect on				Risk Reduction, %		Ref #
	Causes	Aggr	Coag	Fibrin	Stroke	Net	
Potassium	X				40-50	40-50	16-18
Fish oils	X	X	X		40-50	40-50	19,20
Garlic	X	X			50	50	21
Ginkgo biloba	X	X			?	?	
L-arginine	X	X			?	?	
Red wine	X	X	X		45	45	22
Resveratrol	X	X	X		45	45	22
Tea/flavonoids	X				70	70	23
Nattokinase				X	100?	100?	6-9
Aspirin	X	X			30	0	24
Clopidogrel	?	X			40	0	25
Warfarin (a)			X		0	0	26
Warfarin (b)			X		56	57	26
Ximelagatran (b)			X		56	?	27-29
Statin drugs (c)	X	?	?		30	30	30
ACE inhibitors (c)	X	?	?		32	32	31
Exercise	?	?	?	?	50	50	32
No Smoking	?	?	?	?	50	50	33

Causes = Beneficial effect on underlying causes of thrombosis
Aggr = Beneficial effect on platelet aggregation
Coag = Beneficial effect on coagulation process
Fibrin = Beneficial effect of fibrinolysis process
Stroke = Relative reduction in risk of ischemic stroke
Net = Net benefit, ie. Reduction in ischemic stroke risk adjusted for increased risk of major bleeding and hemorrhagic stroke
Ref = Reference number

(a) *In AF patients with no additional risk factors for stroke*
(b) *In AF patients who have suffered a prior stroke*
(c) *In AF patients who have suffered a prior stroke or heart attack*

REFERENCES

1. Sermet, A., et al. Effect of oral pyridoxine hydrochloride supplementation on in vitro platelet sensitivity to different agonists. Arzneimittelforschung, Vol. 45, January 1995, pp. 19-21

2. De, CR, et al. Plasma protein oxidation is associated with an increase of pro-coagulant markers causing an imbalance between pro- and anticoagulant pathways in healthy subjects. Thromb Haemost, Vol. 87, January 2002, pp. 58-67

3. Chesney, CM, et al. Effect of niacin, warfarin, and antioxidant therapy on coagulation parameters in patients with peripheral arterial disease in the Arterial Disease Multiple Intervention Trial (ADMIT). American Heart Journal, Vol. 140, October 2000, pp. 631-36

4. Flaten, H, et al. Fish-oil concentrate: effects of variables related to cardiovascular disease. American Journal of Clinical Nutrition, Vol. 52, 1990, pp. 300-06

5. van Wyk, V, et al. The in vivo effect in humans of pyridoxal-5'-phosphate on platelet function and blood coagulation. Throm Res, Vol. 66, June 15, 1992, pp. 657-68

6. Fujita, M, et al. Thrombolytic effect of nattokinase on a chemically induced thrombosis model in rats. Biol Pharm Bull, Vol. 18, October 1995, pp. 1387-91

7. Suzuki, Y, et al. Dietary supplementation of fermented soybean, natto, suppresses intimal thickening and modulates the lysis of mural thrombi after endothelial injury in rat femoral artery. Life Sciences, Vol. 73, No. 10, July 25, 2003, pp. 1289-98

8. Suzuki, Y, et al. Dietary supplementation with fermented soybeans suppresses intimal thickening. Nutrition, Vol. 19, March 2003, pp. 261-64

9. Cesarone, MR, et al. Prevention of venous thrombosis in long-haul flights with Flite Tabs. Angiology, Vol. 54, No. 5, Sept-Oct, 2003, pp. 531-39

10. Bordia, AK. The effect of vitamin C on blood lipids, fibrinolytic activity and platelet adhesiveness in patients with coronary artery disease. Atherosclerosis, Vol. 35, February 1980, pp. 181-87

11. Bostom, AG, et al. Nonfasting plasma total homocysteine levels and stroke incidence in elderly persons. Annals of Internal Medicine, Vol. 131, September 7, 1999, pp. 352-55

12. Khaw, KT and Woodhouse, P. Interrelation of vitamin C, infection, haemostatic factors, and cardiovascular disease. British Medical Journal, Vol. 310, June 17, 1995, pp. 1559-63

13. Kurl, S, et al. Plasma vitamin C modifies the association between hypertension and risk of stroke. Stroke, Vol. 33, June 2002, pp. 1568-73

14. Stampfer, MJ, et al. Vitamin E consumption and the risk of coronary disease in women and men. New England Journal of Medicine, Vol. 328, May 20, 1993, pp. 1444-56

15. Stampfer, MJ and Rimm, EB. Epidemiologic evidence for vitamin E in prevention of cardiovascular disease. American Journal of Clinical Nutrition, Vol. 62 (suppl), December 1995, pp. 1365S-69S

16. Green, DM, et al. Serum potassium level and dietary potassium intake as risk factors for stroke. Neurology, Vol. 59, August 2002, pp. 314-20

17. Levine, SR and Coull, BM. Potassium depletion as a risk factor for stroke. Neurology, Vol. 59, August 2002, pp. 302-03

18. Ascherio, A, et al. Intake of potassium, magnesium, calcium, and fiber and risk of stroke among US men. Circulation, Vol. 98, September 22, 1998, pp. 1198-1204

19. Iso, H, et al. Intake of fish and omega-3 fatty acids and risk of stroke in women. JAMA, Vol. 285, January 17, 2001, pp. 304-12

20. He, K, et al. Fish consumption and risk of stroke in men. JAMA, Vol. 288, December 25, 2002, pp. 3130-36

21. Siegel, G, et al. Pleiotropic effects of garlic. Wien Med Wochenschr, Vol. 149, No. 8-10, 1999, pp. 217-24 [article in German]
22. Malarcher, AM, et al. Alcohol intake, type of beverage, and the risk of cerebral infarction in young women. Stroke, Vol. 32, January 2001, pp. 77-83
23. Keli, SO, et al. Dietary flavonoids, antioxidant vitamins, and incidence of stroke. Archives of Internal Medicine, Vol. 156, March 25, 1996, pp. 637-42
24. Eidelman, RS, et al. An update on aspirin in the primary prevention of cardiovascular disease. Archives of Internal Medicine, Vol. 163, September 22, 2003, pp. 2006-10
25. CAPRIE Steering Committee. A randomized, blinded, trial of clopidogrel versus aspirin in patients at risk of ischemic events. The Lancet, Vol. 348, November 16, 1996, pp. 1329-39
26. Go, AS, et al. Anticoagulation therapy for stroke prevention in atrial fibrillation. JAMA, Vol. 290, November 26, 2003, pp. 2685-92
27. Stroke prevention with the oral direct thrombin inhibitor ximelagatran compared with warfarin in patients with non-valvular atrial fibrillation (SPORTIF III). The Lancet, Vol. 362, November 22, 2003, pp. 1691-98
28. Halperin, JL, et al. Ximelagatran compared with warfarin for prevention of thromboembolism in patients with nonvalvular atrial fibrillation: rationale, objectives, and design of a pair of clinical studies and baseline patient characteristics (SPORTIF III and V). American Heart Journal, Vol. 146, September 2003, pp. 431-38
29. Haperin, JL. SPORTIF V: Stroke prevention using oral thrombin inhibitor in atrial fibrillation. www.medscape.com/viewarticle/464545
30. Hennekens, CH, et al. Additive benefits of pravastatin and aspirin to decrease risk of cardiovascular disease. Archives of Internal Medicine, Vol. 164, January 12, 2004, pp. 40-44
31. Bosch. J, et al. Use of ramipril in preventing stroke. British Medical Journal, Vol. 324, March 23, 2002, pp. 699-702
32. Kiely, DK, et al. Physical activity and stroke risk: the Framingham Study. American Journal of Epidemiology, Vol. 140, October 1, 1994, pp. 608-20
33. Kawachi, I, et al. Smoking cessation and decreased risk of stroke in women. JAMA, Vol. 269, January 13, 1993, pp. 232-36

Chapter 7

Living with Warfarin

Anticoagulation with warfarin is not recommended for afibbers with no underlying heart disease or other risk factors for stroke.[1,2]   However, in patients with a history of prior stroke or TIA (transient ischemic attack) and in those with prosthetic (artificial) heart valves the use of warfarin is likely to be beneficial overall. Many patients with less serious stroke risk factors such as hypertension and diabetes are also prescribed warfarin although it is somewhat doubtful whether the reduction in ischemic stroke risk outweighs the increase in the risk of serious bleeding and hemorrhagic stroke. A recent study of atrial fibrillation patients on warfarin found that the risk of major bleeding was 2.5% a year in the case of uncontrolled hypertension.[3]   This compares to an ischemic stroke risk of 1.5-2.8% a year when not on warfarin.[4,5] This is not a significant difference.

The study, involving 1604 afibbers released from hospital on warfarin, found that most of the major bleeding events occurred in the gastrointestinal tract (67.3%). Hemorrhagic strokes accounted for 15.3% of the bleeding events, and the remaining 17.3% were in other locations. The seriousness of the bleeds can be judged by the fact that 21.6% of the patients admitted for warfarin-induced bleeding died within 30 days. In comparison, only 6-10% of patients admitted to hospital for ischemic stroke die while in hospital, most of them through errors in the administration of thrombolytic agents.[6]

While it is thus not at all clear that anticoagulation with warfarin produces an overall benefit in the majority of patients, it is nevertheless widely prescribed and many patients need to live with it for the remainder of their lives. For those patients it is clearly important to know what the adverse effects of warfarin are, and how to protect against them.

The most serious adverse effect of warfarin is the potential for major gastrointestinal bleeding and hemorrhagic stroke or bleeding in the brain. A recent study of 1604 afibbers released from hospital on warfarin observed a 5% a year risk of a major bleed and a 21.6% chance of dying from this bleed within 30 days.[3] Warfarin usage has also been linked to arterial calcification (atherosclerosis) and long-term use to an increased risk of osteoporosis. Other less common adverse effects include skin necrosis sometimes requiring amputation, and ocular (eye-related) bleeding.

GASTROINTESTINAL BLEEDING AND HEMORRHAGIC STROKE

Warfarin was originally developed as a rat poison. It works in two ways – in effective doses it increases the permeability of the capillaries (smallest blood vessels) thus allowing blood to seep out of the vessels and into the organs and surrounding body cavity. Secondly, it prevents the vitamin K-dependent clotting activity, which would normally stop the leak until it can be repaired. If nothing is done the animal (or human) will eventually die from loss of blood.[7] To understand the intricacies of this process and find possible ways of preventing it, it is necessary to develop a basic understanding of the function and construction of blood vessels.

Blood vessels

Blood is "the river of life". It carries nutrients to and receives waste from each individual cell in the body. It begins its journey in the main arteries emanating from the heart's left ventricle. As it flows through smaller and smaller arteries it eventually reaches the arterioles, which control the flow of blood to the tissues. Each arteriole, in turn, can serve hundreds of the smallest blood vessel of all, the capillary. The diameter of a capillary is so small that red blood cells can only pass through one at a time. About 10 billion capillaries lace all body tissues bringing blood to within reach of every cell. Capillary walls are highly permeable and while they will not, in normal circumstances, allow the passage of blood itself, they readily allow the transfer of oxygen, nutrients, hormones, carbon dioxide, and waste products between the cell and the blood flowing through the capillary. After the exchange with the cell has taken place the capillaries become part of the venous system with the blood flowing through venules and veins before returning to the right atrium.

In order to achieve the required permeability, the walls of capillaries are, of necessity, very thin. As a matter of fact, they consist of just one layer of epithelial (lining) cells held in place by a "skeleton" of cross-linked collagen fibers embedded in a matrix of laminin which "glues" the lining cells to the collagen "net". The collagen/laminin structure supporting the single layer of epithelial cells is also known as the basement membrane and is a component of all blood vessels whether large or small.

Research involving snake venom and matrix metalloproteinases has clearly shown that hemorrhage (blood seeping out of blood vessels) is caused by destruction of the collagen fibers forming the backbone of the basement membranes.[8] In other words, for red blood cells to be able to get through the collagen "net" it must first be broken. Although I am not aware of any specific research concerning the mechanism by which warfarin causes hemorrhage, it would have to do so by degrading the collagen network and perhaps the laminin matrix as well. Thus, an obvious way of preventing warfarin-induced bleeding would be to strengthen the basement membrane and ensure that the raw materials for repairing it are readily at hand.

Prevention of hemorrhage

Perhaps the most "famous" disease involving internal bleeding is scurvy. Scurvy is now known to be caused by a vitamin C deficiency, but before this was understood scurvy epidemics devastated the ancient populations in Egypt, Greece and Rome, and until the 18th Century caused numerous deaths in Europe as well. In 1536 when the French explorer Jacques Cartier arrived in Newfoundland native Indians advised him to give his men, who were dying from scurvy, a potion made from spruce tree needles. This potion would have been very high in vitamin C and actually cured most of Cartier's crew. In 1742 British naval commander James Lind described the miraculous effects of citrus juice on sailors suffering from scurvy and by the late 1700s all British navy ships carried citrus fruits (especially limes from which the term "limey" originates) to avoid scurvy outbreaks.

There is now substantial evidence that vitamin C works its bleeding preventing magic by promoting the synthesis and deposition of both collagen and laminin.[9-11] There is also direct evidence that vitamin C helps prevent gastrointestinal bleeding resulting from regular aspirin use. German researchers found that combining aspirin (acetylsalicylic acid) with vitamin C (ascorbic acid) significantly reduces the number of microscopic blood leaks normally observed in the stomach when taking aspirin.[12] Another group of German researchers found that aspirin causes gastric mucosal damage and micro-bleeding both before and after *H. pylori* eradication. Buffering the aspirin with vitamin C resulted in significantly less stomach lining damage and bleeding both before and especially after *H. pylori* eradication.[13]

Thus, it would appear that ensuring an adequate daily intake of vitamin C is an important step in reducing and quickly repairing warfarin-induced breakdown of the basement membrane. Since vitamin C is used up and excreted fairly quickly, taking three or four doses of 500 mg of vitamin C throughout the day is the ideal way to ensure a constant and adequate level in the blood stream. Patients with hemochromatosis (iron overload) should only supplement with vitamin C under the supervision of a competent health care provider and should probably limit their intake to 200 mg three or four times daily.

Collagen is the most abundant protein in the human body so it is clearly important to also ensure an adequate intake of the amino acids (lysine, alanine, and proline) that make up the collagen structure. Cheese, eggs, lima beans, potatoes, milk, meat, and brewer's yeast are good sources of lysine, and meats are good sources of proline, which can also be synthesized in the liver from other amino acids. Alanine can be obtained from meat, poultry, fish, eggs, avocado, and dairy products. Lysine, proline and alanine are also available as individual supplements.

Mathias Rath MD, a former associate of the late Linus Pauling, has formulated a supplement specifically designed to ensure optimum collagen production and repair.[14] The formula contains vitamin C and other dietary antioxidants and minerals as well as proline and lysine. Dr. Rath reports that it is effective in preventing and reversing atherosclerosis, but I am not aware of any research that has studied its possible effects in preventing warfarin-induced bleeding.

Green tea and grapeseed extract have also been found to inhibit the collagen-destroying action of metalloproteinases, and green tea on its own has been found to significantly reduce the risk of a certain type of hemorrhagic stroke involving bleeding on the surface of the brain (subarachnoid hemorrhage).[15-16]

There is also some, still controversial evidence, that supplementation with the amino acid arginine may enhance collagen synthesis and deposition.[17-19]

It would thus appear that the risk of warfarin-induced bleeding and hemorrhagic stroke can be materially reduced by supplementing with vitamin C and the amino acids proline and lysine. Green tea may also be helpful because of its significant content of vitamin K, but large amounts should not be consumed without appropriate monitoring of INR.[20,21] There is no evidence that vitamin C interferes with the anticoagulation effect of warfarin.[22] As a matter of fact, low blood levels of vitamin C have been associated with a substantially increased risk of both ischemic and hemorrhagic stroke. Finnish researchers have found that men with a plasma vitamin C level below 28.4 micromol/L have twice the risk of experiencing a stroke (hemorrhagic or ischemic) when compared to men with a level above 65 micromol/L. The association was particularly pronounced among hypertensive men where low vitamin C levels were associated with a 2.6 times higher risk and among overweight men where low levels were associated with a 2.7-fold risk increase.[23] Tissue saturation with vitamin C (about 70 micromol/L in plasma) can be achieved by supplementing with 300-500 mg of vitamin C three times daily.

ARTERIAL CALCIFICATION

Arterial calcification is commonly associated with atherosclerosis and involves the deposition of calcium phosphate (hydroxyapatite) on artery walls. Atherosclerosis is a major risk factor for ischemic stroke so it is indeed ironic that warfarin has been implicated in the formation of arterial calcification. Australian researchers have reported that rats treated with warfarin develop extensive arterial calcification and concluded that, "It is likely that humans on long-term warfarin treatment have extrahepatic vitamin K deficiency and hence are potentially at increased risk of developing arterial calcification."[24] US doctors recently reported the case of an otherwise healthy man who developed extensive calcification of the coronary arteries after long-term warfarin treatment. They conclude that, "physicians prescribing long-term warfarin treatment should consider arterial calcification as one of its potential consequences."[25] Dutch researchers have confirmed that a vitamin K deficiency, such as would be induced by warfarin treatment, increases the risk of arterial calcification and conclude that the current RDA for vitamin K is too low.[26]

Unfortunately, the common advice given by physicians to their warfarin-treated patients is to avoid dark green leafy vegetables (the major dietary source of vitamin K) and to strictly avoid vitamin K-containing supplements – thus guaranteeing a vitamin K deficiency.

Fortunately, this advice may be about to become obsolete. British researchers recently reported that minimizing vitamin K intake while on warfarin might be precisely the wrong thing to do. Their study involved 26 patients (stable) whose INR had remained within the therapeutic range for at least 6 months without a change in warfarin dosage. The daily vitamin K intake of these patients was compared to that of 26 patients (unstable) whose INR had been varying considerably (standard deviation of INR values greater than 0.5) over a 6-month period and thus requiring continuous adjustment of warfarin dosage. All participants carefully weighed their food intake for two 7-day periods and completed detailed food diaries. Analysis of the data showed that the unstable patients had a significantly lower average daily intake of vitamin K (K$_1$) than did stable patients (29 versus 76 micrograms/day). As a matter of fact, the daily vitamin K intake of the unstable patients was significantly lower than the daily intake of 60-80 micrograms estimated for the general UK population. The researchers conclude that INR levels can be stabilized by increasing daily vitamin K intake. They point out that even a daily increase in vitamin K intake of 100 micrograms has comparatively little effect on INR (reduction of about 0.2). While it would be theoretically possible to improve the consistency of daily vitamin K intake through a strictly controlled diet, it is unlikely that this would be a viable solution. The researchers conclude their report with the statement, "Daily supplementation with vitamin K could be an alternative method in stabilizing anticoagulation control, lessening the impact of variable dietary vitamin K intake. We are currently evaluating this possibility."[27]

Johannes Oldenburg, a German medical researcher, concurs and suggests that a continuous low-dose intake of vitamin K may stabilize the INR and subsequently reduce risk of bleeding complications.[28]

Natural vitamin K comes in two forms – phylloquinone (vitamin K1) and menaquinone (vitamin K2). Phylloquinone is found in dark green vegetables like spinach, broccoli and kale. Green, but not black tea is also a rich source of phylloquinone. Menaquinone is found in meats, butter, cheese and fermented foods (especially natto) and can also be produced by conversion of vitamin K1 in the intestinal tract. This conversion, however, is compromised after a course of antibiotics. The RDA for total vitamin K intake is 90 micrograms/day for women and 120 micrograms/day for men, and is essentially the amount required for the synthesis of coagulation factors in the liver. The RDA does not consider that vitamin K (especially K2) is also required outside of the liver (extrahepatic), particularly to ensure healthy bones and blood vessels.[26]

The main role of vitamin K is to act as a cofactor for the conversion of glutamate into gamma-carboxyglutamate. Matrix Gla protein (MGP) is derived from gamma-carboxyglutamic acid residues and is a powerful inhibitor of arterial calcification.[26,27] There is evidence that oxidative stress and warfarin inhibit the synthesis of MGP.[29]

Dutch researchers have observed that vitamin K1 tends to accumulate in the liver where it is used in the synthesis of coagulation factors, whereas K2 preferentially accumulates in the artery walls where it participates in the production of MGP which, in turn, inhibits arterial calcification. Unfortunately, warfarin inhibits the intestinal conversion of K1 to K2, thus explaining why warfarin promotes arterial calcification. The researchers also observed that menaquinone, but not phylloquinone supplementation prevented warfarin-induced arterial calcification in rats.[27]

Another group of researchers from Maastricht University in the Netherlands has reported that a high intake of menaquinone (vitamin K2), but not phylloquinone (vitamin K1) is associated with a significantly reduced risk of arterial (aortic) calcification and coronary heart disease (CHD). The epidemiological study included 4800 participants in the Rotterdam Study. The researchers found that the average daily intake of vitamin K1 was 250 micrograms, while that of vitamin K2 was only about 29 micrograms. Study participants with a vitamin K2 intake of more than 32.7 micrograms/day had a 41% reduced risk of CHD, a 57% reduced risk of dying from CHD, and a 26% reduction in overall mortality when compared to those with an intake below 21.6 micrograms/day. Participants with a high menaquinone intake also had a 52% reduced risk of severe arterial calcification. Phylloquinone intake was not associated with decreased risk of CHD, CHD mortality, overall mortality or arterial calcification.[30]

University of Wisconsin researchers have found that, while warfarin is highly effective in blocking the recycling of vitamin K1, it has little effect on the activity of vitamin K2.[31]

Considering the above findings it is tempting to conclude that daily supplementation with menaquinone (vitamin K2) would be highly beneficial in reducing arterial calcification (whether warfarin-induced or not), CHD, and overall mortality without impacting on warfarin's role in reducing the level of coagulation factors. In other words, supplementing with moderate amounts of vitamin K2 should not affect INR levels. Clinical trials, of course, should and hopefully will be carried out to substantiate or negate this hypothesis.

Vitamin D may also play a role in the prevention of arterial calcification. Researchers at the UCLA School of Medicine have reported that the degree of vascular calcification observed in a group of patients at moderate risk for CHD was inversely proportional to the blood level of 1,25-dihydroxyvitamin D, the active metabolite of vitamin D. They suggest that this form of vitamin D may play a role in inhibiting vascular calcification.[32] Dutch researchers support this observation with their finding that supplementation with vitamin D and vitamin K1 has a beneficial effect on the elastic properties of the arterial vessel wall.[33]

Other researchers have, however, found that very large (20 million IU/day or more) doses of vitamin D may actually induce arterial calcification (at least in rats).[34,35] Thus, it may be best to avoid supplementing with more than the dose known to be free of adverse events (2000 IU/day).

A magnesium deficiency, especially if combined with a high exposure to trans-fatty acids, has been found to increase the risk of arterial calcification in cell culture experiments [36] and supplementation with a combination of magnesium and potassium citrate has been found to reduce arterial calcification in rats.[37]

It would thus appear that supplementation with vitamin K, vitamin D and magnesium and potassium citrate can materially reduce the risk of warfarin-induced arterial calcification. It is, of course, necessary to monitor INR very closely if embarking on vitamin K2 prophylactic therapy and it would also appear wise to limit daily vitamin D intake to 2000 IU or less. The most effective form of vitamin K for prevention of arterial calcification is menaquinone (vitamin K2). However, in view of the finding that supplementing with vitamin K (vitamin K1) may help stabilize INR levels, it may be advisable for warfarin-treated patients to use a 50:50 mixture.

OSTEOPOROSIS

Osteoporosis is characterized by a decrease in bone mass and density, causing bones to become fragile and increasing the risk of fractures. In the United States 26% of women 65 years or older, and more than 50% of women 85 years or older have osteoporosis. Over 1.5 million fractures, requiring about 500,000 hospitalizations and costing the health care system about 12 billion dollars, occur every year as a result of osteoporosis.[38] Men are not immune to osteoporosis, but the incidence is significantly lower than among women.[39]

Vitamin K is a crucial element in the process of bone formation, so it is relevant to ask the question, "Is long-term use of warfarin associated with an increased risk of osteoporotic fractures?" A team of researchers from Washington University School of Medicine and the NYU Medical Center recently investigated the association between osteoporotic fractures and warfarin usage in over 14,000 Medicare beneficiaries who were hospitalized with atrial fibrillation. Most of the study participants (70%) had hypertension, 48% had heart failure, and 35% had a history of stroke. A total of 1005 of the study participants (6.9%) experienced an osteoporotic fracture during the 3-year study period. The researchers found that men who had been taking warfarin for a year or more had a 63% higher relative risk of experiencing an osteoporotic fracture when compared to men not taking warfarin. Hip fractures were most common (65% of all fractures) and were associated with a 30-day mortality of 39%. Men using warfarin for less than a year did not have an increased risk of osteoporotic fractures. Osteoporosis risk was not increased in women irrespective of duration of warfarin usage.

The researchers point out that patients taking warfarin are often advised to limit their intake of vitamin K-rich green vegetables. They believe this may be poor advice and that ensuring an adequate intake of vitamin K-1 (found especially in green vegetables) and vitamin K-2 (present in fermented dairy and soy products, fish, meat, liver and eggs) would be more appropriate. They also caution that avoiding green vegetables may lead to a folic acid deficiency and subsequent high levels of homocysteine, a known promoter of atherosclerosis.[40]

Although this study did not find an increased risk of osteoporosis among female warfarin users, it is possible that an association still exists, but is masked by other, more important, risk factors such as loss of estrogen production after menopause. This hypothesis is supported by the recent finding by Australian researchers that children on long-term warfarin therapy also experience a marked reduction in bone density.[41]

To better understand the role of vitamin K in osteoporosis and to suggest ways of preventing it, it is necessary to first gain a broad understanding of the process of bone formation.

Bone formation

Bones consist of a matrix of hydroxyapatite (calcium phosphate) and other minerals embedded in a cross-linked collagen matrix. The formation and maintenance of the bone structure is an ongoing, dynamic process. Up until the age of about 30 years the process involves mainly bone formation, but after this bone formation and bone resorption develop a delicate balance, which if bone resorption becomes dominant can lead to osteopenia (a forerunner of osteoporosis) and osteoporosis. There are two main types of cells involved in the process – osteoblasts which promote the formation of new bone structure by increasing calcium content, and osteoclasts which promote the resorption (demineralization of old bone) by releasing calcium into the blood circulation. Bone formation and resorption are also known as bone remodelling and take place continuously in the entire skeleton. The concentration of calcium in the blood is maintained within very narrow limits using the bone structure as a reservoir. The hormone calcitonin promotes the transfer of calcium into the bones, while parathyroid hormone (PTH) promotes the release of calcium from the bones.

Vitamin D is important in controlling PTH level with a deficiency leading to higher PTH concentration and subsequent demineralization. There is some evidence that an estrogen deficiency makes the osteoclasts more sensitive to PTH. Vitamin K is important in the synthesis of the gamma-carboxylated protein, osteocalcin. A deficiency of osteocalcin is associated with impaired bone formation (remineralization). Calcium, magnesium, boron, and zinc are all important constituents of the bone matrix with calcium being needed in by far the greatest amounts.

The main effect of warfarin as far as osteoporosis is concerned is that its long-term use leads to impaired remineralization due to its interference with the vitamin K-dependent synthesis of osteocalcin. Thus, the main players in the "osteoporosis drama" are calcium, vitamin D, vitamin K, magnesium, boron, and zinc. Maintaining appropriate levels of these components can go a long way in preventing osteoporosis in both men and women whether on warfarin or not.

Prevention of osteoporosis

Due to the devastating nature of osteoporosis and its enormous cost to the health care system, a great deal of research has gone into finding ways of preventing it. The standard medical approach to osteoporosis prevention and treatment involves the life-long use of bisphosphonates such as etidronate (Didronel), alendronate (Fosamax), and raloxifene (Evista) interspersed with calcium and vitamin D supplementation. These drugs work primarily by decreasing bone resorption, in orders words, they result in "old bones". Bisphosphonate therapy is usually effective, but carries the risk of significant side effects, among them necrosis (rotting) of the jaw bone.[42] Merck & Co., the manufacturer of Fosamax is currently facing several class action suits launched by Fosamax users who developed severe necrosis after undergoing dental work.[43]

Fortunately, it is eminently possible to achieve effective and safe osteoporosis prevention through exercise, proper food choices, and supplementation with natural products.

Exercise

There is little doubt that physical inactivity leads to loss of bone mass – even in highly fit astronauts. There is also evidence that a structured program of load-bearing exercise such as regular walking can help prevent osteopenia and its progression to osteoporosis, especially if accompanied by supplementation with calcium and vitamin D.[44,45] Just recently Dr. Rittweger of the Institute for Biophysical and Clinical Research into Human Movement in the UK suggested that high strain rate exercises (weightlifting), while being beneficial in the prevention of osteopenia, may actually increase the risk of fractures in full-blown osteoporosis.[46] So, while high strain rate exercises may be appropriate for younger people, a more moderate program such as regular walking may be better suited to older people. In any case, the program to be effective needs to be accompanied by a proper diet, judicious supplementation, and avoidance of coffee, alcohol, smoking, and soft drinks (colas) which have all been proven to increase the risk of osteoporosis.[47]

Vitamin D

Several studies have shown that vitamin D deficiency is widespread. Researchers at Boston University School of Medicine found that 52% of postmenopausal women with osteoporosis had abnormally low vitamin D (25-hydroxyvitamin D) levels and commensurate high levels of PTH.[48] Vitamin D deficiency was more prevalent in women whose daily intake of dietary vitamin D was less than 400 IU. Swiss researchers recently reported that 64% of postmenopausal women with osteoporosis had a vitamin D deficiency and elevated PTH.[49]

The connection between vitamin D deficiency and osteoporosis was first reported by Meryl LeBoff and colleagues at Brigham and Women's Hospital in Boston. Their 1999 study found that 50% of women admitted with acute osteoporosis-related hip fracture were vitamin D deficient. They suggested that supplementation with vitamin D and accompanying suppression of PTH may reduce future fracture risk and help the healing of existing fractures. They concluded that vitamin D deficiency among the elderly is entirely preventable and recommended supplementation with calcium and 800 IU/day of vitamin D.[50]

Australian researchers have observed that vitamin D deficiency is also a major cause of osteoporosis and hip fractures among men. Their study involved 41 men (60 years and older) who were admitted with hip fractures. Known risk factors for osteoporosis and hip fracture were determined and compared to those of two control groups – one a group of 41 inpatients, the other a group of 41 outpatients all without hip fractures and aged 60 years or older. The researchers found that men in the hip fracture group had significantly lower blood levels of vitamin D (25-hydroxyvitamin D) than did men in the control group. Sixty-three per cent of the men in the hip fracture group had a subclinical vitamin D deficiency (<50 nmol/L serum 25- hydroxyvitamin D) as compared to only 25 per cent in the control group. The researchers also noted that men with hip fractures and hospital in-patients had lower levels of calcium and testosterone than did the out-patient controls. About 89 per cent of the men with hip fractures and the in-patients were diagnosed with hypogonadism (low testosterone levels). The researchers conclude that a vitamin D deficiency is a major cause of hip fractures in elderly men.[51]

It is clear that vitamin D deficiency, irrespective of calcium status, is critical risk factor for osteoporosis and associated bone fractures. Thus, it is fortunate that several clinical trials have concluded that vitamin D supplementation is effective in fracture prevention. Researchers at Harvard School of Public Health, after evaluating 14 reliable studies of oral vitamin D supplementation, concluded that daily supplementation with 700-800 IU of vitamin D reduced hip fracture risk by 26% and overall non-vertebral fracture rate by 23%. No benefit was observed with a daily dose of 400 IU (current RDA for women under the age of 70 years).[52]

A group of researchers at Harvard Medical School studied over 72,000 postmenopausal nurses for 18 years and found that those whose daily vitamin D intake exceeded 500 IU had a 37% lower risk of hip fracture than did women whose intake was less than 140 IU/day. They found no benefit of a high daily intake of milk or calcium on its own. The researchers point out that about 60% of the women in the survey had vitamin D intakes below those recommended by the Food and Nutrition Board (400 IU for women between the ages of 51 and 70 years and 600 IU for women older than 70 years). They also point out that the amount of vitamin-D produced by exposure to sunlight decreases significantly with age (due to thinning of the skin) and the use of sunscreens. They further suggest that the reason why milk showed no significant protective effect may be due to its content of vitamin A which recently has come under scrutiny in regard to its possible role as a negative factor in bone health. The researchers conclude that women should ensure an adequate daily intake of vitamin D either through the use of supplements or through increased consumption of fish such as salmon or sardines.[53]

The importance of daily supplementation with vitamin D is becoming increasingly clear. A team of American and Swiss researchers recently concluded that a daily intake of at least 1000 IU is required in order to achieve reasonable protection against the risk of osteoporosis, fractures, falls, and colon cancer. They suggest that an increase in the current RDA is warranted.[54] Dr. Reinhold Vieth and colleagues of the University of Toronto go even further. They found that 62% of supposedly healthy Canadians were deficient in vitamin D and that a daily intake of 4000 IU (100 micrograms/day) was needed to bring their level of 25(OH)D, the active metabolite of vitamin D, to the desirable level of 75 nmol/L. The researchers conclude that 4000 IU/day of vitamin D3 is a safe and desirable intake, but very specifically caution that their findings regarding vitamin D3 (cholecalciferol) cannot be applied to the synthetic version of vitamin D2 (ergocalciferol), the form most often used in North America. Vitamin D2 is far more toxic than vitamin D3 and produces unique metabolites not generated by D3. The researchers are very "down" on vitamin D2 and say, "It is an anachronism to regard vitamin D2 as a vitamin."[55]

Vitamin D and calcium
An adequate intake of calcium is clearly essential in achieving and maintaining sufficient bone mass due to the simple fact that calcium, in the form of hydroxyapatite, constitutes the major part of the bone structure. In combination with vitamin D it is effective in preventing bone loss and fractures. Ten years ago French researchers discovered that daily supplementation with 1200 mg of calcium and 800 IU of vitamin D3 (cholecalciferol) for 3 years reduced the number of hip fractures in a group of 3270 elderly women by 23%. The researches also noted that the bone density in calcium/vitamin D supplemented women increased by 2.7% over an 18-month period, while it decreased by 4.6% in the placebo group.[56] Since 1996 several other studies have verified the benefits of supplementation with calcium and vitamin D. In 1998 researchers at Johns Hopkins Medical School concluded that, "Optimal intakes of both calcium and vitamin D are relatively cost-effective, safe, and easily implemented approaches to maintain existing bone mass and assist in the prevention of fractures."[57]

Dutch researchers report that 1000-1200 mg/day of calcium (elemental) plus 800 IU/day of vitamin D is effective in the prevention and treatment of osteoporosis.[58] German researchers, after evaluating several randomized, prospective, placebo-controlled clinical trials, conclude that supplementation with 800-1500 mg/day of calcium plus 400-1200 IU/day of vitamin D reduces the risk of falls and fall-related fractures in the elderly.[59] Indeed, the evidence that supplementation with calcium and vitamin D is beneficial in preventing and treating osteoporosis is incontrovertible.

It is, however, becoming increasingly clear that a supposedly adequate calcium intake does not guarantee the absence of osteoporosis. The calcium must not only be ingested, it must also be absorbed and its excretion minimized. In other words, it is not the calcium intake per se that is important, but rather how much of it is actually retained in the body. Researchers at the University of Pittsburgh have found that the intake of fat and fiber significantly influences calcium absorption. Their study involved 142 healthy pre-menopausal white women who had enrolled in the Women's Healthy Lifestyle Project in 1995-96. The women had blood samples drawn three hours after consuming apple juice containing labeled (isotope) calcium. The blood samples were analyzed for calcium, 1,25 dihydroxyvitamin D (the active from of vitamin D), and PTH. The researchers found that about 35% (17-58%) of the labeled calcium had been absorbed. It was clear that women with a higher fat intake and a lower intake of fiber absorbed significantly more calcium than did women with less fat and more fiber in their diet. Women with high blood levels of vitamin D also showed increased absorption while women who consumed alcohol had decreased absorption. There is also some indication that a higher total calcium intake is associated with a lower rate of absorption. The researchers caution that it may only be certain types of fiber (eg. wheat bran) that inhibit calcium absorption. Fiber found in green leafy vegetables such as kale, broccoli, and bok choy may not be detrimental to absorption. They found no indication that genetic differences among the women were in any way related to calcium absorption. The researchers express the hope that their findings will encourage a second look at the current standard recommendation to emphasize a low-fat, high-fiber diet.[60]

The rate of excretion of calcium is also an important factor in determining its effectiveness in osteoporosis prevention. Dr. Christopher Nordin of Australia's Institute of Medical and Veterinary Science points out that is not the total calcium intake which determines bone strength (density), but rather the difference between what is taken in and what is excreted. Research has shown that for each gram of animal protein consumed one milligram of calcium is lost in the urine. This means that a 40-gram reduction in animal protein intake reduces the urinary calcium loss by 40 mg which, in turn, corresponds to a reduction in calcium requirements of 200 mg (assuming an absorption of 20%). A reduction in sodium (salt) intake of 2.3 grams also reduces urinary calcium loss by 40 mg lowering requirements by another 200 mg. So a person with a low intake of protein and salt might have half the calcium requirements of a person eating a typical North American diet. This and the fact that developing countries generally get more sunshine (vitamin D) than developed countries go a long way towards explaining the difference in the incidence of osteoporosis and bone fractures between different cultures and individuals. Dr. Nordin concludes that there is no single, universal calcium requirement, only a requirement linked to the intake of other nutrients especially animal protein and sodium.[61]

Dairy products like milk, cheese and yogurt are the richest sources of calcium followed by collards, spinach, beans, sardines and canned salmon. There is some indication that milk may not be an optimum source of calcium for older people. Researchers at the Boston University School of Medicine have studied the effectiveness of various sources of supplemental calcium in preventing bone loss in older women. Their study involved 60 postmenopausal women aged 65 years or older who did not suffer from osteoporosis and whose daily calcium intake from their regular diet was less than 800 mg/day. The women were randomly assigned to three groups. Group 1 supplemented with four 8-ounce glasses of vitamin D-fortified milk per day, group 2 took a 500 mg calcium carbonate supplement twice a day with meals, and group 3 took a placebo twice a day with meals. Bone density measurements of the spine (L2-L4) and thighbone (greater trochanter [GT]) were done at six-month intervals for a two-year period. After two years women in the placebo group (average daily calcium intake was 683 mg) had lost an average of 3% of their baseline bone mineral density in the trochanter area. This loss occurred exclusively during the winter months. Women in the milk group had an average daily calcium intake of 1028 mg and lost 1.5% of their bone density in the GT area. Women who supplemented with calcium carbonate tablets increased their daily intake to 1633 mg and suffered no bone loss in the GT area. The women in the supplement group also increased the bone density in their spine and femoral neck area by about 3%, while the placebo group women lost about 0.3%, and the milk group about 1.8%. The researchers conclude that 1000 mg/day of supplemental calcium is required in order to prevent bone loss in older women living in northern latitudes. They also point out that an adequate vitamin D intake (600-700 IU/day) is essential in order to prevent bone loss during the winter.[62]

Other researchers, however, have found that calcium is equally well absorbed from skim milk, calcium-fortified orange juice, and calcium carbonate tablets.[63] The most commonly used calcium supplements are calcium carbonate and calcium citrate. A comprehensive study comparing the bioavailability of calcium carbonate and calcium citrate found that calcium citrate was consistently better absorbed whether taken on an empty stomach or with a meal.[64] Other research has shown that calcium carbonate is extremely poorly absorbed by people with low stomach acid even if taken with meals.[47] Inasmuch as low stomach acid (achlorhydria) is a common condition among older people, calcium citrate, calcium malate or calcium fumarate are all much better choices than calcium carbonate. Natural oyster shell calcium, dolomite, and bone-meal products should be avoided due to the potential for lead contamination and poor absorbability.[47]

As an added bonus, supplementation with vitamin D and calcium has also been found to reduce systolic blood pressure by about 10%.[65] Calcium citrate supplementation is also effective in reducing LDL cholesterol (the "bad" kind) and increase HDL cholesterol (the "good" kind").[66] LAF Survey 3 observed that some vagal afibbers who supplemented with calcium experienced longer episodes than average.[67] Thus, vagal afibbers may have to experiment with calcium sources and dosages to find a protocol that works for them.

Calcium
The evidence that calcium supplementation on its own (without vitamin D) increases bone mass and helps prevent osteoporosis is somewhat sparser and more controversial. A 1998 study at the Boston University School of Medicine concluded that 2 x 500 mg of calcium carbonate taken with meals for two years improved bone density in the spine and femoral neck area by about 3%.[62] However, researchers at the Harvard Medical School found no benefit of calcium supplementation on its own.[47] It is quite likely that vitamin D status could explain the differences and also quite conceivable that an adequate

vitamin D intake is actually more important than an increased calcium intake. However, as far as I know, no clinical trials have addressed this question.

In any case, there would seem to be little advantage in consuming more than the RDA (1200 mg/day) of calcium and a great advantage in ensuring that this intake is accompanied by a vitamin D3 intake of at least 1000 IU/day.

Magnesium

Magnesium is a hugely important mineral, especially for afibbers. Its many vital functions have been discussed in detail in Conference Room Sessions 14 and 14A and will not be repeated here.[68,69] Suffice it to say that calcium and magnesium are intimately linked and that a high calcium to magnesium ratio can be detrimental and lead to hypertension and other conditions involving the cardiovascular system.[70]

Legumes, tofu, seeds, nuts, whole grains, and green leafy vegetables are good sources of magnesium. Magnesium glycinate (chelated magnesium) is the most bioavailable and best tolerated supplement. Magnesium citrate is also highly available, but may cause loose stools. The common form of magnesium used in supplements, magnesium oxide, is essentially useless in that only about 4% of the ingested amount is actually absorbed.[71]

About half of the body's magnesium stores can be found in bones, so it is clearly a very important mineral as far as osteoporosis prevention is concerned. Magnesium deficiency is, unfortunately, very common. A recent study found that 74% of a cohort of 2000 elderly men and women did not consume the recommended 400 mg/day. This same study also concluded that a high magnesium intake is associated with a significantly higher bone density in older white men and women. Every 100 mg/day extra intake of magnesium was found to correspond to a 2% increase in whole-body bone mass. This compares to an approximate 2% increase per 400-mg/day increase in calcium consumption. It is thought that magnesium may act as a buffer for the acid produced by the typical Western diet and may also replace calcium in the hydroxyapatite part of bone, thus resulting in a stronger structure.[72] There is also evidence that magnesium suppresses bone resorption (demineralization) at least in younger people.[73]

Other minerals

A high salt diet has been found to significantly increase urinary calcium excretion and bone loss. Supplementing with 90 mmol/day of **potassium** citrate (3500 mg of elemental potassium) will prevent this detrimental effect.[74]

Boron is also a very important mineral in osteoporosis prevention. Researchers at the U.S. Department of Agriculture found that women who supplemented with 3 mg of boron daily reduced the amount of calcium excreted in their urine by 44%. The conclusion of the study was that boron improves the metabolism of calcium and magnesium.[75]

A low dietary intake of <u>**zinc**</u> and accompanying low blood levels has been associated with an increased risk of osteoporosis in women. Researchers at the University of California have found that an adequate zinc intake is equally important for men. Their study involved 396 men aged between 45 and 92 years who had their bone mineral density (BMD) measured at baseline (in 1988-1992) and 4 years later. Plasma zinc level correlated well with the total intake from diet and supplements. The average daily intake was 11.2 mg and the mean plasma zinc concentration was 12.7 micromol/L. The researchers observed that men with a low zinc intake and plasma concentration were significantly more likely to have osteoporosis of the hip and spine.[76]

Vitamin K
Vitamin K is essential in the synthesis of osteocalcin, the hormone that promotes bone formation. Several epidemiological studies have concluded that a vitamin K deficiency (such as would be induced by warfarin therapy) causes reductions in bone mineral density and increases the risk of fractures. Other studies have shown that the concurrent use of menaquinone (vitamin K2) and vitamin D substantially reduces bone loss. There is evidence that the average dietary intake of vitamin K is insufficient to ensure optimum osteocalcin production and that the RDA should be increased.[77] Supplementation with vitamin K (preferably K2) would, thus, be important for afibbers on warfarin.

Conclusion
Osteoporosis is widespread and of particular concern for afibbers on warfarin. It is clear that moderate exercise combined with an appropriate intake of vitamin D, calcium, magnesium, boron, zinc, and vitamin K can substantially reduce the risk of bone loss and fractures.

SKIN NECROSIS

Warfarin-induced skin necrosis is a rare, but serious disorder which primarily affects middle-aged, obese women. The disorder has a prevalence of less than 0.1%. Skin necrosis usually appears in breast, buttocks or thighs of women and on the penis of men. If it is going to occur it would usually do so within the first 3 to 6 days after starting warfarin therapy. It is thought to be associated with a sharp drop in protein C and factor VII experienced in some patients following initiation of therapy. The disorder manifests itself by large bleeding skin eruptions and may require extensive surgery and even amputation. The risk of skin necrosis can be reduced by avoiding large initial doses of warfarin and by increasing dosages slowly. In some cases, it is possible to reverse the condition with rapid intervention with vitamin K infusions. Skin necrosis is a serious condition and its symptoms and the symptom of its close cousin, "purple toes" should not be ignored.[78]

EYE DAMAGE

Massive bleeding in the eye in patients with age-related macular degeneration (AMD) is a devastating event. Dutch researchers have found that warfarin treatment increases the risk of serious bleeding in AMD patients and recommend that warfarin therapy for such patients only be prescribed when absolutely essential.[79]

INR CONTROL

An obvious way of improving the safety and efficacy of warfarin therapy is to control the INR within close limits. Doing this, by going to a clinic or medical laboratory weekly or more frequently, is clearly inconvenient, time-consuming and expensive. Fortunately, there are now several home testing kits that provide quick and accurate results for INR and prothrombin time. *INRatio* by HemoSense is probably the most reliable and accurate. It must be prescribed by a physician and its cost may be reimbursed by Medicare in the US (http://www.hemosense.com).

SUMMARY

Warfarin (Coumadin) is an effective anticoagulant, but has the potential for serious adverse effects – notably internal bleeding, hemorrhagic stroke, arterial calcification, osteoporosis, and skin necrosis. Fortunately, as detailed in this report, it is possible to greatly reduce the risk of adverse events by judicious supplementation, avoidance of drugs and herbs that interact with warfarin, and maintaining close control of INR through monitoring at home.

SUPPLEMENTATION

The most important supplements for patients on long-term warfarin therapy are:

Supplement	Suggested intake
Vitamin C	500 mg 3-4 times daily with meals
Vitamin D3 (1)	2000-4000 IU daily
Vitamin K*(2)	100 micrograms daily
Magnesium (elemental) (3)	100-200 mg 3 times daily
Calcium (elemental) (4)	200 mg 3 times daily
Potassium (elemental) (5)	2-3 grams daily
Boron	3 mg daily
Zinc	15 mg daily
Proline	500 mg daily [18]
Lysine	500 mg daily [18]
Green tea*(6)	4-6 cups daily

* These supplements should only be taken with a doctor's approval and require close INR monitoring.

(1) Please note that many supplements such as multivitamins, calcium, magnesium and vitamin K also contain vitamin D. Total intake from all sources should not exceed 4000 IU/day.

(2) The preferred form of vitamin K is vitamin K2 (menaquinone). However, if the intake of green leafy vegetables is low and INR is fluctuating significantly then a mixture of vitamin K1 (phylloquinone) and vitamin K2 is preferable.

(3) Taurine (3 x 1000 mg/day) may be helpful in ensuring optimum efficacy of magnesium. Magnesium supplementation is not advised in patients with kidney failure.

(4) Total daily calcium intake from diet and supplements should not exceed 1200-1500 mg.

(5) This amount can be obtained from 6-7 daily servings of fruits and vegetables. Supplementation is not advised in patients with kidney failure.

(6) It is likely, but not proven, that a similar benefit can be obtained through supplementing with green tea extract in capsules.

REFERENCES

1. Fuster, V, et al. ACC/AHA/ESC Guidelines for the Management of Patients with Atrial Fibrillation: Executive Summary. Circulation, Vol. 104, October 23, 2001, pp. 2118-50
    http://circ.ahajournals.org/cgi/content/full/104/17/2118

2. Fuster, V, et al. ACC/AHA/ESC Guidelines for the Management of Patients with Atrial Fibrillation: Executive Summary. Circulation, Vol. 114, August 15, 2006, pp. 700-52
    http://circ.ahajournals.org/cgi/reprint/CIRCULATIONAHA.106.177031v1

3. Gage, BF, et al. Clinical classification schemes for predicting hemorrhage: results from the National Registry of Atrial Fibrillation (NRAF). American Heart Journal, Vol. 151, March 2006, pp. 713-19

4. Gage, BF, et al. Validation of clinical classification schemes for predicting stroke: results from the National Registry of Atrial Fibrillation. JAMA, Vol. 285, June 13, 2001, pp. 2864-70

5. Go, AS, et al. Anticoagulation therapy for stroke prevention in atrial fibrillation: how well do randomized trials translate into clinical practice? JAMA, Vol. 290, November 26, 2003, pp. 2685-92

6. Dubinsky, R and Lai, SM. Mortality of stroke patients treated with thrombolysis: analysis of nationwide inpatient sample. Neurology, Vol. 66, No. 11, June 13, 2006, pp. 1742-44

7. Brown, AE. Mode of action of structural pest control chemicals. Pesticide Information Leaflet No. 41, June 2006, University of Maryland, Dept. of Entomology. http://www.entmclasses.umd.edu/peap/leaflets/PIL41.pdf

8. Paulsson, M. Basement membrane proteins: structure, assembly, and cellular interactions. Critical Reviews in Biochemistry and Molecular Biology, Vol. 27, Issue 1, 1992, pp. 93-127

9. Graham, MF, et al. Role of ascorbic acid in procollagen expression and secretion by human intestinal smooth muscle cells. Journal of Cellular Physiology, Vol. 162, February 1995, pp. 225-33

10. Perrin, A, et al. Stimulating effect of collagen-like peptide on the extracellular matrix of human skin: histological studies. International Journal of Tissue React., Vol. 26, No. 3-4, 2004, pp. 97-104

11. Marionnet, C, et al. Morphogenesis of dermal-epidermal junction in a model of reconstructed skin: beneficial effects of vitamin C. Experimental Dermatology, Vol. 15, August 2006, pp. 625-33

12. Dammann, HG, et al. Effects of buffered and plain acetylsalicylic acid formulations with and without ascorbic acid on gastric mucosa in healthy subjects. Aliment Pharmacol Ther., Vol. 19, No. 3, February 1, 2004, pp. 367-74

13. Konturek, PC, et al. Effect of vitamin C-releasing acetylsalicylic acid on gastric mucosal damage before and after Helicobacter pylori eradication therapy. European Journal of Pharmacology, Vol. 506, No. 2, December 15, 2004, pp. 169-77

14. Rath, Matthias. Why Animals Don't Get Heart Attacks – but People Do. Health Now Inc., 387 Ivy Street, San Francisco, CA 94102, 1997

15. Katiyar, SK. Matrix metalloproteinases in cancer metastasis: molecular targets for prostate cancer prevention by green tea polyphenols and grape seed proanthocyanidins. Endocr Metab Immune Disord Drug Targets, Vol. 6, No. 1, March 2006, pp. 17-24

16. Okamoto, K. Habitual green tea consumption and risk of an aneurismal rupture subarachnoid hemorrhage: a case-control study in Nagoya, Japan. European Journal of Epidemiology, Vol. 21, No. 5, May 2006, pp. 367-71

17. Williams, JZ, et al. Effect of a specialized amino acid mixture on human collagen deposition. Annals of Surgery, Vol. 236, No. 3, September 2002, pp. 369-75

18. Kirk, SJ, et al. Arginine stimulates wound healing and immune function in elderly human beings. Surgery, Vol. 114, No. 2, August 1993, pp. 155-60

19. Stechmiller, JK, et al. Arginine supplementation and wound healing. Nutr Clin Practice, Vol. 20, No. 1, February 2005, pp. 52-61

20. Taylor, JR and Wilt, VM. Probable antagonism of warfarin by green tea. Annals of Pharmacotherapy, Vol. 33, April 1999, pp. 426-28

21. Izzo, AA, et al. Cardiovascular pharmacotherapy and herbal medicines: the risk of drug interaction. International Journal of Cardiology, Vol. 98, January 2005, pp. 1-14

22. Fugh-Berman, A. Herb-drug interactions. The Lancet, Vol. 355, January 8, 2000, pp. 134-38

23. Kurl, S, et al. Plasma vitamin C modifies the association between hypertension and risk of stroke. Stroke, Vol. 33, June 2002, pp. 1568-73

24. Howe, AM and Webster, WS. Warfarin exposure and calcification of the arterial system in the rat. Int J Exp Pathol., Vol. 81, No. 1, February 2000, pp. 51-56

25. Schori, TR and Stungis, GE. Long-term warfarin treatment may induce arterial calcification in humans: case report. Clin Invest Med., Vol. 27, No. 2, April 2004, pp. 107-09

26. Schurgers, LJ, et al. Role of vitamin K and vitamin K-dependent proteins in vascular calcification. Z Kardiol., Vol. 90, Suppl. 3, 2001, pp. 57-63

27. Sconce, E, et al. Patients with unstable control have a poorer dietary intake of vitamin K compared to patients with stable control of anticoagulation. Thrombosis and Haemostasis, Vol. 93, May 2005, pp. 872-75

28. Oldenburg, J. Vitamin K intake and stability of oral anticoagulant treatment. Thrombosis and Haemostasis, Vol. 93, May 2005, pp. 799-800

29. Wallin, R, et al. Arterial calcification: a review of mechanisms, animal models, and the prospects for therapy. Medicinal Research Reviews, Vol. 21, No. 4, 2001, pp. 274-301

30. Geleijnse, JM, et al. Dietary intake of menaquinone is associated with a reduced risk of coronary heart disease: the Rotterdam Study. Journal of Nutrition, Vol. 134, 2004, pp. 3100-05

31. Reedstrom, CK and Suttie, JW. Comparative distribution, metabolism, and utilization of phylloquinone and menaquinon-9 in rat liver. Proc Soc Exp Biol Med., Vol. 209, No. 4, September 1995, pp. 403-09

32. Watson, KE, et al. Active serum vitamin D levels are inversely correlated with coronary calcification. Circulation, Vol. 96, 1997, pp. 1755-60 http://circ.ahajournals.org/cgi/content/full/96/6/1755

33. Braam, LA, et al. Beneficial effects of vitamins D and K on the elastic properties of the vessel wall in postmenopausal women: a follow-up study. Thrombosis and Haemostasis, Vol. 91, February 2004, pp. 373-80

34. Price, PA, et al. Warfarin-induced artery calcification is accelerated by growth and vitamin D. Arteriosclerosis, Thrombosis, and Vascular Biology, Vol. 20, February 2000, pp. 317-27 http://atvb.ahajournals.org/cgi/content/full/20/2/317

35. Fleckenstein-Grun, G, et al. Progression and regression by verapamil of vitamin D3-induced calcific medial degeneration in coronary arteries of rats. Journal of Cardiovascular Pharmacology, Vol. 26, No. 2, August 1995, pp. 207-13

36. Kummerow, FA, et al. Effect of trans-fatty acids on calcium influx into human arterial endothelial cells. American Journal of Clinical Nutrition, Vol. 70, 1999, pp. 832-88

37. Schwille, PO, et al. Media calcification, low erythrocyte magnesium, altered plasma magnesium, and calcium homeostasis following grafting of the thoracic aorta to the infrarenal aorta in the rate: differential preventive effects of long-term oral magnesium supplementation alone and in combination with alkali. Biomed Pharmacother., Vol. 57, No. 2, March 2003, pp. 88-97

38. Gass, M and Dawson-Hughes, B. Preventing osteoporosis-related fractures: an overview. American Journal of Medicine, Vol. 119, Suppl 1, April 2006, pp. S3-S11

39. Wright, VJ. Osteoporosis in men. J Am Acad Orthop Surg., Vol. 14, June 2006, pp. 347-53

40. Gage, BF, et al. Risk of osteoporotic fracture in elderly patients taking warfarin: results from the National Registry of Atrial Fibrillation 2. Archives of Internal Medicine, Vol. 166, January 23, 2006, pp. 241-46

41. Barnes, C, et al. Reduced bone density in children on long-term warfarin. Pediatric Research, Vol. 57, No. 4, 2005, pp. 578-81

42. Farrugia, MC, et al. Osteonecrosis of the mandible or maxilla associated with the use of new generation bisphosphonates. Laryngoscope, Vol. 116, January 2006, pp. 115-20

43. http://www.yourlawyer.com/topics/overview/Fosamax

44. American College of Sports Medicine position stand: osteoporosis and exercise. Med Sci Sports Exerc., Vol. 27, April 1995, pp. i-vii

45. Borer, KT. Physical activity in the prevention and amelioration of osteoporosis in women: interaction of mechanical, hormonal and dietary factors. Sports Medicine, Vol. 35, No. 9, 2005, pp. 779-830

46. Rittweger, J. Can exercise prevent osteoporosis? J Musculoskelet Neuronal Interact., Vol. 6, No. 2, June 2006, pp. 162-66

47. Murray, Michael T and Pizzorno, Joseph E. Encyclopedia of Natural Medicine. Prima Publishing, PO Box 1260K, Rocklin, CA 95677. Revised 2nd edition, 1998, pp. 706-14

48. Holick, MF, et al. Prevalence of vitamin D inadequacy among postmenopausal North American women receiving osteoporosis therapy. Journal of Clinical Endocrinology and Metabolism, Vol. 90, June 2005, pp. 3215-24

49. Rizzoli, R, et al. Risk factors for vitamin D inadequacy among women with osteoporosis: an international epidemiological study. International Journal of Clinical Practice, Vol. 60, August 2006, pp. 1013-19

50. LeBoff, MS, et al. Occult vitamin D deficiency in postmenopausal US women with acute hip fracture. JAMA, Vol. 281, April 28, 1999, pp. 1505-11

51. Diamond, T, et al. Hip fracture in elderly men: the importance of subclinical vitamin-D deficiency and hypogonadism. Medical Journal of Australia, Vol. 169, August 3, 1998, pp. 138-41

52. Bischoff-Ferrari, HA, et al. Fracture prevention with vitamin D supplementation: a meta-analysis of randomized controlled trials. JAMA, Vol. 293, May 2005, pp. 2257-64

53. Feskanich, D, et al. Calcium, vitamin D, milk consumption, and hip fractures: a prospective study among postmenopausal women. American Journal of Clinical Nutrition, Vol. 77, February 2003, pp. 504-11

54. Bischoff-Ferrari, HA, et al. Estimation of optimal serum concentrations of 25-hydroxyvitamin D for multiple health outcomes. American Journal of Clinical Nutrition, Vol. 84, 2006, pp. 18-28

55. Vieth, R, et al. Efficacy and safety of vitamin D intake exceeding the lowest observed adverse effect level. American Journal of Clinical Nutrition, Vol. 73, February 2001, pp. 288-94

56. Meunier, P. Prevention of hip fractures by correcting calcium and vitamin D insufficiencies in elderly people. Scandinavian Journal of Rheumatology Supplement, Vol. 103, 1996, pp. 75-80

57. O'Brien, KO. Combined calcium and vitamin D supplementation reduces bone loss and fracture incidence in older men and women. Nutrition Reviews, Vol. 56, May 1998, pp. 148-58

58. Boonen, S, et al. Calcium and vitamin D in the prevention and treatment of osteoporosis: a clinical update. J Intern Med., Vol. 259, June 2006, pp. 539-52

59. Pfeifer, M and Minne, HW. The role of vitamin D in the treatment of osteoporosis in the elderly. Med Klin (Munich), Vol. 101, Suppl, June 2006, pp. 15-19 [article in German – English abstract only]

60. Wolf, RL, et al. Factors associated with calcium absorption efficiency in pre- and perimenopausal women. American Journal of Clinical Nutrition, Vol. 72, August 2000, pp. 466-71

61. Nordin, B.E. Christopher. Calcium requirement is a sliding scale. American Journal of Clinical Nutrition, Vol. 71, June 2000, pp. 1381-83

62. Storm, D, et al. Calcium supplementation prevents seasonal bone loss and changes in biochemical markers of bone turnover in elderly New England women: a randomized placebo-controlled trial. Journal of Clinical Endocrinology and Metabolism, Vol. 83, November 1998, pp. 3817-25

63. Martini, L and Wood, RJ. Relative bioavailability of calcium-rich dietary sources in the elderly. American Journal of Clinical Nutrition, Vol. 76, December 2002, pp. 1345-50

64. Sakhaee, K, et al. Meta-analysis of calcium bioavailability: a comparison of calcium citrate with calcium carbonate. American J Ther., Vol. 6, No. 6, November 1999, pp. 313-21

65. Pfeifer, M, et al. Effects of short-term vitamin D3 and calcium supplementation on blood pressure and parathyroid hormone levels in elderly women. Journal of Clinical Endocrinology and Metabolism, Vol. 86, April 2001, pp. 1633-37

66. Reid, IR, et al. Effects of calcium supplementation on serum lipid concentrations in normal older women: a randomized controlled trial. American Journal of Medicine, Vol. 112, April 1, 2002, pp. 343-47

67. Larsen, Hans R. Lone Atrial Fibrillation: Towards A Cure. International Health News, Victoria, BC, Canada, 2006, p. 103

68. http://www.afibbers.org/conference/session14.pdf

69. http://www.afibbers.org/conference/PCMagnesium.pdf

70. Murray, Michael T. Encyclopedia of Nutritional Supplements. Prima Publishing, PO Box 1260K, Rocklin, CA 95677, 1996, pp. 159-75

71. Firoz, M and Graber, M. Bioavailability of US commercial magnesium preparations. Magnesium Research, Vol. 14, No. 4, December 2001, pp. 257-62

72. Ryder, KM, et al. Magnesium intake from food and supplements is associated with bone mineral density in healthy older white subjects. Journal of the American Geriatrics Society, Vol. 53, November 2005, pp. 1875-80

73. Dimai, HP, et al. Daily oral magnesium supplementation suppresses bone turnover in young adult males. Journal of Clinical Endocrinology and Metabolism, Vol. 83, August 1998, pp. 2742-48

74. Sellmeyer, DE, et al. Potassium citrate prevents increased urine calcium excretion and bone resorption induced by a high sodium chloride diet. Journal of Clinical Endocrinology and Metabolism, Vol. 87, May 2002, pp. 2008-12

75. Nielsen , FH. Effect of dietary boron on mineral, estrogen, and testosterone metabolism in postmenopausal women. FASEB Journal, Vol. 1 (5), November 1987, pp. 394-7

76. Hyun, TH, et al. Zinc intakes and plasma concentrations in men with osteoporosis: the Rancho Bernardo Study. American Journal of Clinical Nutrition, Vol. 80, September 2004, pp. 715-21

77. Adams, J and Pepping, J. Vitamin K in the treatment and prevention of osteoporosis and arterial calcification. Am J Health Syst Pharm., Vol. 62, No. 15, August 1, 2005, pp. 1574-81

78. Warfarin-induced skin necrosis. University of Cincinnati, Dept. of Pathology and Laboratory Medicine, Lab Lines, Vol. 7, No. 6, November/December 2001

79. Tillanus, MA, et al. Relationship between anticoagulant medication and massive intraocular hemorrhage in age-related macular degeneration. Graefes Arch Clin Exp Ophthalmol., Vol. 238, June 2000, pp. 482-85

Chapter 8

Warfarin Interactions

Warfarin (Coumadin) is prescribed for the prevention of ischemic stroke and deep venous thrombosis in patients with atrial fibrillation, prosthetic heart valves, venous thromboembolism, and coronary artery disease. The major potential adverse effects of warfarin are hemorrhagic stroke and internal bleeding. The blood level of warfarin must be controlled within very narrow limits in order to ensure that clots don't form while avoiding internal bleeding. The efficacy and safety of warfarin therapy depends on maintaining a reasonably constant **INR** (International Normalized Ratio) between 2.0 and 3.0. An INR below 2.0 is less effective in preventing ischemic stroke and at an INR of 3.0 or higher the risk of a hemorrhagic stroke outweighs the risk of an ischemic stroke [1]. Numerous drugs, herbs, and foods affect the action of warfarin by either increasing or decreasing its anticoagulation effect. It is clearly important to be aware of these interactions so as to avoid large swings in INR and the accompanying risks of over- or under-coagulation.

Researchers at Harvard Medical School reported that the incidence of warfarin-related major bleeding and intracranial hemorrhage (hemorrhagic stroke) among patients admitted to the Brigham and Women's Hospital has increased substantially from the 4-year period 1995-1998 to the 4-year period 1999-2002. Among the highlights of the findings are:

- The annual incidence of warfarin-related bleeding increased by 22% between the two time periods.
- The proportion of patients with major bleeding increased from 20.2% to 33.3% and that of intracranial bleeding from 1.9% to 7.8%.
- The proportion of warfarin-treated patients who had an INR value higher than the intended range was 57% in the first time period and 59% in the second.

Sixty-two per cent of the warfarin-treated patients also received medications that are known to potentiate the effect of warfarin. Among the more common ones were quinolone antibiotics (32%), levothyroxine (15%), simvastatin (10%), and amiodarone (10%). The use of more than one potentiating medication increased from 24% in the first period to 41% in the second period. If aspirin, clopidogrel and other antiplatelet agents and anticoagulants are included, then a full 86.6% of warfarin-treated patients received one or more medications that would increase the effect of warfarin and make them susceptible to major bleeding [1].

A team of researchers from Germany, Sweden and Switzerland studied 4152 afib patients who were on warfarin therapy for non-valvular atrial fibrillation. During follow-up (for an average of 11 months) 133 patients died from internal bleeding and another 432 were hospitalized with serious bleeding. This corresponds to a warfarin-associated mortality rate of 3.5% a year and a serious bleeding rate of 12% a year. The researchers observed that 58% of all patients on warfarin had also been prescribed one or more of 88 specific drugs that are known to interact with warfarin. They also found that patients who were taking potentially interacting drugs experienced a 3.4-fold increased risk of serious bleeding. The use of a combination of warfarin and aspirin (75-325 mg/day) was associated with a 4.5-fold risk increase, while the concomitant use of acetaminophen (Tylenol, Paracetamol) was associated with a 3.8-fold increased risk at doses between 885-2900 mg/day taken for at least 4 weeks. Other particularly detrimental drugs were allopurinol (Zyloprim), amiodarone (Cordarone), levothyroxine (Synthroid), Metronidazole, Miconazole, and omeprazole (Prilosec). Taking Metronidazole or Miconazole during warfarin therapy was associated with a 40-fold increase in the risk of a serious bleeding event.

The researchers conclude that drug interactions are an independent risk factor for serious bleeding in patients on long-term warfarin therapy. They also point out that the practice of prescribing potentially interacting drugs is widespread. [2]

A team of Canadian medical doctors and pharmacists recently reviewed the medical literature from 1993 to March 2004 in order to compile a verified list of important interactions between warfarin and foods, supplements, and other drugs. The most probable and best-verified interactions are presented below [3].

INTERACTIONS THAT <u>POTENTIATE</u> WARFARIN'S EFFECT

Highly Probable	Probable
Acetaminophen (Tylenol)	Amoxicillin
Ciprofloxacin	NSAIDs
Citalopram	COX-2 inhibitors
Diltiazem	Fluorouracil
Entacapone	Fluvastatin
Fenofibrate	Fluvoxamine
Micronazole	Gemcitabine
Sertraline	
Voriconazole	
Zileuton	
Bold/fenugreek	Danshen
Fish oil	Dong quai
Mango	Grapefruit juice
Quilinggao	

INTERACTIONS THAT <u>INHIBIT</u> WARFARIN'S EFFECT

Highly Probable	Probable
Cholestyramine	Azathioprine
Mercaptopurine	Bosentan
Mesalamine	Dicloxacillin
Ribavirin	Ritonavir
Trazodone	Ginseng

According to the Canadian researchers there are no credible studies supporting an interaction between warfarin and the following drugs and foods – alcohol, antacids, atenolol, clopidogrel, fluoxetine (Prozac), metoprolol, naproxen, psyllium, ranitidine, vitamin E, atorvastatin (Lipitor), coenzyme Q10, ginkgo biloba, ibuprofen, and influenza vaccine.

The researchers point out that there are now so many potential interactions between warfarin and other drugs that it would be impossible for a physician or pharmacist to remember them all. They recommend that doctors prescribing other drugs to patients on warfarin keep in mind that many drugs in the following groups can potentiate or inhibit the effect of warfarin:

- Antibiotics and antifungal agents
- Cardiovascular drugs (including propafenone, amiodarone, and cholesterol-reducing drugs)
- Painkillers
- Anti-inflammatories
- Central nervous system drugs (citalopram, sertraline)
- Gastrointestinal drugs (cimetidine, omeprazole)
- Anabolic steroids

It is clear that the potential for interactions between warfarin and other drugs is very substantial and that supplementing with certain herbs may also be a problem as may chelation therapy [4]. Although the Canadian study discussed above did conclude that fish oil may potentiate the effect of warfarin this conclusion is by no means unanimous.

WARFARIN AND FISH OILS

Background

An increased intake of oily fish and long-chain polyunsaturated omega-3 fatty acids (fish oils) is generally beneficial and reduces the risk of ischemic stroke. For people on warfarin it is clearly important to know if it is safe to take both fish oils and warfarin.

Warfarin works by inhibiting the activation of vitamin K-dependent coagulation Factors V, VII and X in the extrinsic and common pathways of the coagulation cascade. Fish oil works primarily by inhibiting platelet aggregation, stabilizing atherosclerotic plaque, and reducing fibrinogen level, but there is some evidence that it also reduces Factors V and VII in both men and women and Factor X in women [5, 6].

There is no evidence that fish oil causes hemorrhagic stroke or internal bleeding, while there is abundant evidence that warfarin does [7-11]. Warfarin was originally developed as a rat poison and has two effects – it damages the integrity of blood vessel walls and inhibits the normal blood clotting action which would prevent the rat from bleeding to death. It would seem that a similar mechanism operates in humans.

The purpose of anticoagulants like warfarin and fish oil is to prevent blood from forming a clot or at least significantly increase the length of time it takes before a clot is formed in response to trauma or stagnation. There are several different tests for measuring clotting tendency, and it is somewhat unfortunate that the test in general use today, the prothrombin time (INR), is not an absolute measure of the blood's tendency to form a clot (thrombus), but rather a measure of the blood level of those coagulation factors that depend on vitamin K for their synthesis and the factors they, in turn, activate. In other words, the universal test today is primarily designed to measure blood level of warfarin. Aspirin, vitamin E, garlic and other natural antiplatelet/anticoagulant agents generally have no or very little effect on INR – and yet, these substances all have proven preventive effects against thrombus formation.

The problem is that the INR test only measures blood coagulation time in the extrinsic and common pathways. Retardation of the coagulation sequence by antiplatelet aggregation medications (aspirin, clopidogrel, ticlopidine), for example, will not affect INR because the sequence is halted in the intrinsic pathway before vitamin K-dependent coagulation factors become involved. Similarly, if the coagulation process is initiated via the intrinsic pathway and prekallikrein, Factor VIII or von Willebrand Factor are blocked, the thrombus formation sequence will not proceed either, but the INR test, because it bypasses the intrinsic pathway, will not show that you are protected even though you clearly are.

It is clear that both fish oil and warfarin are effective anticoagulants and it is thus likely that taking both would be superior to either agent alone in preventing ischemic stroke. The question is, "Would taking both increase the risk of hemorrhagic stroke and internal bleeding?" As far as I know only three studies have investigated the possible interaction between warfarin and fish oil.

Clinical Studies

A group of Norwegian medical researchers found that fish oil supplementation did not increase the bleeding tendency in heart disease patients receiving aspirin or warfarin. The study involved 511 patients who had undergone coronary artery bypass surgery. On the second day after the operation half the patients were assigned in a random fashion to receive 4 grams of fish oil per day (providing 2 g/day of eicosapentaenoic acid, 1.3 g/day of docosahexaenoic acid, and 14.8 mg/day of vitamin E). At the same time the patients were also randomized to receive either 300 mg of aspirin per day or warfarin aimed at achieving an INR of 2.5-4.2. The patients were evaluated every 3 months and questioned about bleeding episodes for the duration of the 9-month study.

The researchers concluded that fish oil supplementation did not result in a statistically significant increase in bleeding episodes in either the aspirin group or in the warfarin group. Nosebleeds were somewhat more common in the fish oil + warfarin group, while gastrointestinal bleeding was more common in the warfarin group. None of the differences were statistically significant. They also found no significant long-term effects of fish oil on common parameters of coagulation and fibrinolysis – including bleeding time. They noted that the blood levels (serum phospholipid levels) of eicosapentaenoic acid and docosahexaenoic acid increased by 140% and 14% respectively in the patients taking fish oil. The serum triglyceride levels decreased by 19.1% in the fish oil group while no significant change was observed in the remainder of the patients [12].

Researchers at the University of Texas Health Sciences Center have addressed the question, "Does fish oil supplementation change INR in patients on warfarin?" Their placebo-controlled, randomized, double-blind study included 11 patients with prosthetic heart valves, cardiomyopathy or deep vein thrombosis who were taking warfarin and had achieved stable INR values for at least 4 weeks. The participants were assigned to receive a placebo, 3 grams/day of fish oil (*MaxEPA*), or 6 grams/day of fish oil for a 4-week period. Their INR was measured twice weekly during the study period. INR values remained steady in all groups and there were no significant differences in INR values between the groups during the trial. The researchers conclude that, *"there does not appear to be a clinically significant interaction between warfarin and up to 6 grams/day of the fish oil supplement MaxEPA in terms of INR changes and bleeding incidence."*[13]

Mitchell Buckley and colleagues at the Shawnee Mission Medical Center in Kansas recently reported the case of a 67-year-old woman whose INR increased significantly after she increased her daily dose of fish oil from 1 gram to 2 grams. The woman had serious health problems (TIAs, hypothyroidism, hyperlipidemia, osteopenia, and coronary artery disease) and had experienced a heart attack necessitating angioplasty. She was taking several medications including warfarin, aspirin, levothyroxine, atorvastatin, bisoprolol, lisinopril, and conjugated estrogens. She was also supplementing with 400 IU a day of vitamin E and 1 gram a day of fish oil. The patient had been stable for a 5-month period at an INR of between 2 and 3 taking 1.5 mg a day of warfarin. In March 2002 she increased her fish oil dosage to 2 grams a day and a week later her INR measured 4.1. Upon returning to 1 gram a day of fish oil her INR dropped to 1.6. The researchers conclude that the higher dose of fish oil could have provided additional anticoagulation as expressed in a higher INR. There was no indication that the INR was affected by 1 gram a day of fish oil [14].

Conclusion

There is no evidence that taking both warfarin and fish oil increases the incidence of bleeding. However, there is no clear consensus as to whether fish oil affects INR. One small study found that 3 and 6 grams a day of fish oil had no significant effect on INR, whereas a single case study found that 2 grams a day increased INR significantly. Thus, it would appear that supplementing with 1 gram a day of fish oil while on warfarin is safe and does not affect INR.

It is not clear whether higher fish oil intakes may affect INR, so it is advisable to increase INR monitoring frequency when changing one's daily fish oil intake. It is possible, but certainly not proven, that taking fish oil and warfarin together may reduce the amount of warfarin required to keep the INR in the therapeutic range.

REFERENCES

1. Kucher, N, et al. Time trends in warfarin-associated hemorrhage. American Journal of Cardiology, Vol. 94, August 1, 2004, pp. 403-06
2. Gasse, C, et al. Drug interactions and risk of acute bleeding leading to hospitalisation or death in patients with chronic atrial fibrillation treated with warfarin. Thrombosis and Haemostasis, Vol. 94, September 2005, pp. 537-43
3. Holbrook, AM, et al. Systematic overview of warfarin and its drug and food interactions. Archives of Internal Medicine, Vol. 165, May 23, 2005, pp. 1095-1106
4. Grebe, HB and Gregory, PJ. Inhibition of warfarin anticoagulation associated with chelation therapy. Pharmacotherapy, Vol. 22, August 2002, pp. 1067-69
5. Oosthuizen, E, et al. Both fish oils and olive oil lowered plasma fibrinogen in women with high baseline fibrinogen levels. Throm. Haemost., Vol. 72, No. 4, October 1994, pp. 557-62
6. Flaten, H, et al. Fish-oil concentrate: effects of variables related to cardiovascular disease. American Journal of Clinical Nutrition, Vol. 52, 1990, pp. 300-06
7. Iso, H, et al. Intake of fish and omega-3 fatty acids and risk of stroke in women, JAMA, Vol. 285, January 17, 2001, pp. 304-12
8. He, K, et al. Fish consumption and risk of stroke in men. JAMA, Vol. 288, December 25, 2002, pp. 3130-36
9. Warfarin versus aspirin for prevention of thromboembolism in atrial fibrillation: Stroke Prevention in Atrial Fibrillation II study. The Lancet, Vol. 343, March 19, 1994, pp. 687-91
10. Go, AS, et al. Anticoagulation therapy for stroke prevention in atrial fibrillation. JAMA, Vol. 290, November 26, 2003, pp. 2685-92
11. Warfarin of only modest benefit. Circulation, Vol. 108, No. 17, October 28, 2003, p. IV-757, abstract #3419
12. Eritsland, J., et al. Long-term effects of n-3 polyunsaturated fatty acids on haemostatic variables and bleeding episodes in patients with coronary artery disease. Blood Coagulation and Fibrinolysis, Vol. 6, 1995, pp. 17-22

13. Bender, NK, et al. Effects of marine fish oils on the anticoagulation status of patients receiving chronic warfarin therapy. Journal of Thrombosis and Thrombolysis, Vol. 5, July 1998, pp. 257-61

14. Buckley, MS, et al. Fish oil interaction with warfarin. Annals of Pharmacotherapy, Vol. 38, January 2004, pp. 50-53

Other sources of information regarding warfarin interactions

- Chung, MK. Vitamins, supplements, herbal medicines, and arrhythmias. Cardiology in Review, Vol. 12, No. 2, March-April 2004, pp. 73-84

- Heck, AM, et al. Potential interactions between alternative therapies and warfarin. American Journal of Health-System Pharmacology, Vol. 57, No. 13, July 1, 2000, pp. 1221-27

- Fugh-Berman, A. Herb-drug interactions. The Lancet, Vol. 355, January 8, 2000, pp. 134-38

- Canadian Pharmacists Association. Compendium of Pharmaceuticals and Specialties, 35th edition, 2000

- Kim, JM and White, RH. Effect of vitamin E on the anticoagulant response to warfarin. American Journal of Cardiology, Vol. 77, No. 7, March 1, 1996, pp. 545-54

- Wintrobe's Clinical Hematology, 9th edition, 1993, Lea & Fibiger, Philadelphia, p. 1530

Chapter 9

Stroke Risk Factors

LAF does not increase stroke risk

Researchers at the *Mayo Clinic* have published a very important study regarding the correlation between lone atrial fibrillation (LAF) and stroke risk and overall mortality. The study is remarkable in that it followed the participants for 30 years and thus gives a good indication of the long-term prognosis for untreated LAF. The study involved 46 residents of Olmsted County who were diagnosed with LAF at an average age of 45.8 years (range of 34-58 years). None of the participants had coronary artery disease, hypertension, diabetes, mitral valve prolapse, congestive heart failure, or any other condition that would increase their risk of ischemic stroke (cerebral infarction). None of the participants were treated with warfarin. They were followed until death or July 1, 2002. At time of last follow-up the average age was 74 years (range of 63-85 years). At the beginning of the study 76% of participants had paroxysmal afib and 24% had the persistent variety; this changed to 59% paroxysmal and 41% persistent by the end of the study period. All participants were Caucasians and 83% were men.

The Mayo researchers made the following important observations:

1. The observed mortality rate among the afibbers over a 25-year period was substantially lower (15.9%) than the mortality expected in a group of age- and sex-matched white Minnesotans (32.5%).

2. The incidence of ischemic stroke (cerebral infarction) in the afib group was no greater (0.5%/person-year) than in the general population. The researchers conclude that, "This observation indicated that the pathophysiological mechanisms responsible for the development of a cerebrovascular event were unrelated to the continued presence of AF." In other words, LAF as such is not associated with an increased risk of stroke.

3. The volume of the left atrium (LAV) is an important indicator of the risk of adverse events such as stroke, heart attack (myocardial infarction), and congestive heart failure. A LAV (indexed for age and body mass) equal to or greater than 32 mL/m^2 was associated with a 4.46-fold increase in the probability of experiencing an adverse event.

4. All cerebral infarctions occurred in participants whose LAV prior to the incident was greater than 32 mL/m^2.

5. No correlation between age or the number of years afib had been present (duration) and LAV was observed; however, there was a highly significant correlation between persistent afib and enlarged LAV.

6. The average age at which a stroke occurred in the LAF group was 77 years, not significantly different from that observed in the general population.

7. Eighteen participants died during the study; 9 of cardiovascular disease, 4 of cancer, and 4 of a respiratory tract infection.

The researchers conclude that LAV is an important predictor of the likelihood that lone afibbers will suffer adverse events (stroke, heart attack, etc) during their lifetime. It is far more important than age and left ventricular ejection fraction. They suggest that only afibbers with a LAV less than 32 mL/m² should be classified as "lone". These afibbers had a benign clinical course during follow-up, while afibbers with an elevated LAV at diagnosis or later during follow-up experienced adverse events.[1]

The findings of the Mayo study are indeed encouraging. They confirm my long-held conviction that otherwise healthy lone afibbers are at no greater risk of stroke than is the general population and therefore does not warrant warfarin therapy. It is encouraging that the mortality among lone afibbers over 25 years of the study was less than half that found in the general population. The observation that left atrial volume (LAV) is an important predictor of future adverse events is intriguing. Hopefully, it will eventually lead to LAV being measured as part of the routine examination of afibbers.

Blood viscosity and stroke risk

There is evidence that a high blood viscosity (thick blood) may increase the risk of ischemic stroke. Blood viscosity, as a whole, affects the ease of general circulation, while erythrocyte (red blood cell) deformability affects circulation through the capillaries. Because red blood cells can only flow through a capillary (the smallest diameter blood vessels involved in nutrient and waste exchange with individual cells) one at a time and even then must be elongated to do so, it is clearly advantageous to have a high erythrocyte deformability index. Research has shown that endurance athletes have significantly higher erythrocyte deformability indices than do sedentary people. The main reason for this is that red blood cells in endurance athletes tend to be replaced quicker than they are in sedentary people, thus creating a population of younger, more deformable cells.

Italian researchers have reported on a study to determine if afibbers and afibbers who have suffered a stroke or TIA ("mini-stroke") have higher blood viscosity and lower erythrocyte deformability than does a control population of non-afibbers without cardiovascular disease. Their study involved 42 afibbers who had suffered an ischemic stroke, 20 who had suffered a TIA, 94 afibbers who had not suffered a stroke or TIA, and 130 age- and gender-matched healthy volunteers. About 60% of the afibbers were hypertensive and about 25% had coronary artery disease and/or left ventricular dysfunction. Average age of the study participants was 73 years and all afibbers were on oral anticoagulation.

After adjusting for gender, age, hypertension, left ventricular dysfunction, coronary artery disease, diabetes, elevated cholesterol level, smoking, hematocrit, fibrinogen, and C-reactive protein levels (hs-CRP), the researchers concluded that healthy controls had a significantly lower whole blood viscosity (at a shear rate of 94.5 seconds^{-1}) and a significantly higher erythrocyte deformability index than did afibbers who had not suffered a stroke. Afibbers who had not suffered a stroke, in turn, had a lower blood viscosity and higher erythrocyte deformability than did those afibbers who had suffered a stroke or TIA.

The researchers also noted a correlation between hypertension and reduced erythrocyte deformability, but observed no effect of ACE inhibitors, beta-blockers, diuretics, and calcium channel blockers on deformability. This would indicate that treating hypertension does not reduce the stroke risk attributable to reduced erythrocyte deformability. The researchers speculate that reduced erythrocyte deformability may be partly caused by a lack of nitric oxide availability and perhaps by inflammation or oxidative stress resulting in "premature aging" of red blood cells. They also suggest that adding a small dose of aspirin to oral anticoagulants in high-risk patients may be beneficial since aspirin has been found to improve erythrocyte deformability.[2]

A large epidemiological study has shown that drinking 5 or more glasses of water every day cuts the risk of coronary artery disease in half as compared to drinking only 2 or fewer glasses of water every day. It is likely that this beneficial effect of adequate water intake is closely linked to the fact that water, but not necessarily other fluids, reduces blood viscosity. It is also of interest that NO-ASA, a recently developed nitrogen oxide-releasing version of aspirin, has been found to reduce thrombosis (blood clotting).

Embolic risk markers in LAF patients

The presence of SEC (spontaneous echocardiographic contrast) in a transesophageal echocardiogram has been shown to predict the ischemic stroke risk in patients with AF. A team of *French and Italian* researchers has completed a study aimed at determining the extent of SEC and other thromboembolic risk markers in patients with AF. Their study included 82 patients with lone atrial fibrillation (LAF) and 289 patients with AF and underlying heart disease. The definition of LAF used by the researchers differed somewhat from the conventional one in that it excluded AF with any of the following features – a history of stroke, coronary artery disease, congestive heart failure, valvular heart disease, cardiomyopathy, cardiomegaly, hypertension (controlled or uncontrolled), hyperthyroidism, diabetes, chronic obstructive pulmonary disease (emphysema and chronic bronchitis). The definition of LAF also excluded AF occurring only during trauma, surgery, or an acute medical illness. The definition used for persistent AF was AF that required electrical or pharmacologic cardioversion or lasted more than 7 days.

Paroxysmal AF was defined as episodes that self-terminated within 48 hours or lasted less than 7 days. Left atrial appendage (LAA) abnormalities were defined as a LAA area greater than 5 square centimeters, an emptying or filling velocity less than 25 cm/second, or the presence of a clot (thrombus) in the LAA or left atrium. All patients underwent conventional transthoracic echocardiography as well as transesophageal echocardiography (TEE) in which the ultrasound probe is placed in the esophagus rather than on the outside chest wall.

The researchers found that 29.3% of LAF patients showed signs of SEC as compared to 49.8% of non-LAF patients. They also observed that LAF patients over the age of 60 years were more likely to have SEC (39.5%) than were patients 60 years or younger (17.9%). Paroxysmal LAF patients were least likely to show SEC (5.9%), while 45.8% of persistent LAF patients had signs of SEC. It was also clear that paroxysmal LAF patients had a significantly smaller left atrial diameter (37.4 mm) than did persistent lone afibbers (40.9 mm). In general, the researchers found the lowest incidence of thromboembolic risk markers in paroxysmal lone afibbers below the age of 60 years. Older age, persistent afib, and the presence of cardiovascular disease or other risk factors markedly increased the incidence of SEC and LAA abnormalities.[3]

Stroke risk in AF patients correlates with CRP levels
C-reactive protein (CRP) or, more specifically, high sensitivity CRP has emerged as an important indicator of systemic inflammation. A study of 5000 healthy individuals found that values varied between 0.01 mg/dL (0.1 mg/L) and 0.38 mg/dL (3.8 mg/L) with a median of 0.16 mg/dL (1.6 mg/L). CRP values tend to increase with age and are generally higher in men than in women. Typical normal values are 0.06 mg/dL for men between the ages of 20-29 years and 0.17 mg/dL for men aged 70-79 years. Corresponding values for women are 0.032 mg/dL and 0.13 mg/dL respectively.

A value higher than 0.38 mg/dL (3.8 mg/L) is generally considered an indication of a systemic inflammation. (For a thorough discussion of CRP please see http://www.yourhealthbase.com/heart_CRP.htm).

British researchers reported an association between the presence of blood clots (thrombi) in the left atrium and high CRP levels in AF patients. Researchers at the *Cleveland Clinic* now confirm these observations and add the important finding that high CRP levels are generally associated with an increased risk of ischemic stroke. The Cleveland study involved 104 afibbers who underwent transesophageal echocardiography (TEE) and had their CRP levels measured within 1 week of the TEE. The researchers observed significantly higher CRP levels in men (median 0.59 mg/dL), patients with hypertension (median 0.48 mg/dL), patients with coronary artery disease (median 0.78 mg/dL), and in patients with severe mitral regurgitation (median 0.67 mg/dL). Afibbers with significant TEE risk factors (presence of thrombi in left atrium, severe spontaneous echo contract or inadequate blood flow from left atrial appendage [emptying velocity of 20 cm/sec or less]) were found to have an average (median) CRP value of 1.0 mg/dL, while those without TEE risk factors had a median value of 0.30 mg/dL. The researchers also found a strong correlation between CRP levels and overall stroke risk (according to SPAF criteria). Patients with an average CRP level of 0.21 mg/dL (0.08 to 0.68) had a low stroke risk, those with an average level of 0.47 mg/dL an intermediate risk, and those with a level of 1.21 mg/dL had a high risk.

The researchers conclude that high CRP levels (greater extent of systemic inflammation) are associated with a greater risk of ischemic stroke and a greater chance of finding thromboembolic abnormalities on a TEE. They speculate that, apart from being an indicator of systemic inflammation, high levels of CRP in themselves can increase the synthesis of tissue factor, an important initiator of blood coagulation.[4]

The finding that afibbers with a CRP level of 0.2 mg/dL or lower have a low risk of ischemic stroke and a low risk of thrombus formation in the left atrium is of significant importance. My own CRP level is 0.03 mg/dL, thus supporting my decision to forego warfarin therapy. Maintaining a CRP level at or below 0.2 mg/dL is clearly important for afibbers. Fortunately, there are many effective, natural approaches for accomplishing this.

Stroke risk linked to cognitive decline

Hypertension, diabetes, smoking, cardiovascular disease, and elevated cholesterol levels are among the major risk factors for ischemic stroke. Researchers at *Boston University* now report that a decline in cognitive function is also associated with an increased risk of experiencing a stroke within 10 years of assessment. The researchers tested the cognitive performance level of 2175 members of the Framingham Offspring Study. The tests included visual-spatial memory, attention, organization, scanning, abstract reasoning, and verbal learning and memory. After adjusting for other known stroke risk factors the researchers conclude that a significant decline in cognitive function is associated with an increased 10-year risk of stroke. They speculate that the mechanism underlying cognitive decline is related to the mechanism causing an increased risk of stroke.[5]

Heavy exercise may increase stroke risk in afibbers

German researchers have completed a study aimed at determining if physical exercise affects platelet aggregation and blood coagulation in people with persistent lone atrial fibrillation (LAF). An increase in either parameter could translate into an increased risk of ischemic stroke. The study involved 13 persistent afibbers and 13 matched controls in normal sinus rhythm. The LAF patients were all effectively anticoagulated with warfarin. All participants underwent bicycle ergometry using a respiratory gas exchange technique for 20 minutes at one-third of their age adjusted maximal workload (moderate exercise). The workload was then increased until maximum exercise capacity was achieved (heavy exercise). The following markers were determined in all participants throughout the study:

- Von Willebrand factor (a marker of endothelial dysfunction)
- Platelet factor-4 (a marker of platelet activation)

- Beta-thromboglobulin (a marker of platelet activation)
- Prothrombin fragments 1 and 2 (a coagulation marker)
- Fibrinogen levels.

The researchers found that levels of platelet factor-4 and beta-thromboglobulin increased significantly in LAF patients during heavy exercise, but not during moderate exercise. Exercise, whether moderate or heavy, had no significant effect on platelet activation in participants in normal sinus rhythm. The level of von Willebrand factor increased by about 24% in all participants during maximal exercise while the level of prothrombin fragments 1 and 2 only increased in the patients in sinus rhythm, thus indicating that warfarin does effectively interfere in the final step of the coagulation pathway.

The researchers conclude that heavy exercise increases platelet activity and von Willebrand factor levels during atrial fibrillation, but that moderate exercise has no detrimental effect on platelet activation or coagulation. They recommend further studies to determine whether heavy physical exercise is a risk factor for stroke in patients with AF.[6]

The finding that vigorous physical exercise increases platelet activation and thus possibly the risk of stroke in patients with persistent LAF points to the advisability of going easy on the exercise when in afib. Heavy physical exercise also increases cortisol levels and vagal tone, so moderation is also important in avoiding afib episodes, especially among vagal afibbers.

Risk of stroke after TIA

It is estimated that about 15% of ischemic strokes are preceded by a TIA (transient ischemic attack) or a minor stroke. A TIA may produce symptoms similar to that of a stroke, but lasts only a few minutes. It is important that TIAs and minor strokes be diagnosed quickly and preventive treatment initiated as soon as possible after the event. North American guidelines recommend that assessment and investigation be completed within one week of the event, while British guidelines allow two weeks for assessment to take place.

Researchers at *Radcliffe Infirmary* report that the risk of another stroke during the first weeks after a TIA is much higher than previously assumed (1-2% at 7 days and 4% at 1 month). Their study included 87 patients who had experienced a TIA and 87 who had suffered a minor stroke. Forty-one per cent of the TIA patients had already experienced a previous TIA or stroke, 55% were being treated for hypertension, and 32% had high cholesterol levels – so these patients were by no means healthy. It is of interest to note that 51% of them had taken aspirin or other antiplatelet agents prior to suffering the TIA indicating that these agents provide limited protection.

The researchers found that 8% of patients suffered a minor or major stroke within 7 days of the first event, 11.5% experienced another stroke within the first month, and 17.3% did so within 3 months. Of the 15 strokes suffered by TIA patients within the 3-month follow-up period 10 were minor strokes and 2 were fatal. Of the 16 strokes suffered by patients with minor stroke as the baseline event 4 were fatal and 2 resulted in increased disability at 3 months. The researchers conclude that the 2-week guideline for assessment after a TIA or minor stroke is unacceptable and that patients need to be examined as soon as possible after the event.[7]

Hypertension and stroke

Hypertension (high blood pressure) is a potent risk factor for stroke. It is, however, not clear whether the risk increases more with rising blood pressure in the case of ischemic stroke (stroke caused by a blood clot) or in the case of hemorrhagic stroke (stroke caused by a burst blood vessel). Researchers at the *Seoul National University* have released a report which throws considerable light on this question. Their study involved 955,000 public servants and teachers who were followed through biennial health examinations for 10 years. During the 9.5 million person-years of observation 14,057 strokes occurred. Of these, 10,716 had complete diagnostic information; 2695 strokes were classified as hemorrhagic, 5326 as ischemic, 964 as subarachnoid hemorrhage (bleeding into the space surrounding the brain and spinal cord), and 1731 were of undetermined origin.

The researchers noted that the increase in stroke incidence with increasing blood pressure was much steeper for hemorrhagic stroke than for ischemic stroke. Participants with stage 1 hypertension (140-159/90-99 mm Hg) were 2.76 times more likely to suffer an ischemic stroke than were participants with normal blood pressure (less than 140/90 mm Hg). However, participants with stage 1 hypertension were 4.9 times more likely to suffer a hemorrhagic stroke than were those with normal blood pressure. Participants with stage 3 hypertension (greater than 180/110 mm Hg) were 9.56 times more likely to suffer an ischemic stroke, but 28.83 times more likely to suffer a hemorrhagic stroke than were participants with normal blood pressure.[8]

The finding that the risk of hemorrhagic stroke increases much more sharply with an increase in blood pressure (above normal) than does the risk of ischemic stroke is of considerable interest when considering the use of warfarin in stroke prevention. The use of warfarin in patients with stage 2 (160-179/100-109 mm Hg) or stage 3 hypertension may be counterproductive because warfarin therapy markedly increases the risk of hemorrhagic stroke, which is already high in this group of patients.

Atrial thrombus formation in AF patients

A blood clot formed in the left atrium or the left atrial appendage (LAA) is a significant source of ischemic stroke in afibbers with underlying heart disease or heart failure. The presence of clots in the atrium or LAA can be determined through transesophageal echocardiography (TEE). TEE differs from the normal transthoracic echocardiography in that the ultrasound probe is positioned in the esophagus rather than on the outside of the chest wall. TEE cannot only pick up clots, but can also be used to give an indication of the extent of dense spontaneous echo contrast (SEC). Dense SEC, in turn, is considered an indication of the likelihood that a clot will form. TEE is increasingly used in preparation for cardioversion and pulmonary vein ablation.

British researchers set out to determine the factors influencing the presence of dense SEC and actual clots in patients with permanent (chronic) atrial fibrillation and risk factors such as heart disease, heart failure, diabetes, prior stroke, or hypertension. All the patients had been on warfarin (INR=2.0-3.0) for at least 3 weeks prior to the study. The researchers found that 3 out of 37 patients had a blood clot in the LAA and 22 had dense SEC. The patients all had significantly elevated levels of C-reactive protein (CRP) and tissue factor when compared to healthy controls. CRP, soluble P-selectin, and hematocrit levels were higher among AF patients with dense SEC than in those without. Twenty-eight patients (76%) had one or more risk factors for thromboembolism (dense SEC, plaque in the descending aorta, LAA thrombus or slow emptying velocity of the LAA).

Upon considering all their findings, the researchers concluded that an elevated hematocrit level was the only variable which was significantly related to the presence of one or more risk factors and to the presence of dense SEC. The risk of dense SEC increased by 40% for each 1% increase in hematocrit. Hematocrit or packed cell volume is determined as the volume of red cells (erythrocytes) in the blood expressed as a percent of total blood volume. The researchers speculate that increased hematocrit may increase dense SEC directly due to increased concentration of erythrocytes or indirectly by promoting blood stagnation.[9]

The fact that over two-thirds of the patients had blood clots or dense SEC after at least 3 weeks of warfarin treatment does not speak highly of warfarin's efficacy in protecting against embolism in the left atrium. It is quite likely that nattokinase would be equally or more effective. There is no evidence that lone afibbers with no other risk factors for stroke have an elevated risk of clot formation in the left atrium or LAA. Nevertheless, the findings concerning CRP and hematocrit levels are intriguing. Low levels of these factors would seem to be protective against embolism (and possibly stroke). It is likely that CRP levels can be reduced by the use of natural anti-inflammatories and high hematocrit levels may respond to increased water intake.

Lifestyle and stroke risk

There is overwhelming evidence that maintaining a healthy lifestyle (not smoking, eating a healthy diet, engaging in regular, moderate exercise, and maintaining optimal body weight) can reduce the risk of cancer, diabetes, and cardiovascular disease more than any other intervention.

Researchers at *Harvard Medical School* report that a healthy lifestyle also materially reduces the risk of suffering a stroke, particularly one caused by a blood clot or the rupture of atherosclerotic plaque (ischemic stroke). The Harvard researchers describe a low-risk lifestyle as:

- Not smoking
- A body mass index < 25 kg/m2
- At least 30 minutes/day of moderate physical activity

- Modest alcohol consumption (5-30 g/day for men, 5-15 g/day for women)
- Scoring within the top 40% of a healthy diet score.

A healthy diet was defined as follows:

- High intake of vegetables, fruits, nuts, soy and cereal fiber
- High ratio of chicken plus fish to red meat
- High ratio of polyunsaturated to saturated fat
- Low intake of trans-fatty acids
- Daily supplementation with multivitamins for 5 years or more.

The Harvard lifestyle/stroke risk study is a very large one involving 43,685 men enrolled in the Health Professionals Follow-up Study (begun in 1986) and 71,243 women from the Nurses' Health Study (begun in 1976). All participants were free of cancer and cardiovascular disease at baseline. The mean age at baseline (study entry) was 50 years for women and 54 years for men.

During follow-up, a total of 994 strokes (600 ischemic, 161 hemorrhagic [caused by a burst blood vessel], and 233 of unknown type) were documented among male participants. A total of 1559 strokes (853 ischemic, 278 hemorrhagic, and 428 of unknown type) were documented among female participants. Women with all 5 low-risk factors as defined above were found to have an 81% lower risk of suffering a stroke (79% lower risk of suffering an ischemic stroke) compared with women who had none of these low-risk factors, i.e. a highly unhealthy lifestyle. Corresponding risk reductions for men were 69% for total stroke and 80% for ischemic stroke. Unfortunately, only 2% of women and 4% of men had all 5 low-risk factors. Heavy smoking was, by far, the most significant risk factor for stroke followed by obesity (BMI over 30 kg/m2), lack of exercise, and excessive alcohol consumption.

Adherence to a healthy diet was clearly more important for women than for men with the very worst diet increasing total stroke risk by 47%, ischemic stroke risk by 33%, and hemorrhagic stroke risk by 70% among women. Corresponding figures for men were 16%, 16%, and 10%. The researchers conclude that 47% of all strokes (54% of ischemic strokes) among women can be attributed to lack of adherence to a low-risk lifestyle. Corresponding figures for men are 35% and 52%.[10,11]

It is not clear how many person-years were involved in these follow-up studies. However, assuming that follow-up was completed in 2006 (last dietary evaluation was in 2002) would result in a maximum follow-up for women (nurses) of 2.14 million (30 x 71,243) person-years and 0.87 million (20 x 43,685) persons-years for men (health professionals). Thus, total stroke rates would be 0.11%/year for men and 0.07% for women. These are indeed very low rates when compared to the oft-quoted rate of 1%/year among the general US population. I noticed this discrepancy in a 14-year follow-up study of the health professionals published in 2003. Following is an explanation provided by Dr. Ka He, the lead author (personal communication to me, November 30, 2003):

The annual incidence of new and recurrent stroke in the US is about 700,000 according to the American Stroke Association. Based on a population of 270,000,000 the annual rate is 0.26 per 100 person-years, or 0.26% per year. Stroke risk, of course, increases with age so it would clearly be higher if, for example, only people over 50 years of age were considered. Says Dr. He, "In our study, we only count the first event not recurrent stroke. Also, the participants are all healthcare professionals. They are health-conscious and relatively healthy (they were free from any CVD and diabetes). I would not be surprised if there is relatively low rate of stroke in our cohort."

Platelet activation in acute atrial fibrillation

It is not known whether atrial fibrillation as such results in a hypercoagulable state that could increase the risk of ischemic stroke. A group of cardiovascular researchers at *Loyola University Medical Center* now provides an intriguing insight into this question. Their study involved 22 patients with paroxysmal afib who were scheduled to undergo radiofrequency catheter ablation. The patients did not have left ventricular dysfunction, rheumatic valve disease, mitral valve prolapse, or any significant valvular regurgitation; however, about 30% had hypertension and about 14% had diabetes. The study participants were divided into two groups of 14 (Group A) and 8 patients (Group B) respectively. The only statistically significant difference between the two groups was a greater preponderance of men (93%) in Group A than in Group B (50%).

All patients were in sinus rhythm when the study began and had sheaths (tubes) inserted in the femoral veins and coronary sinus (via the right internal jugular vein) for collection of blood samples. Atrial fibrillation was induced for 15 minutes by burst pacing (330 bpm or a cycle length of 180 ms) in Group A resulting in a ventricular rate (heart beat) of 121 bpm. In Group B atrial pacing to achieve a ventricular rate at 120 bpm without going into afib was applied for 15 minutes. Analysis of blood samples taken at the coronary sinus in Group A revealed increased platelet activation and thrombin generation as well as reduced nitrogen oxide production when compared with Group B. The blood sample (systemic) taken from the femoral vein did not change with pacing indicating that the effect is localized to the heart – at least for the first 15 minutes.

The researchers conclude that their findings may help explain why short episodes of atrial fibrillation predispose to stroke, especially in patients with underlying vascular disease such as diabetes and hypertension.[12]

Obviously, an important question is "Do these findings apply to lone afibbers without hypertension and diabetes?" Unfortunately, the researchers did not separate out the effects due to hypertensive/diabetic subjects vs. those with no stroke risk factors, so it is impossible to say and, in all fairness, the study population really was not large enough to allow such a separation. However, the results of this study would certainly support the supplementation with natural antiplatelet agents such as vitamins C, E, B3 and B6, and fish oils, some of which would also have an inhibitory effect on the formation of prothrombin. Nattokinase would not have any effect on platelet activation or prothrombin or thrombin formation, but would be effective in increasing fibrinolytic actively and thereby prevent blood clots from forming.

LAA thrombi rare in PVI patients

Suffering a stroke during or after a pulmonary vein isolation (PVI) procedure is fairly rare (approximately 1.5% incidence rate), but obviously constitutes a serious complication. To avoid stroke during the procedure, patients are usually pre-screened for clots in the left atrium (LA) and left atrial appendage (LAA) using CT scanning and/or transesophageal echocardiography (TEE). In addition, heparin is used during the procedure and warfarin after to avoid post-procedural stroke. It is not known just how frequent LA or LAA clots are found in patients prior to their PVI.

Electrophysiologists at the *Cleveland Clinic* have published the results of a study involving 1221 afibbers who underwent a pulmonary vein antrum isolation during the period 2000-2004. All patients underwent a pre-procedure CT scan and 60 also underwent a TEE. Nine patients were found to have a thrombus (clot) in the LAA as per the CT scan; however, when checked with TEE only three were actually clots, while the remaining 6 were smoke-like echo.

Two of the 3 patients had permanent afib with an average left ventricular ejection fraction (LVEF) of 48%, while the sole paroxysmal afibbers with a clot had an ejection fraction of only 25%. Thus, no paroxysmal afibbers with an ejection fraction of 50% or greater (normal) experienced LAA thrombi. Inasmuch as lone afibbers, by definition, have normal LVEFs (50% or greater), there were no incidences of LAA clots in paroxysmal, lone afibbers. It is likely that the two permanent afibbers had underlying heart disease (average LVEF was 48%), so it is probably safe to assume that even permanent, lone afibbers would be very unlikely to have thrombi in the LAA.

The Cleveland EPs conclude that a pre-procedure CT scan may be all that is required and that the use of TEE may not be needed in the case of paroxysmal afibbers with normal (50% or greater) LVEF. [13]

This is good news indeed and confirms earlier research that lone afibbers are not prone to clot development in the LAA. As far as the CT scan or TEE is concerned, if given the choice, I would personally prefer the TEE so as to avoid the radiation inherent in CT scanning and the potential adverse effects of the contrast medium (x-ray dye) used during the scan.

Incidence of thrombi prior to ablation

Catheter ablation for atrial fibrillation (AF) carries a low (0.3 – 0.7%), but still significant, risk of ischemic stroke and transient ischemic attack (TIA). The two major causes of stroke or TIA occurring during the procedure are the formation and subsequent embolization (blocking of a blood vessel) of char or thrombi (blood clots) formed on the ablation catheter and the disturbance of existing thrombi in the left atrium or left atrial appendage (LAA). This disturbance can be caused by catheter manipulation or be related to the more forceful heart beat accompanying restoration of normal sinus rhythm. The risk of a stroke or TIA during the procedure can clearly be reduced by ensuring that there are no clots in the left atrium or LAA prior to starting the procedure. This is the reason why most major ablation centers insist that patients scheduled for an ablation undergo a TEE (transesophageal echocardiogram) shortly before the procedure. A TEE is the "gold standard" for determining if clots are present in the left atrium or LAA, but the procedure is invasive, uncomfortable for the patient and relatively costly. Thus, researchers at *Johns Hopkins University School of Medicine* undertook a study to determine if all afib patients scheduled for ablation actually needed a pre-procedural TEE.

Their study involved 585 patients who underwent a total of 732 ablation procedures (repeat rate of 25%). All patients were anticoagulated with warfarin for at least 4 weeks prior to their procedure except for the last 5 days when warfarin was replaced by enoxaparin (a low molecular weight heparin). All patients also underwent a TEE within 24 hours prior to the procedure. The researchers found thrombi in the LAA in 12 cases (1.6%) requiring cancellation of the procedure. All 12 patients had been on warfarin for at least 6 months prior to the procedure and all had a left atrial diameter equal to or greater than 4.5 cm (45 mm). Nine of the patients had persistent afib and 3 had paroxysmal AF.

Analysis of all the TEE data collected revealed that the risk of finding a clot in the left atrium or LAA was significantly associated with left atrial diameter and stroke risk as measured with the CHADS2 score. NOTE: The CHADS2 score assigns a risk of 1 point each for congestive heart failure, hypertension, age 75 years or older and diabetes, and 2 point score if having suffered a previous stroke or TIA. Thrombi were present in 0.3%, 1.4% and 5.3% in patients with CHADS2 scores of 0, 1 and 2 or greater. None of the cases where thrombi were observed had a left atrial diameter less than 4.5 cm. In contrast, no thrombi were observed in patients with a CHADS2 score of 0 and a left atrial diameter of less than 4.5 cm.

The researchers suggest that a pre-procedural TEE may be unnecessary in this group of patients provided they have been properly anticoagulated prior to the procedure.[14, 15]

This study confirms that warfarin is by no means 100% effective in preventing clot formation in the left atrium and, on a more positive note, that healthy afibbers with no stroke risk factors and a left atrial diameter less than 4.5 cm have a very low risk of forming clots in the left atrium.

Mitral regurgitation and stroke risk

Extensive research has shown that the main factor determining left atrium clot formation and associated stroke risk is the rate at which blood flows in and out of the left atrial appendage (LAA). If this rate is high then the formation of a clot or the precursors of a clot (smoke-like echoes [spontaneous echo contrast or SEC] on a transesophageal echocardiogram) is very unlikely.

Factors that can reduce the flow rate through the LAA include aging, congestive heart failure, poor left ventricular ejection fraction, elevated levels of hematocrit or von Willebrand factor, and a prior ischemic stroke or transient ischemic attack (TIA). Fortunately, a recent Japanese study concluded that lone afibbers and patients with atrial flutter are at very low risk for thrombus formation in the LAA. Now a group of researchers from *Toyama University* in Japan report that the presence of severe mitral regurgitation (MR), including mitral valve prolapse, increases the flow of blood in and out of the LAA and thus is associated with a substantially lower risk of clot formation.

Their study included 271 patients (average age of 67 years) with permanent atrial fibrillation who underwent both transthoracic and transesophageal echocardiography (TEE) and also had blood samples taken to measure markers of blood clotting, notably D-dimer. NOTE: Fibrin monomers and dimers polymerize into blood clots through the action of activated coagulation factor XIII. The patients investigated were by no means lone afibbers – about 40% had hypertension, 25% had heart failure, 25% had a history of stroke or TIA, and 56% were on warfarin. Of the 271 patients, 20 (7%) had severe MR including 9 patients with mitral valve prolapse, 45 (17%) had moderate MR, and 92 (34%) had mild MR as determined with TEE. The TEE study found that patients with severe MR had a higher average LAA peak flow velocity (35.2 cm/s) than did those with no or only mild MR (25.5 cm/s). In addition, the severity of SEC was significantly lower in patients with severe MR (0.7) than in those with moderate (1.7), mild (2.2) or no MR (1.9). The level of D-dimer was surprisingly low (0.76 mcg/mL) in patients with severe MR and highest (1.72) in those with moderate MR. Patients with no MR had an average D-dimer level of 0.82. Warfarin therapy had no effect on d-dimer levels or presence of SEC.

The Japanese researchers conclude that patients with severe MR, including mitral valve prolapse, have a lower thromboembolic risk than do those with mild or moderate MR. They speculate that the more "chaotic" blood flow resulting from severe MR helps prevent blood stasis in the LAA. They suggest that the increased D-dimer levels found among patients with moderate MR may be associated with their heart failure, but caution that the higher D-dimer levels and SEC values found among these patients could increase their risk of thromboembolism.[16]

In an earlier LAF survey 7% of respondents reported that they had been diagnosed with mitral valve prolapse, while 14% had mild regurgitation. Although there is no evidence that lone afibbers with a normal left ventricular ejection fraction are at increased risk for LAA blood stasis, SEC or thrombus formation, it is comforting to learn that the presence of severe mitral valve regurgitation, including mitral valve prolapse, does not increase stroke risk, but is actually protective against thromboembolism.

Plasma von Willebrand factor and stroke risk

Platelet activation and aggregation is a crucial first step in the formation of blood clots (thrombi) that may cause an ischemic stroke. Platelets, like red and white blood cells, are an integral part of normal blood. In spite of their small size they contain an amazing variety of enzymes that interact with other plasma components crucial to the formation of blood clots. Among the more significant of these components are thromboxane A2, ADP (adenosine diphosphate) and von Willebrand factor (vWF). The first step in the platelet aggregation process involves the adherence of platelets to sub-endothelial tissue or a foreign object. Von Willebrand factor is the main "glue" involved in platelet sticking to each other and to the vessel wall.

There is evidence that thrombosis in the left atrial appendage (LAA) may be related to elevated levels of vWF. There is also evidence that a high plasma level of vWF increases the risk of stroke and cardiovascular events in non-anticoagulated atrial fibrillation (AF) patients. A group of researchers from the *University of Birmingham* and the *University of Murcia* in Spain reports that high vWF levels are also associated with an increased risk of stroke, cardiovascular events, bleeding, and death in AF patients on warfarin therapy.

The study included 829 older patients with permanent (long-standing persistent) AF (50% male with a median age of 76 years) who were on warfarin therapy and had maintained an INR between 2.0 and 3.0 for at least 6 months prior to having their medical history recorded and blood samples drawn for the measurement of plasma concentration of vWF and D-dimer. The study participants were, not unexpectedly, an unhealthy lot. Eighty-two percent had hypertension, 37% had heart failure, 31% had high cholesterol levels, 25% had diabetes, and 18% had a history of stroke or TIA (transient ischemic attack).

The patients were followed for an average of 2 years. During this time, 32 (1.7% per year) suffered a stroke or TIA, 36 (1.9% per year) experienced acute coronary syndrome events (heart attack, unstable angina, etc), 27 (1.5% per year) had acute heart failure, and 68 (3.6% per year) suffered a major bleeding event. Sixty-nine patients (3.7% per year) died during follow-up of which 25 deaths (1.13% per year) were related to cardiovascular causes. Multivariate Cox regression analysis showed that patients 75 years and older had a two-fold increase in risk of an adverse cardiovascular event (stroke/TIA, acute coronary syndrome, acute heart failure, peripheral embolism, and cardiac death). A history of stroke or heart failure was associated with an 80% increased risk of an adverse cardiovascular event, while a vWF level at or above 221 IU/dL was associated with an almost three-fold (HR = 2.71) increase in risk. The association between stroke risk and vWF level was particularly pronounced with a level at 221 IU/dL or above associated with a five-fold increase in stroke risk.

A high vWF level was also associated with a four-fold (HR = 4.47) increase in the risk of major bleeding, a three-fold increase in the risk of cardiovascular death and a doubling of all-cause mortality. Age of 75 years or older, current smoking, and diabetes were also major risk factors for increased overall mortality. High cholesterol levels, on the other hand, were associated with a significantly lower risk of cardiovascular death (HR = 0.27) and overall mortality (HR = 0.46). Somewhat surprisingly, vWF level was significantly more predictive of the risk of cardiovascular events, bleeding and death than were the commonly used risk scores of $CHADS_2$, CHA_2DS_2VASc, and HAS-BLED. The authors of the study conclude that the addition of vWF level to these risk scores will materially increase their predictive ability. [17]

Although the patient population in the study bears no resemblance to a group of otherwise healthy lone afibbers, it may nevertheless be a good idea to have a vWF measurement. It is surprising, or maybe not, that the authors do not suggest that it may be a good idea for afibbers with a high vWF level to take steps to reduce it. There is ample evidence that this can be accomplished by supplementation with vitamin C and vitamin E. [18-20]

Stroke risk and vitamin D intake

There is, by now, ample evidence that vitamin D deficiency is associated with many disease conditions including hypertension, insulin resistance, diabetes, infections, influenza, autoimmune diseases, cancers, cardiovascular disease, stroke, and heart failure. A study carried out by a group of researchers at *Harvard Medical School* concluded that having a low blood plasma level of 25[OH]D – the first metabolite of vitamin D – increases the risk of suffering an ischemic stroke (stroke caused by a blood clot) by between 50 and 100%.

A group of researchers from the *University of Hawaii* reports that a low dietary intake of vitamin D is associated with an increased risk of suffering an ischemic stroke. Their study included 7385 Japanese-American men who were 45 to 68 years old when enrolled in the Honolulu Heart Program between 1965 and 1968. At time of enrolment, all study participants completed a detailed food frequency questionnaire. Dietary intake of vitamin D ranged from 0 to 212 micrograms/day (0 – 8500 IU/day) with the average being 3.62 micrograms/day (145 IU/day).

Over the 34 years following enrolment, 960 study participants suffered a stroke, of which, 651 were ischemic (thromboembolic), 269 were hemorrhagic (caused by a burst blood vessel), and 40 were of unknown type. The incidence of stroke in the lowest quartile of dietary vitamin D intake (0 – 45 IU/day) was 0.64%/year as compared to 0.51%/year in the highest quartile (165 – 8500 IU/day). After adjusting for potential confounding variables including age, total daily food consumption, body mass index, hypertension, diabetes, smoking, physical activity, cholesterol level and alcohol intake, the researchers conclude that a low dietary vitamin D intake is associated with a 27% increased risk of suffering an ischemic stroke. No association was found between vitamin D intake and the risk of suffering a hemorrhagic stroke. The researchers suggest that vitamin D supplementation may be beneficial for stroke prevention. [21]

This study confirms the importance of vitamin D as an integral part of a stroke prevention program. The Nurses' Health Study observed a 2-fold reduction in the risk of suffering an ischemic stroke at a 25[OH]D plasma level of 95 nmol/L (38 ng/mL) as compared to a level of 50 nmol/L (20 ng/mL). To reach a level of 95 nmol/L would, for most people, require supplementation with about 4000 IU/day. Vitamin D comes in two different forms – vitamin D2 (ergocalciferol) and vitamin D3 (cholecalciferol). Vitamin D2 is found in poorly formulated multivitamins, as an additive to some foods, and is the form preferably prescribed by many physicians. Unfortunately, it is about 10 times less effective than vitamin D3 and is, by some researchers, considered toxic. [22]

Seasonal variation in AF-related stroke

There is evidence that hospital admissions for certain cardiovascular diseases such as heart attack, sudden death, and heart failure are substantially higher during the winter than during the rest of the year. A similar trend has been reported for hospital admissions related to atrial fibrillation (AF), which seem to be inversely associated with outdoor temperatures. Now a team of *Danish and New Zealand* researchers reports a significant seasonal variation in hospitalizations for AF-related stroke.

Their study involved 243,000 Danish men and women (48% female) diagnosed with AF during the period 1980 to 2008, and 51,500 New Zealand men and women (48% female) diagnosed with AF during the period 1991 to 2008. The median age at diagnosis was 75 years for men and 78 years for women in the Danish cohort, and 76 years for men and 78 years for women in the NZ cohort. About 33% of Danish study participants and 53% of NZ participants had one or more comorbid conditions with congestive heart failure at 28% being the most common amongst New Zealanders and hypertension at 11.5% being most common amongst Danes.

Hospitalization rate for AF was significantly higher amongst study participants above 65 years of age than for younger ones. It is also clear that the incidence (new cases on an annual basis) of AF-related hospital admissions increased significantly during the study period – about 5% annually in Denmark and 2.6% in NZ for patients older than 65 years. Corresponding numbers for younger participants were 5.4% in Denmark and 0.2% in NZ.

During follow-up, 36,000 Danish study participants and 7,518 NZ participants (54.6% females) were hospitalized with stroke. The risk of stroke was found to be 22% higher in winter than in summer in Denmark, and 27% higher in NZ. The risk of dying within 30 days of suffering a stroke was about 20% in both countries as measured during the period 2000 to 2008.

The researchers conclude that the incidence of AF is increasing significantly and that the incidence of AF-related stroke peaks during the winter season in both Denmark and New Zealand. [23]

The finding that the incidence of AF-related stroke peaks in winter is intriguing. The authors suggest that climate factors such as ambient temperature, humidity, and hours of sunshine may play a role. There is evidence that hypertension is more pronounced during winter and that the degree of blood pressure elevation is directly related to blood viscosity and fibrinogen level. Thus it would seem plausible that the observed increase in stroke rate during winter time is related to increased blood viscosity.

Long-term outcome following ischemic stroke

There is still no consensus as to whether type of atrial fibrillation (paroxysmal, persistent or permanent) affect the risk of suffering an ischemic stroke, although the preponderance of evidence points to the risk being similar for all three types, with permanent AF perhaps having a slightly higher risk. A group of Greek physicians at the *Alexandra Hospital* in Athens now reports on a study aimed at determining the association between AF type and the long-term outcome (recurrence rate and mortality) in patients with non-valvular AF who had suffered an ischemic stroke.

The study involved 811 patients (52% women) of which 34.2% had paroxysmal AF, 20.3% had persistent, and the remaining 45.5% had permanent AF. Patients with permanent AF were older (mean age of 77 years), 77% had hypertension, 14% had heart failure, and 20% were on warfarin or other vitamin K antagonists when they suffered a first ischemic stroke. In contrast, patients with paroxysmal AF were younger (mean age of 74 years), and were less likely to have hypertension (69%) and heart failure (8%). Patients were followed for an average of about 3 years. Stroke recurrence during the first 30 days was 4.3% for paroxysmal AF vs. 11.9% for permanent AF. Ten-year recurrence rate (estimated from Kaplan-Meyer curves) was 33.5% for paroxysmal AF vs. 41.4% for permanent AF. Similarly, 10-year overall survival rate was more than twice as high amongst paroxysmal afibbers (34.6%) than amongst permanent afibbers (15.8%).

The researchers speculate that the lower rate of stroke recurrence in paroxysmal AF could be explained by the concept that thromboembolic risk in AF depends on the duration of the episode. They also point out that stroke severity and subsequent disability were significantly lower amongst paroxysmal afibbers and suggest that the reason for this is that short, paroxysmal episodes lead to the formation of thrombi of relatively smaller size compared to those formed in permanent AF. They conclude that paroxysmal afibbers have lower rates of recurrence and mortality compared to those with permanent AF.[24]

Although the patients involved in this study were by no means lone afibbers (about 20% had coronary artery disease and about 10% had heart failure), it would seem reasonable to assume that lone afibbers with paroxysmal AF who suffer an ischemic stroke have a better long-term prognosis than do those with permanent AF.

Left atrial appendage and risk of stroke

Although lone atrial fibrillation (LAF) as such is not a risk factor for ischemic stroke, the likelihood of suffering a stroke or transient ischemic attack (TIA) increases if the LAF is accompanied by heart disease, presence of prosthetic heart valves, hypertension (blood pressure greater than 160/90 mm Hg), diabetes, low left ventricular ejection fraction (< 45%) or a history of stroke, TIA, heart attack or peripheral vascular embolism.

A group of *Italian* medical researchers have found that an elevated level of the inflammation marker C-reactive protein (CRP) and a reduced blood flow through the left atrial appendage (LAA) are associated with an increased risk of forming blood clots (thrombi) in the left atrium. Their study included 150 patients (46% men, age ranging between 53 and 77 years) with persistent, non-valvular atrial fibrillation (AF). Prior to their scheduled electrical cardioversion, all patients underwent transesophageal echocardiography (TEE) and had blood samples drawn for later analysis. Examination of the echocardiograms revealed the existence of dense spontaneous echo contrast (SEC) in 52 patients. SEC is considered to be the origin of thrombi and is seen as a swirling pattern (fog) on the TEE; the denser the pattern the more likely it is that a clot will eventually develop. Nine patients were found to have a thrombus in the LAA and were excluded from further evaluation. The remaining 98 patients had no dense SEC. It is interesting that 85% of study participants were on warfarin, which is supposed to prevent clot formation.

Analysis of blood samples drawn prior to cardioversion showed that the presence of dense SEC was directly associated with elevated levels of C-reactive protein, D-dimer and fibrinogen. Examination of the echocardiogram revealed that the presence of dense SEC was strongly associated with a low velocity of blood flow in the LAA and significantly related with an enlarged left atrium. Somewhat surprisingly, left ventricular ejection fraction did not seem to affect LAA flow velocity. After correcting for possible confounders, a multivariate analysis showed that only LAA flow velocity and CRP level were associated with the presence of dense SEC at a level achieving statistical significance.

The researchers conclude that patients with low LAA velocity (less than 0.25 m/sec) have a 19-fold increased risk of harboring dense SEC as compared to those with normal flow velocity. Similarly, a CRP level above 3 mg/L (0.3 mg/dL) was associated with a 3.4-fold increased risk of dense SEC. [25]

The finding that a low LAA flow velocity is associated with a greater risk of forming dense SEC and blood clots is not surprising. Blood stasis, such as also found in deep vein thrombosis, is an obvious incubator of thrombi. What is somewhat surprising is the finding that left ventricular ejection fraction is not associated with SEC formation. Seeing that the left ventricle abuts the LAA, one would expect that a more forceful left ventricular ejection would result in a greater LAA emptying velocity. The finding that a high CRP level (inflammation) is associated with an increased risk of dense SEC, once again emphasizes the importance of knowing one's CRP level and, if necessary, reduce it through the use of natural anti-inflammatories.

Mitral regurgitation and lone atrial fibrillation

Mitral regurgitation (MR) is defined as an abnormal reversal of blood flow from the left ventricle to the left atrium. The most common causes of MR are mitral valve prolapse (MVP), rheumatic heart disease, and ischemic heart disease. A group of researchers from *Bakersfield Heart Hospital* have found that MR is significantly more prevalent in patients with lone atrial fibrillation (LAF) than in patients without this condition.

Their study involved 57 patients with LAF who underwent transesophageal echocardiography (TEE) prior to cardioversion and 100 patients without LAF who underwent TEE for various other reasons. All of the study participants had structurally normal mitral valves. LAF was defined as AF without concomitant heart disease, hypertension or diabetes, and age less than 60 years.

The researchers found that LAF patients were far more likely to exhibit moderate MR than were controls (66% vs 6%). Mild MR was found in 18% of LAF patients vs 31% in controls, and absence of MR was noted in 16% of LAF patients vs 63% of controls. Left ventricular ejection fraction and left atrial diameter did not differ between the two groups, but the diameter of the mitral annulus was significantly greater in the LAF group.

The researchers conclude that moderate MR may be a risk factor for the development of LAF primarily by causing mechanical stretch of the left atrium or conversely, that LAF may predispose to the development of MR over time. They also suggest the possibility that the observed MR may be a transient phenomenon that resolves once normal sinus rhythm is restored. [26]

The finding that mitral regurgitation and lone atrial fibrillation are somehow connected is most interesting. It is not clear from the study which is cause and which is effect, although the authors clearly lean toward the hypothesis that moderate MR is the forerunner for LAF. Another possibility obviously has to be that MR and LAF have the same origin. If this is indeed the case, then magnesium deficiency is likely to be the common factor since both LAF and mitral valve prolapse have been found to be associated with magnesium deficiency [27, 28]

REFERENCES

1. Osranek, M, et al. Left atrial volume predicts cardiovascular events in patients originally diagnosed with lone atrial fibrillation: three-decade follow-up. European Heart Journal, Vol. 26, 2005, pp. 2556-61
2. Cecchi, E, et al. Hyperviscosity as a possible risk factor for cerebral ischemic complications in atrial fibrillation patients. American Journal of Cardiology, Vol. 97, June 15, 2006, pp. 1745-48

3. Di Angelantonio, E, et al. Comparison of transesophageal echocardiographic identification of embolic risk markers in patients with lone versus non-lone atrial fibrillation. American Journal of Cardiology, Vol. 95, March 1, 2005, pp. 592-96

4. Thambidorai, SK, et al. Relation of C-reactive protein correlated with risk of thromboembolism in patients with atrial fibrillation. American Journal of Cardiology, Vol. 94, September 15, 2004, pp. 805-07

5. Elias, MF, et al. Framingham stroke risk profile and lowered cognitive performance. Stroke, Vol. 35, February 2004, pp. 404-09

6. Goette, A, et al. Effect of physical exercise on platelet activity and the von-Willebrand-factor in patients with persistent lone atrial fibrillation. J Interv Card Electrophysiol, Vol. 10, No. 2, April 2004, pp. 139-46

7. Coull, AJ, et al. Population based study of early risk of stroke after transient ischemic attack or minor stroke: implications for public education and organization of services. British Medical Journal, Vol. 328, January 26, 2004

8. Song, YM, et al. Blood pressure, hemorrhagic stroke, and ischemic stroke: the Korean national prospective occupational cohort study. British Medical Journal, Vol. 328, February 7, 2004, pp. 324-25

9. Conway, DSG, et al. Relation of interleukin-6, C-reactive protein, and the prothrombotic state to transesophageal echocardiographic findings in atrial fibrillation. American Journal of Cardiology, Vol. 93, June 1, 2004, pp.1368-73

10. Chiuve, SE, et al. Primary prevention of stroke by healthy lifestyle. Circulation, Vol. 118, August 26, 2008, pp. 947-54

11. Gorelick, PB. Primary prevention of stroke – Impact of health lifestyle. Circulation, Vol. 118, August 26, 2008, pp. 904-06 (editorial)

12. Akar, JG, et al. Acute onset human atrial fibrillation is associated with local cardiac platelet activation and endothelial dysfunction. Journal of the American College of Cardiology, Vol. 51, May 6, 2008, pp. 1790-93

13. Khan, MN, et al. Low incidence of left atrial or left atrial appendage thrombus in patients with paroxysmal atrial fibrillation and normal EF who present for pulmonary vein antrum isolation procedure. Journal of Cardiovascular Electrophysiology, Vol. 19, April 2008, pp. 356-58

14. Scherr, D, et al. Incidence and predictors of left atrial thrombus prior to catheter ablation of atrial fibrillation. Journal of Cardiovascular Electrophysiology, Vol. 20, April 2009, pp. 379-84

15. Cappato, R. Searching for left atrial thrombi prior to catheter ablation of atrial fibrillation. Journal of Cardiovascular Electrophysiology, Vol. 20, April 2009, pp. 385-87

16. Fukuda, N, et al. Relation of the severity of mitral regurgitation to thromboembolic risk in patients with atrial fibrillation. International Journal of Cardiology, August 5, 2009 [Epub ahead of print]

17. Roldan, V, Lip, GYH, et al. Plasma von Willebrand factor levels are an independent risk factor for adverse events including mortality and major bleeding in anticoagulated atrial fibrillation patients. Journal of the American College of Cardiology, Vol. 57, No. 25, June 21, 2011

18. Antoniades, C., et al. Effects of antioxidant vitamins C and E on endothelial function and thrombosis/fibrinolysis system in smokers. Thromb Haemost, Vol. 89, June 2003, pp. 990-95

19. Tousoulis, D, et al. Vitamin C affects thrombosis/fibrinolysis system and reactive hyperemia in patients with type 2 diabetes and coronary artery disease. Diabetes Care, Vol. 26, October 2003, pp. 2749-53

20. Huang, N, et al. Alpha-tocopherol, a potent modulator of endothelial cell function. Thromb Res, Vol. 50, No. 4, May 1988, pp. 547-57

21. Kojima, G, et al. Low dietary vitamin D predicts 34-year incident stroke. Stroke, Vol. 43, August 2012, pp. 2163-67

22. Armas, LAG, et al. Vitamin D2 is much less effective than vitamin D3 in humans. Journal of Clinical Endocrinology & Metabolism, Vol. 89, No. 11, 2004, pp. 5387-91

23. Christensen, AL, et al. Seasonality, incidence and prognosis in atrial fibrillation and stroke in Denmark and New Zealand. BMJ Open, Vol. 2, No. 4, August 24, 2012

24. Ntaios, G, et al. The type of atrial fibrillation is associated with long-term outcome in patients with acute ischemic stroke. International Journal of Cardiology, May 16, 2012 [Epub ahead of print]

25. Cianfrocca, C, Santini, M, et al. C-reactive protein and left atrial appendage velocity are independent determinants of the risk of thrombogenesis in patients with atrial fibrillation. International Journal of Cardiology, Vol. 142, 2010, pp. 22-28

26. Sharma, S, et al. Clinically unrecognized mitral regurgitation is prevalent in lone atrial fibrillation. World Journal of Cardiology, Vol. 4, May 26, 2012, pp. 183-87

27. Khan, AM, et al. Low serum magnesium and the development of atrial fibrillation in the community. Circulation, Vol. 127, January 1, 2013, pp. 33-38

28. Bobkowski, W, et al. The importance of magnesium status in the pathophysiology of mitral valve prolapse. Magnesium Research, Vol. 18, No. 1, March 2005, pp. 35-52

Chapter 10

Stroke and Bleeding Risk Estimates

STROKE RISK

It is a well-established fact that atrial fibrillation is associated with an increased risk of ischemic stroke. However it was only in 2001 that it was realized that the risk of stroke differed from patient to patient. This realization led to the development of the *National Registry of Atrial Fibrillation Scheme* for predicting stroke risk also known as the CHADS$_2$ scheme. The CHADS$_2$ scheme assigns a score of zero to atrial fibrillation patients with no additional risk factors. One point is added for the presence of worsening congestive heart failure, hypertension, age 75 years or older, and diabetes (1 point for each) and 2 points for a history of stroke or TIA (transient ischemic attack).

CHADS$_2$ Risk Score

Risk Factor	Points
75 years of age or older	1
Hypertension [1]	1
Diabetes [2]	1
Congestive heart failure [3]	1
Stroke or TIA [4]	2

[1] Treated hypertension or blood pressure above 140/90 mm Hg
[2] Diagnosis of diabetes or fasting glucose level above 126 mg/dL
    (7 mmol/L)
[3] Congestive heart failure that had worsened recently
[4] Having experienced an ischemic stroke or transient ischemic attack (TIA)

By 2009 it became apparent that the CHADS$_2$ scheme could be further refined by adding female gender, vascular disease, and age above 65 years as additional risk factors. This led to the development of the *Birmingham Stroke Risk Schema* also known as the CHA$_2$DS$_2$-VASc score. The original intent behind the new scheme was to be able to better classify atrial fibrillation patients who were at such a low risk for stroke that they did not need anticoagulation with warfarin or one of the newer anticoagulants (NOACs).

The *2016 ESC guidelines for the management of atrial fibrillation* classify such patients as those having a CHA$_2$DS$_2$-VASc score of 0 for men or 1 for women. Men with a score of 1 and women with a score of 2 are classified as being of moderate risk and anticoagulation is optional. However, for men with a score of 2 or higher and for women with a score above 2 anticoagulation is recommended. The CHA$_2$DS$_2$-VASc scheme clearly would recommend anticoagulation for far more patients than would the original CHADS$_2$ score in that women and men over 65 years of age with just one other risk factor would automatically be prescribed anticoagulation.

CHA$_2$DS$_2$-VASc Risk Score

Risk Factor	Points
Age below 65 years	0
Age 65-74 years	1
Age 75 years or older	2
Female gender	1
Congestive heart failure (1)	1
Diabetes (2)	1
Hypertension (3)	1
Vascular disease (4)	1
Previous ischemic stroke or TIA	2

(1) Congestive heart failure that had worsened recently
(2) Diagnosis of diabetes or fasting glucose level above 126 mg/dL (7 mmol/L)
(3) Treated hypertension or blood pressure above 140/90 mm Hg
(4) Peripheral artery disease, previous heart attack, aortic plaque

Comparison of stroke risk estimates

The two stroke risk estimates, CHADS$_2$ and CHA$_2$DS$_2$-VASc have been validated in several relatively small studies, but it is still not entirely clear how well they correlate with events in the "real world". Medical doctors at *Copenhagen University Hospital* have investigated the correlation between stroke risk as predicted by the two schemes and the actual incidence of thromboembolism (ischemic stroke, pulmonary embolism, and peripheral artery embolism). The annual incidence of thromboembolism was calculated 1, 5 and 10 years after discharge from hospital in a group of 73,538 patients with non-valvular atrial fibrillation. The majority (60%) of patients were 75 years of age or older, 34% had high blood pressure (hypertension), 51% were female, 18% had suffered a previous stroke, and 43% had been prescribed digoxin. None of the patients had been prescribed warfarin at discharge.

At year 5 of follow-up, the actual incidence of thromboembolism corresponding to the risk scores was as shown below. Please note that the risk scores are not directly comparable. As an example, a 70 year-old woman with diabetes and hypertension would have a risk score of 2 according to the CHADS$_2$ scheme, but a risk score of 4 according to the CHA$_2$DS$_2$-VASc scheme. Thus for this women the annual risk of thromboembolism would be 5.58% if evaluated with the CHADS$_2$ scheme and 6.69% if evaluated with the CHA$_2$DS$_2$-VASc scheme.

Similarly, for a 70 year-old man with hypertension the CHADS$_2$ risk score would be 1 while the CHA$_2$DS$_2$-VASc score would be 2. Corresponding annual risk of thromboembolism would be 3.7% and 3.01%.

Comparison of Thromboembolism Risk Estimates

CHADS$_2$ Score	Incidence %/year	CHA$_2$DS$_2$-VASc Score	Incidence %/year
0	1.28	0	0.69
1	3.70	1	1.51
2	5.58	2	3.01
3	10.29	3	4.41
4	14.00	4	6.69
5	12.98	5	10.42

It is clear that the stroke risk in afibbers with a score of 0, that is, no accompanying risk factors, is low according to both schemes. However, as stroke risk factors are added, incidence increases significantly. In the CHADS$_2$ score, having experienced a previous thromboembolic event was the most significant risk factor, followed by a combination of diabetes and heart failure, and age 75 years or older. In the CHA$_2$DS$_2$-VASc score, a previous thromboembolism was also the most significant risk factor, followed by age of 75 years or older, and a combination of diabetes and heart failure.

The researchers conclude that male afibbers with a CHA$_2$DS$_2$-VASc score of 0 and female afibbers with a score of 1 are truly at very low risk and do not require nor benefit from antithrombotic therapy. [1]

This study lends credence to my long-held belief that atrial fibrillation, in itself, is a minor component in overall stroke risk. For example, the risk of experiencing a stroke more than doubles each decade after the age of 55, irrespective of whether AF is also present. Hypertension alone doubles stroke risk, and diabetes is associated with a 2- to 5-fold increase in stroke risk. Furthermore, it should also be kept in mind that only about 15% of all ischemic strokes are cardioembolic – those caused by a clot originating in the left atrium or atrial appendage.

Finally, while the CHADS$_2$ and the CHA$_2$DS$_2$-VASc scores were developed to predict the risk of ischemic stroke only, the Danish researchers used them to predict not only the estimated risk of ischemic stroke, but also the risk of pulmonary embolism and peripheral artery embolism, thus increasing the incidence of events associated with a specific risk score beyond what would have been observed if only ischemic stroke had been considered.

Stroke risk and afib episode duration
There is evidence that the risk of stroke among atrial fibrillation patients with underlying heart disease increases with the duration of episodes. A team of

cardiologists at *S. Anna Hospital* in Como, Italy have combined $CHADS_2$ score and episode duration into a new scheme aimed at further improving stroke risk prediction.

Their one-year study included 568 AF patients (aged between 60 and 80 years with 49% being male) who had had a pacemaker (Medtronic AT500) implanted to deal with sinus node disease (bradycardia/tachycardia syndrome). About half the patients had hypertension, a third were over the age of 75 years, 8% had diabetes, 1.5% had congestive heart failure, and 1.4% had suffered a previous stroke or TIA. Nineteen percent were taking a daily aspirin for stroke prevention, while 25% were on warfarin. Thus, just over half the group did not receive anti-platelet therapy (aspirin) or anticoagulation (warfarin). Beta-blockers were prescribed for 10% of patients and antiarrhythmics for 46%.

Study participants who had been afib-free or experienced no more than one episode (lasting less than 5 minutes) over the one-year monitoring period were considered afib-free (group A). Patients with one episode lasting more than 5 minutes, but less than 24 hours were stratified as group B, while those with one or more episodes lasting more than 24 hours were classified as group C. (NOTE: This group would presumably include permanent afibbers).

The overall annual incidence of stroke in the group with a $CHADS_2$ score of 0 was 0%, although 1.1% did suffer a TIA. The annual incidence of stroke in the groups with $CHADS_2$ scores of 1, 2, and 3 or greater was 0.7%, 2.7%, and 18% respectively. Considering afib status, the annual stroke rate was 1.2% in the afib-free (group A), 0% in group B, but a rather high 2.6% in group C. By combining $CHADS_2$ score and afib duration, the researchers uncovered two distinctly different "populations". The first consisted of afib-free individuals (group A) with a $CHADS_2$ score of 2 or less, group B members with a $CHADS_2$ score of 1 or less, and group C members with a $CHADS_2$ score of 0. In this group the average annual stroke risk was 0.8% - actually somewhat lower than what is considered normal for an age-matched population. Study participants not meeting the above criteria had an average annual stroke risk of 5%.

As a separate part of the study, the Italian group simulated the results of 24-hour, 7-day, and 30-day Holter monitoring and found that this type of monitoring, in general, only picks up about 50% of the afib events actually occurring. The researchers conclude that using both $CHADS_2$ score and afib duration to determine the need for anticoagulation would result in a much better management of stroke prevention. [2]

This study confirms that afibbers with no risk factors for stroke have a very low risk of ischemic stroke, irrespective of the duration of their episodes. As a matter of fact, this particular study found an annual stroke risk of 0% among participants with a $CHADS_2$ score of 0. Even those with a $CHADS_2$ score of 1, only had an average annual stroke risk of 0.7%.

Stroke-associated mortality

Statisticians at *Technical University of Denmark* have completed a major study to determine the risk factors, severity and incidence of ischemic and hemorrhagic stroke in Denmark. Their study involved almost 40,000 patients who had suffered a stroke in the period from March 2001 to February 2007. Of these patients 25,123 had complete data including CT or MRI scans, admission stroke severity as measured by the Scandinavian Stroke Scale (SSS), risk factors, and ultimate outcome (survival or death). The highlights of the study are:

- Ten percent of the strokes recorded were hemorrhagic and these tended to be considerably more severe than the ischemic strokes.
- The risk of dying from a hemorrhagic stroke was 13% during the first 7 days, 20% during the 30 days following the stroke, and 25% during the 90 days following. Corresponding mortality rates for ischemic strokes were 1.8%, 4.8%, and 11%. All told, 49% of hemorrhagic stroke victims died during the follow-up as compared to 26% in the ischemic stroke group.
- The major risk factors favoring ischemic stroke over hemorrhagic stroke were intermittent arterial claudication, a previous stroke or heart attack, diabetes, and atrial fibrillation.
- The major risk factors favoring hemorrhagic stroke were smoking and heavy alcohol consumption.
- There was no difference in gender, age and prevalence of hypertension between patients with ischemic stroke and those with hemorrhagic stroke.

The researchers conclude that hemorrhagic strokes are generally more severe and have a poorer outcome than do ischemic strokes. [3]

It is unfortunate that the Danish statisticians did not include an evaluation of the relative risk of ischemic versus hemorrhagic stroke in patients taking warfarin or aspirin. Both drugs are acknowledged as important risk factors for hemorrhagic stroke. Nevertheless, it is of considerable interest to establish that the risk factors favoring one type of stroke over the other are different. In considering the above results, it should be kept in mind that atrial fibrillation on its own is not a risk factor for ischemic stroke. It only becomes so when accompanied by other risk factors such as hypertension or heart disease.

Predicting risk of cardioembolic stroke

About 50% of strokes occurring in atrial fibrillation (AF) patients are cardioembolic in nature and usually related to thrombus (blood clot) formation in the left atrial appendage (LAA). Such strokes are best prevented by anticoagulation with warfarin. The other 50% of strokes are either thrombotic (most often involving rupture of atherosclerotic plaque) or hemorrhagic in nature. The optimum way of preventing thrombotic stroke is through the use of antiplatelet agents such as aspirin or clopidogrel. Thus, it is important to know if a patient is at increased risk of cardioembolic stroke and thus may need warfarin, or has no increased risk in which antiplatelet therapy may be a better choice.

The presence of thrombi in the LAA can be established with reasonable accuracy by doing a transesophageal echocardiography (TEE) in which the ultrasound probe is placed in the esophagus rather than on the chest as is the case in standard transthoracic echocardiography. TEE will show the presence of existing thrombi and will also detect spontaneous echocardiographic contrast (SEC) – a pattern of "smoke-like", slow-swirling, echo densities in the LAA or left atrium. SEC is believed to be the genesis of thrombi.

Electrophysiologists at the *Mayo Clinic* have developed a scoring system which would predict the likelihood of finding thrombi in the LAA. Their study involved 110 patients with nonvalvular AF (not on warfarin) in whom thrombi had been detected in the LAA (cases) and 387 patients with nonvalvular AF (not on warfarin) in whom no thrombi had been detected during TEE (controls). Statistically significant differences between the two groups included the following:

Conditions	Cases	Controls
Permanent AF	43%	11%
AF duration >1 year	55%	11%
Congestive heart failure	64%	21%
Diabetes	31%	16%
Prior TIA/Stroke	39%	13%
Presence of SEC	92%	41%

The average CHADS$_2$ score was also significantly higher among cases (mean = 2.8) than among controls (mean = 1.6). The incidence of LAA thrombi was not related to age, gender or the presence of hypertension. Thus, while age above 75 years is considered a risk factor in the CHADS$_2$ score, there was no indication that advanced age is associated with an increased risk of LAA thrombi. Based on their findings, the Mayo researchers propose a new algorithm for predicting the presence of LAA thrombi and resulting risk of cardioembolic stroke or TIA.

A prior stroke or TIA, permanent AF, diabetes, and AF duration longer than 48 hours would each be allocated 1 point, while the presence of SEC, congestive heart failure, and AF duration longer than one year would be allocated 2 points each. Therefore, LAA thrombi risk would be graded from 0 to 10 by this new system which has yet to receive a catchy acronym. A separate analysis showed the presence of SEC and congestive heart failure to be, by far, the most predictive of LAA thrombi (odds ratios of 9.68 and 5.12 respectively). The Mayo researchers point out that prior research has shown that if TEE detects no thrombi in the LAA the risk of a cardioembolic stroke is pretty close to zero. [4]

Increased stroke risk for older women

Researchers at *McGill University Health Center* in Montreal, Canada have found that older women with recently diagnosed AF have a significantly higher risk of stroke than do recently diagnosed older men. Their study included 39,398 men and 44,115 women admitted to hospital with AF as a primary diagnosis (24%) or with coronary artery disease, valvular heart disease, heart attack, chronic kidney disease, or high cholesterol as the primary diagnosis and AF as the secondary diagnosis (76%). The average age of the male study participants was 77 years and that of the female participants was 80 years. The average $CHADS_2$ score for men was 1.7 vs 2.0 for women. The percentage of women and men diagnosed with the individual components of the $CHADS_2$ score were:

Component	Women	Men
Congestive heart failure	27.8%	28.9%
Hypertension	63.9%	51.3%
Age 75 years or older	74.2%	61.4%
Diabetes	22.1%	24.6%
History of stroke or TIA	8.0%	6.9%

Warfarin was prescribed at discharge from hospital for 60.6% of women and 58.2% of men. The study participants were followed for 1 year during which a total of 2570 strokes (2.02%/year) occurred among the women and 1696 (1.61%/year) occurred among the men. NOTE: Stroke was defined as ischemic stroke (cerebral thrombosis), embolism, artery occlusion, transient ischemic stroke, or retinal infarction. The rates of hemorrhagic stroke (intracerebral hemorrhage) were 1.42% among men and 1.33% among women.

Stroke risk was found to increase significantly with age, rising from 1.05%/year among women aged 65 to 69 years (corresponding figure for men was 1.17%/year) to 2.38%/year for women aged 75 years or older (corresponding figure for men was 1.95%/year). Not surprisingly, stroke risk also increased significantly with increasing $CHADS_2$ score from 1.03%/year for women with a score of 0 (corresponding number for men was 0.86%/year) to 4.91%/year for women with a score of 5 (corresponding number for men was 4.88%/year). NOTE: Only 0.17% of the total patient population had a $CHADS_2$ score of 5 or higher, so it would seem to be gross exaggeration to claim that all AF patients have a 5-fold increased risk of stroke.

As shown below, it is clear that women aged 75 years or older have a higher risk of stroke than do age-matched men, and that this excess risk is reduced by the use of warfarin.

Stroke Incidence - Below age of 75 years

	No Warfarin	Warfarin
Women	1.47%/year	1.10%/year
Men	1.48%/year	1.04%/year

Stroke Incidence - At or above 75 years

	No Warfarin	Warfarin
Women	2.91%/year	2.05%/year
Men	2.20%/year	1.78%/year

The authors conclude that the risk of stroke among older women with recently diagnosed AF is greater than that of age-matched men irrespective of whether warfarin therapy is implemented. [5]

It is unfortunate that the authors of the Montreal report did not provide details of the distribution of hemorrhagic strokes other than to say that most of them occurred in patients on warfarin. However, based on results from similar studies, it is likely that about two-thirds of hemorrhagic strokes occurred in the warfarin group. Thus, the incidence of hemorrhagic stroke would be 0.44%/year in women not on warfarin and 0.89%/year for women on warfarin. The corresponding numbers for men would be 0.47%/year and 0.95%/year.

It is now well established that the benefits of warfarin are, often to a considerable extent, reduced by its inherent propensity to cause intracranial bleeding (hemorrhagic stroke). A recent study has used the concept of Net Clinical Benefit (NCB) to determine the real, overall benefit of warfarin therapy. NCB considers both the benefit (reduction in ischemic stroke) and harm (increase in hemorrhagic stroke) in administering the drug. NCB is defined as: [6]

NCB = (TE rate off warfarin – TE rate on warfarin) – W x (ICH rate on warfarin – ICH rate off warfarin)

TE rate is the annualized rate of thromboembolic events (ischemic stroke and systemic emboli).
W is a weighting factor designed to reflect the fact that the consequences of a hemorrhagic stroke (intracranial bleeding) are far more serious than that of an ischemic stroke. W is usually assumed to be 1.5.
ICH rate is the annualized rate of intracranial bleeding (incl. hemorrhagic stroke).

Using the above formula, and assuming that hemorrhagic stroke incidence is independent of age, the following NCBs can be calculated.

NCB of Warfarin Therapy

	Below age of 75 years	Age 75 years or older
Women	-0.31%/year	+0.18%/year
Men	-0.24%/year	-0.26%/year

The above calculation shows that the average NCB of warfarin therapy in recently diagnosed female afibbers, at or above the age of 75 years, is indeed slightly beneficial at 0.18%/year. It would appear to be detrimental for men at all ages, and for women below the age of 75 years. Of course, these numbers are average and whether or not warfarin therapy would be beneficial for an individual afibber would clearly depend on his or her age and CHADS$_2$ score. Thus, warfarin therapy would likely be beneficial for an older woman (age 75 years or older) with a CHADS$_2$ score of 3 or higher, but would almost certainly be detrimental for women with a CHADS$_2$ score below 3 unless the reason for their CHADS$_2$ score of 2 was a history of stroke or TIA. The same cut-off points would apply to men.

The ATRIA scheme for stroke risk prediction

The commonly used schemes for estimating stroke risk in atrial fibrillation patients have only moderate ability to predict which patients will actually suffer an ischemic stroke. AF specialists at *Massachusetts General Hospital, University of California San Francisco, Stanford University School of Medicine,* and *Kaiser Permanente of Northern California* have developed a new scheme (ATRIA) which is superior in its ability to predict stroke risk, particularly for patients in the low and high risk categories.

The scheme is based on data collected in the Anticoagulation and Risk Factors in Atrial Fibrillation (ATRIA) study involving 10,927 atrial fibrillation patients not on warfarin. The patients were adult members of Kaiser Permanente Northern California who had an outpatient diagnosis of AF between July 1, 1996 and December 31, 1997. Study participants were followed through December 2003 during which time 685 thromboembolic events (TEs) were recorded for an annualized rate of 2.1%. The majority (643) of events were verified ischemic strokes and the remaining 42 events were other TEs (sudden occlusion of an artery to a visceral organ or extremity). Based on the collected data the researchers developed the ATRIA Stroke Risk Scoring System.

ATRIA Stroke Risk Scoring System

Risk Factor	Points without prior stroke	Points with prior stroke
Age less than 65	0	8
Age 65 to 74	3	7
Age 75 to 84	5	7
Age 85 or older	6	9

ATRIA Stroke Risk Scoring System [continued]

Risk Factor	Points without prior stroke	Points with prior stroke
Female gender	1	1
Diabetes	1	1
CHF (1)	1	1
Hypertension	1	1
Proteinuria (2)	1	1
eGFR <45 or ESRD (3)	1	1

(1) CHF = Congestive heart failure
(2) Proteinuria (urine dipstick)
(3) eGFR <45 ml/min/per 1.73 m² or end stage kidney disease requiring dialysis

It is interesting that the ATRIA scheme, in contrast to CHA_2DS_2-VASc scheme, did not find the presence of coronary disease to be a significant risk factor.

ATRIA Point Score vs. Annual Stroke Risk

Points	Stroke Risk %	Points	Stroke Risk %
0	0.08	7	2.50
1	0.43	8	3.86
2	0.99	9	4.33
3	0.73	10	6.35
4	0.64	11	6.18
5	0.99	12	10.95
6	1.91	13	7.52

The score was collapsed into low (0 to 5 points), moderate (6 points), and high (7-15 points) risk to fit annualized event rates (stroke risk) of 1%, 1% to <2%, and TEs equal to or greater than 2%. The ATRIA score categorized 47% of study participants as low risk, 13% as moderate risk and 40% as high risk. In contrast, the CHADS2 score categorized 50% as low risk, 45% as moderate risk, and only 5% as high risk while the CHA_2DS_2-VASc score placed 81% in the high risk category. The ATRIA scheme was validated in a separate study of 25,306 patients who were off warfarin for a year. The overall TE rate in this group was 1.9%.

The authors of the report conclude that the ability of the ATRIA score to accurately predict stroke risk is superior to that of the CHADS2 and CHA_2DS_2-VASc scores. The ATRIA score also identified a substantially larger fraction of patients at low risk and was particularly accurate in predicting severe strokes. [7]

It is to be hoped that the ATRIA scheme becomes the standard stroke risk prediction scheme as it is more accurate than currently used schemes and vastly reduces the number of patients that are prescribed anticoagulants as compared to the CHA₂DS₂-VASc scheme which would require 81% of afib patients to be on anticoagulants.

Anticoagulation detrimental in low-risk patients

Most guidelines for the management of atrial fibrillation suggest that patients with a CHADS₂ score of zero do not need anticoagulation. However, ESC (European Society of Cardiology) guidelines prefer anticoagulation with a CHA₂DS₂-VASc score of 1 which would include 65- to 74-year-olds with a CHADS₂ score of zero.

Cardiologists at *Washington University* and *New York University School of Medicine* now provide convincing evidence that anticoagulating 65- to 74-year-olds with a CHADS₂ score of zero is detrimental. Their study involved 478 atrial fibrillation patients (age between 65 and 74 years) who had a CHADS₂ score of zero and an average CHA₂DS₂-VASc score of 1.95. The group was followed for 10 months during which time the stroke rate (ischemic and hemorrhagic) was 2.6%/year for patients on warfarin and 2.9% for non-anticoagulated patients (control group). The annual rate of ischemic stroke was 1.7% and that of hemorrhagic stroke 0.6% in the warfarin group vs. 2.9% and 0% in the control group resulting in a net clinical benefit of 0.3%/year. However, the rate of major bleeding (extracranial hemorrhage) was significantly higher in the warfarin group (21.1%/year) then in the control group (7.4%/year) with gastrointestinal bleeding being the most common type of hemorrhage.

The cardiologists point out that 333 patients would have to be treated with warfarin to avoid one stroke. However, anticoagulating 333 patients would be expected to cause 44 extracranial hemorrhages of which 3 would be fatal. The authors conclude that *"By expanding warfarin use to 65-to 74-year-olds with a CHADS₂ score of zero, rates of hemorrhages would rise without a significant reduction in stroke equivalents."* [8]

The conclusion from this study must surely be that a CHADS₂ score of zero is truly low risk and that being in the age group 65-74 years does not increase that risk.

Improved stroke risk score needed for atrial fibrillation

The CHADS₂ and CHA₂DS₂-VASc schemes for estimating the risk of ischemic stroke were originally developed for atrial fibrillation patients and were only validated in populations of afib patients. Since then these schemes have been evaluated in several populations with heart-related problems excluding atrial fibrillation and have been found to have good predictive capability. [9]

This leads one to the conclusion that the CHADS$_2$ and CHA$_2$DS$_2$-VASc schemes are not specific to atrial fibrillation and may not be that indicative of stroke risk associated with cardioembolic stroke.

A group of medical doctors at *Brown University* and *Cornell Medical College* believes that an improved risk scheme is required and have developed a list of risk factors specific to afib-related strokes and provided an estimate of the hazard ratio of these factors. It is clear that the shape (morphology) of the left atrial appendage (LAA) and the flow velocity of blood entering and leaving the LAA are critical factors in predicting stroke risk. NOTE: A hazard ratio of 2.0 means that stroke risk is doubled.

Risk Factor	Hazard Ratio
High level of cardiac troponin	2.0
High level of NT-pro BNP	2.4
High level of inflammatory cytokine IL-6	2.0
Left atrial diameter >45 mm	1.7
LAA flow velocity <20 cm/s	2.6
Unfavourable morphology of LAA (Windsock)	4.5

The authors urge clinical trials to determine whether therapeutic strategies based on afib-specific risk markers can improve stroke prevention compared to the current approach of tailoring therapy based on clinical risk scores applicable to the general population. [10]

Value of stroke risk scores in anticoagulated patients

Medical doctors at *University of Bologna* and *Azienda Ospedaliero-Universitaria Careggi* in Florence report the results of a study aimed at determining the value of stroke risk classification schemes in predicting stroke risk in already anticoagulated AF patients. Their study included 662 AF patients (64% male) with an average age of 74 years. The study participants had several stroke risk factors such as hypertension (64%), previous stroke/TIA (31%), and coronary artery disease or heart failure (45%).

During the follow-up period of 3.6 years, a total of 32 thromboembolic events occurred corresponding to an annual incidence rate of 1.3%. Neither the CHADS$_2$ nor CHA$_2$DS$_2$-VASc scores were particularly effective in predicting stroke risk since the only risk factor that actually did confer an increased risk of stroke (5.6-fold) was a previous history of stroke, TIA or other systemic embolism. Age, hypertension, diabetes, heart failure, female gender, and low left ventricular ejection fraction did not increase the risk of stroke in this elderly, anticoagulated group of AF patients. The authors conclude that current stroke risk scores have modest ability to predict stroke risk in anticoagulated patients. [11, 12]

First off, it should be kept in mind that cardioembolic strokes constitute only about 15% of all strokes, so protecting against this form of stroke by no means guarantees that one will not suffer an ischemic or hemorrhagic stroke. It would seem that warfarin therapy is not adequate to protect afibbers with a history of TIA, stroke or other embolic events against a repeat of these. On the other hand, having diabetes, heart failure, hypertension, or being over the age of 75 years do not increase stroke/TIA risk in anticoagulated AF patients.

BLEEDING RISK

Anticoagulation with drugs such as warfarin (Coumadin) and dabigatran (Pradaxa) and antiplatelet therapy with aspirin or clopidogrel treads a fine line between benefit and risk. While anticoagulation and, to a much lesser extent, antiplatelet therapy can reduce the risk of ischemic stroke in atrial fibrillation (AF) patients with coexisting risk factors, these therapies also significantly increase the risk of hemorrhagic stroke and major internal bleeding. While there now are two commonly used schemes (CHADS$_2$ and CHA$_2$DS$_2$-VASc) for predicting stroke risk, there is no universally accepted scheme for predicting risk of major bleeding.

A team of researchers from the *University of Maastricht* and the *University of Birmingham* has now developed a simple, quite accurate bleeding risk score called HAS-BLED where the letter in the acronym and their assigned risk scores are as follows:

H = Hypertension - 1 point
A = Abnormal kidney and liver function - 1 point each
S = Stroke (previous ischemic) - 1 point
B = Bleeding (previous event/events) - 1 point
L = Labile INRs (difficulty maintaining stable INR) - 1 point
E = Elderly - 1 point
D = Drug or alcohol use - 1 point each

The research team applied the HAS-BLED risk score to a group of 3,456 patients with AF without structural heart disease (non-valvular AF). The average age of the group was 67 years and 39% were women. At discharge from hospital, 52% of patients were prescribed an anticoagulant (most likely warfarin), 12.8% were prescribed anticoagulant + aspirin and/or clopidogrel, 24% received antiplatelet therapy (aspirin or clopidogrel) on its own, and the remaining 10.2% received no antithrombotic therapy. The most common reason for prescribing therapy was age over 65 years, although the researchers point out that the biological age of an elderly patient is probably more relevant to bleeding risk than is the chronological age.

During a 1-year follow-up, 52 patients (1.56%) experienced a major bleeding event (requiring hospitalization and/or blood transfusion). The annual risk (%/year) of a bleeding event increased with increasing HAS-BLED score as shown below.

HAS-BLED Score vs. BLEEDING INCIDENCE

HAS-BLED Score	Bleeds/patient-year, %
0	1.13
1	1.02
2	1.88
3	3.74
4	8.70
5	12.50

The overall annual bleeding rate was highest for patients treated with anticoagulants (1.75%/year) followed by those receiving no antithrombotic treatment (1.42%/year), and those on antiplatelet therapy alone (0.97%/year). Anticoagulation and antiplatelet therapy is not recommended for afibbers with a $CHADS_2$ score of zero and thus the HAS-BLED score is not really relevant here. However, in the case of a $CHADS_2$ score of 1, the researchers suggest that the HAS-BLED score must exceed 2 in order for the risk of anticoagulation to offset its benefits. For a $CHADS_2$ score of 2 or higher, they suggest that the risk of bleeding outweighs the potential benefits of anticoagulation if the HAS-BLED score exceeds the $CHADS_2$ score. The researchers acknowledge the limitation of not including INR variation in their evaluation. [13]

Anticoagulation and antiplatelet therapy are double-edged swords, in that benefits and risks must be carefully weighed for the individual patient before being prescribed. Until now, only schemes dealing with stroke risk have been employed with no or little attention paid to bleeding risk. Hopefully, this will change with the widespread use of the HAS-BLED scheme.

A team of researchers from *England, Sweden and the United States* reports their evaluation of the validity of the scheme in a group of 7,329 AF patients at moderate to high risk of stroke who were anticoagulated with warfarin (3,665 patients) or ximelagatran (no longer available). They compared the HAS-BLED scheme to four other less well known schemes and found HAS-BLED to be superior.

In looking at the actual risk factors in the overall group (warfarin and ximelagatran), they found (in multivariate analysis) that the following factors were independent predictors of an increased risk of bleeding when being anticoagulated.

- Concomitant aspirin use – increased bleeding risk by 92%
- Kidney dysfunction – increased bleeding risk by 90%
- Age 75 years or greater – increased bleeding risk by 71%
- Diabetes – increased bleeding risk by 36%
- Left ventricular dysfunction – increased bleeding risk by 31%.

Applying the HAS-BLED scoring system to the whole patient group resulted in the following annual risk (%/year) of suffering a major bleed when on warfarin or ximelagatran.

HAS-BLED Score	Entire Group, %/year	Warfarin Only, %/year
0	1.2	0.9
1	2.8	3.4
2	3.6	4.1
3	6.0	5.8
4	9.5	8.9
5	7.4	9.1

The most important risk factors for bleeding events as predicted by HAS-BLED were:

- Labile (varying) INR – increased risk by 105% (106%)
- Use of aspirin or NSAIDs – increased risk by 85% (96%)
- Kidney dysfunction – increased risk by 77% (NS)
- Age above 75 years at entry increased risk by 76% (82%)

NOTE: Numbers in brackets indicate risk increases for warfarin group only.

The authors conclude that the HAS-BLED scheme may provide a useful assessment of bleeding risk in AF patients in everyday clinical practice. [14, 15]

Inadequate control of INR is clearly the most important factor in estimating the risk of bleeding when anticoagulated. Concomitant use of aspirin, kidney dysfunction, and age of 75 years or older are also important factors, although the authors emphasize that, "bleeding in elderly patients with AF is more related to biological age rather than chronological age." It would also seem that it may be wise to add diabetes and left ventricular dysfunction to the factors that can increase bleeding risk. Finally, the huge importance of adequate INR control may make the use of an INR home testing kit a worthwhile investment for afibbers on warfarin.

The ATRIA scheme for predicting bleeding risk

Medical doctors at *Massachusetts General Hospital, University of California San Francisco, Stanford University School of Medicine*, and *Kaiser Permanente of Northern California* have developed a scheme (ATRIA) to predict the risk of serious bleeding in patients anticoagulated with warfarin.

The scheme is based on data collected in the Anticoagulation and Risk Factors in Atrial Fibrillation (ATRIA) study involving 9186 atrial fibrillation patients anticoagulated with warfarin. The patients were adult members of Kaiser Permanente Northern California who had an outpatient diagnosis of AF between July 1, 1996 and December 31, 1997. Study participants were followed through December 2003 during which time 461 validated major hemorrhages (intracranial and extracranial) occurred corresponding to an annual incidence rate of 1.4%. Based on the collected data the researchers developed the ATRIA Bleeding Risk Model Point Scoring System shown below:

ATRIA Bleeding Risk Scoring System

Risk Factor	Points
Hypertension	1
Prior hemorrhage diagnosis	1
Age 75 years or older	2
Anemia	3
Severe renal disease	3

Severe renal disease defined as eGFR<30 mL/min or dialysis-dependent.

The annual rate of serious bleeding (hemorrhage) for the various risk categories expressed as %/year were as follows:

ATRIA Point Score vs. Annual Bleeding Risk

Points	Bleeding Risk %	Points	Bleeding Risk %
0	0.40	5	5.65
1	0.55	6	4.95
2	0.97	7	5.17
3	1.01	8	9.61
4	2.62	9	12.43

The score was collapsed into low (0 to 3 points), intermediate (4 points), and high (5-10 points) risk to fit average annualized event rates (bleeding risk) of 0.8%, 2.6%, and 5.8%. Overall, 83% of study participants fell in the low risk category while only 10% fell in the high risk category. However, 43% of major hemorrhages occurred in the high risk group. [16]

It is unfortunate that the authors of the study do not provide any guidance as to the level of bleeding risk at which warfarin therapy becomes counterproductive.

REFERENCES

1. Olesen, JB, et al. Validation of risk stratification schemes for predicting stroke and thromboembolism in patients with atrial fibrillation: nationwide cohort study. British Medical Journal, Vol. 342, January 28, 2011
2. Botto, GL, et al. Presence and duration of atrial fibrillation detected by continuous monitoring: crucial implications for the risk of thromboembolic

events. Journal of Cardiovascular Electrophysiology, Vol. 20, March 2009, pp. 241-48

3. Andersen, KK, et al. Hemorrhagic and ischemic strokes compared: stroke severity, mortality, and risk factors. Stroke, Vol. 40, June 2009, pp. 2068-72

4. Wysokinski, WE, et al. Predicting left atrial thrombi in atrial fibrillation. American Heart Journal, Vol. 159, April 2010, pp. 665-71

5. Avgil Tsadok, M, et al. Sex differences in stroke risk among older patients with recently diagnosed atrial fibrillation. Journal of the American Medical Association, Vol. 307, No. 18, May 9, 2012, pp. 1952-58

6. Singer, DE, et al. The net clinical benefit of warfarin anticoagulation in atrial fibrillation. Annals of Internal Medicine, Vol. 151, September 1, 2009, pp. 297-305, pp. 355-56

7. Singer, DE, et al. A new risk scheme to predict ischemic stroke and other thromboembolism in atrial fibrillation: the ATRIA study stroke risk score. Journal of American Heart Association, June 21, 2013

8. Andrade, AA, et al. Clinical Benefit of American College of Chest Physicians versus European Society of Cardiology Guidelines for Stroke Prophylaxis in Atrial Fibrillation. Journal of General Internal Medicine, Vol. 30, No. 6, June 2015, pp. 77-82

9. Mitchell, LB, et al. Prediction of stroke or TIA in patients without atrial fibrillation using CHADS2 and CHA2DS2-VASc scores. Heart, Vol. 100 , No. 19, October 2014, pp. 1525-30

10. Yaghi, S and Kamel, H. Stratifying stroke risk in atrial fibrillation. Stroke, Vol. 48, No. 10, October 2017, pp. 2665-2670

11. Poli, D, et al. Stroke risk stratification in a "real-world" elderly anticoagulated atrial fibrillation population. Journal of Cardiovascular Electrophysiology, Vol. 22, January 2011, pp. 25-30

12. Boriani, G, et al. The challenge of preventing stroke in elderly patients with atrial fibrillation. Journal of Cardiovascular Electrophysiology, Vol. 22, January 2011, pp. 31-33

13. Pisters, R, et al. A novel user-friendly score (HAS-BLED) to assess 1-year risk of major bleeding in patients with atrial fibrillation. Chest, Vol. 138, No. 5, November 2010, pp. 1093-1100

14. Lip, GYH, et al. Comparative validation of a novel risk score for predicting bleeding risk in anticoagulated patients with atrial fibrillation. Journal of the American College of Cardiology, Vol. 57, No. 2, January 11, 2011, pp. 173-80

15. Hohnloser, SH. Stroke prevention versus bleeding risk at atrial fibrillation. Journal of the American College of Cardiology, Vol. 57, No. 2, January 11, 2011, pp. 181-83

16. Fang, MC, et al. A new risk scheme to predict warfarin-associated hemorrhage: The ATRIA (Anticoagulation and Risk Factors in Atrial Fibrillation) Study. Journal of the American College of Cardiology, Vol. 58, No. 4, July 19, 2011, pp. 395-401.

Chapter 11

Alternative Approaches To Stroke Prevention

Most ischemic strokes are thrombotic and involve the formation of atherosclerotic plaque and subsequent narrowing and clot (thrombus) formation at the point of obstruction. Afibbers with common stroke risk factors such as hypertension or atherosclerosis are at risk for such strokes, but are particularly at risk for cardioembolic stroke caused by the formation of a blood clot in the heart (usually in the left atrial appendage) and its subsequent migration to the brain.

The mechanism involved in a thrombotic stroke is different from the mechanism involved in a cardioembolic stroke so it follows that natural approaches to their prevention are different. Most natural stroke prevention protocols with the exception of vitamin C, vitamin B6, and nattokinase are aimed only, or at least primarily, at preventing thrombotic strokes.

VITAMINS B AND C

An elevated blood level of homocysteine, a sulfur-containing amino acid, is strongly associated with an increased risk of thrombotic stroke. A "cocktail" of **vitamins B6**, **vitamin B12**, and **folic acid** has been found to effectively lower homocysteine levels and thus reduce stroke risk. The vitamin "cocktail" also imparts its stroke preventing effect by reducing endothelial dysfunction, inflammation, and platelet aggregation and by inhibiting the conversion of prothrombin to thrombin.

Vitamin B6, or rather its metabolite pyridoxal-5-phosphate, is also effective on its own in lowering homocysteine levels and reducing endothelial dysfunction, inflammation, and platelet aggregation . There is also evidence that it is effective in preventing deep vein thrombosis. It is highly likely that the mechanism (blood coagulation or inadequate fibrinolysis) involved in deep vein thrombosis is very similar to the mechanism involved in thrombus formation in the left atrial appendage. Thus, if vitamin B6 is protective against deep vein thrombosis, it may also be protective against thrombosis and stroke in atrial fibrillation.

Vitamin C is a powerful, water-soluble antioxidant and as such helps to prevent oxidative stress, a major underlying cause of thrombosis and reperfusion injury. Vitamin C also helps prevent stroke by reducing endothelial dysfunction, reducing the levels of von Willebrand factor and plasminogen activation inhibitor 1 (PAI-1), and by inhibiting blood coagulation by reducing the level of intrinsic pathway factors VIII, IX, XI, and XII.

Low intakes of B-vitamins and vitamin C and stroke risk

Researchers in South Korea report that a high intake of fruits, vegetables, vitamin C and folate is associated with a reduced risk of ischemic stroke. Their study included 60 patients who had suffered an ischemic stroke and 60 age and sex-matched controls. Stroke patients had higher waist hip ratios, lower HDL cholesterol, higher fasting blood glucose, and greater prevalence of hypertension and diabetes. They were also substantially less likely to engage in regular exercise – only 23% of stroke patients had done so before their stroke, compared to 88% of controls. While 95% of controls reported that they ate regular meals only 60% of stroke victims did. Stroke patients were also significantly more likely to dine out 3-4 times/week than were controls.

The daily intake of fruits and vegetables, vitamin C, vitamin E, vitamin B6, and folate were significantly lower in stroke patients than in controls. [1]

Average Dietary Intake in Stroke Patients and Controls

Diet Component	Controls	Stroke Patients
Fruits	230 g/day	73 g/day
Vegetables	562 g/day	221 g/day
Vitamin C	191 mg/day	118 mg/day
Vitamin E	25.6 mg/day	19.1 mg/day
Vitamin B6	2.4 mg/day	1.8 mg/day
Folate	809 micrograms/day	595 micrograms/day

Supplementation with B vitamins reduces stroke risk

A team of medical researchers from *University of Toronto and McMaster University* reports that supplementation with folic acid, vitamin B6, and vitamin B12 reduces the risk of stroke. Their clinical trial involved 5522 men and women most of whom had coronary artery disease (83%), hypertension (56%) and/or diabetes (40%). The mean age of the participants was 69 years, 72% were men and 72% were living in North America. Participants were randomized to receive placebo or 2.5 mg/day of folic acid, 50 mg/day of vitamin B6 and 1 mg/day of vitamin B12 for 5 years.

During the trial period the incidence of stroke was 0.88%/year in the supplement group and 1.15%/year in the placebo group corresponding to a relative risk reduction of 25%. The relative risk reduction increased to 29% when adjusting for the use of medications known to be protective against ischemic stroke. It is also of interest to note that the average level of homocysteine dropped by 2.2 micromol/L to an average of 9.3 micromol/L in the supplement group while in the placebo group it increased by 0.80 micromol/L to 13.3 micromol/L or a relative decrease of 24% associated with vitamin B supplementation. The decrease in homocysteine level was particularly noteworthy among participants having a high level at entry to the study. [2]

Vitamin C protects against stroke

Researchers at *Cambridge University* have confirmed that high blood levels of vitamin C (ascorbic acid) protect against stroke. Their study involved 20,649 men and women between the ages of 40 and 79 years when enrolled during the period 1993-1997. None of the participants had suffered a prior stroke. Blood samples were drawn and analyzed for ascorbic acid content at baseline and participants were then followed for an average of 10 years. During this time a total of 448 strokes occurred corresponding to an average annual stroke rate of 0.2%.

After adjusting for the possible effects of gender, age, smoking, BMI, blood pressure, cholesterol, physical activity, diabetes, heart attack, social class, alcohol consumption, and supplement use the researchers conclude that study participants whose blood plasma levels of vitamin C were above 66 micromol/L had a 42% lower <u>relative</u> risk of stroke than did those whose levels were below 41 micromol/L. They also observed a 17% reduction in stroke for every 20-micromol/L increase in plasma vitamin C concentration. A 20-micromol/L increase in plasma vitamin C concentration can be achieved by adding one additional serving of fruit and vegetables daily.

It is also of interest to note that six times as many study participants in the high plasma vitamin C group were supplementing with vitamin C as compared to those in the low plasma vitamin C group (10.5% vs 1.9%). [3]

An average <u>relative</u> reduction in stroke risk of 42% is indeed impressive and compares favourably with the 25-30% relative risk reduction often quoted for aspirin, and the 50-55% reduction attributed to warfarin, especially since increasing one's vitamin C intake is not associated with any adverse effects. The Cambridge researchers point out that vitamin C has a very short half-life in the blood (about 30 minutes), so spreading one's intake (whether through foods or supplements) throughout the day is essential.

Stroke prevention with vitamin C

Investigators involved with the *Japan Public Health Center-based Prospective Study* report that dietary vitamin C intake is associated with a reduced risk of stroke among non-smokers.

Their study involved 82,000 Japanese men and women between the ages of 40 and 69 years at entry to the study. The participants were relatively healthy with about 6% having diabetes, about 23% having hypertension and between 30 and 40% being current smokers. During the 10 year follow-up period the investigators confirmed 3451 total strokes (0.36%/year) of which 2138 (0.22%/year) were ischemic strokes.

The intake of antioxidant vitamins (alpha-carotene, beta-carotene, alpha-tocopherol, and vitamin C) was determined from food frequency questionnaires completed every year during the 10-year study period. While no correlations were found between stroke risk and the intake of alpha-carotene, beta-carotene, and alpha-tocopherol there was a clear association between vitamin

C intake and stroke risk in non-smokers. Non-smokers with an average (mean) vitamin C intake of 246 mg/day had a 25% lower risk (<u>relative</u>) of any stroke than did non-smokers with an average daily intake of only 69 mg/day when adjusted for age and gender. The <u>relative</u> risk decrease for ischemic stroke was 28%. There was no significant association between vitamin C intake and stroke risk in current smokers. The investigators suggest that this lack of association is related to the fact that smoking consumes vitamin C. [4]

The official recommended daily allowance for vitamin C is 90 mg/day for non-smoking men and 75 mg/day for non-smoking women. The actual average daily intake in the US is 105 mg for adult men and 84 mg for adult women. Clearly not enough to provide any meaningful stroke protection. Good food sources of vitamin C are red, green, and yellow peppers (about 100 mg per ½ cup), kiwi fruits (about 85 mg in a large fruit) and oranges (about 70 mg in a medium orange). However, the simplest way of ensuring an adequate vitamin C intake is to supplement with 200-500 mg three times a day.

Vitamin C and warfarin

The evidence regarding a possible interaction between warfarin (Coumadin) and vitamin C is conflicting. A reduction in INR was noted in 2 separate cases involving patients supplementing with 2 grams/day of vitamin C and an unspecified amount respectively. In contrast, a trial in which 5 patients supplemented with 1 gram/day for 14 days revealed no effect of vitamin C on INR. Another trial involving patients given 1 gram/day of vitamin C for 6 months demonstrated no change in required warfarin dosage compared with control patients not supplementing with vitamin C.

Another trial involving 19 warfarin-treated patients given 3, 5, or 10 grams of vitamin C for 7 days showed no clinically important changes in INR, but did result in a 17.5% drop in total plasma warfarin concentration. The researchers involved in this study attribute the decreased absorption of warfarin to the loose stools or diarrhea often accompanying high vitamin C intakes.

A group of researchers at the *University of Newcastle* reported that normal dietary intakes of vitamin C (20-600 mg/day; 92 mg/day average) has no effect on warfarin clearance from the blood and thus is unlikely to affect INR. Their study involved 57 patients (31 males) who were receiving warfarin. [5]

The evidence regarding a possible effect of vitamin C on warfarin clearance and INR is clearly mixed. It would seem though that, while relatively small doses would be expected to have no effect, large doses (3-10 grams/day) may decrease plasma concentrations of warfarin and thus could potentially lead to a drop in INR. From the sparse data available, it would appear that the drop would be relatively minor (from 2.5 to 2.1, for example) and could safely be compensated for by a slight increase in warfarin dosage. In my opinion, continuing supplementation (on a steady basis) with 3 x 500 mg/day of vitamin C when on warfarin would be more beneficial than detrimental.

VITAMINS D AND E

Vitamin D deficiency is widespread even in southern latitudes. A deficiency is linked to osteoporosis, colon cancer and other cancers, hypertension, diabetes, and cardiovascular disease. It is likely that that the role of vitamin D in stroke prevention is due mainly to its ability to lower blood pressure and reduce inflammation.

Vitamin E is a powerful, fat-soluble antioxidant that is effective in preventing heart disease and ischemic stroke. It helps prevent and reduce endothelial dysfunction and inhibits platelet aggregation by inhibiting the release of thromboxane A2 and by suppressing the negative effect of protein kinase C. There is also evidence that vitamin E decreases the levels of von Willebrand factor and prothrombin fragments 1 and 2. The bottom line is that vitamin E, especially *gamma*-tocopherol, is effective in preventing thrombosis related to platelet aggregation, is safe, does not cause bleeding, and does not interact with warfarin except possibly in some patients with specific coagulation disorders.

Vitamin D protects against stroke

There is convincing evidence that vitamin D, a hormone primarily involved in regulating calcium metabolism, reduces the risk of hypertension and diabetes. Since both of these conditions increase the risk of stroke, it is tempting to speculate that an adequate vitamin D status may also reduce the risk of stroke. A group of researchers from *Harvard School of Public Health* now confirms that low vitamin D levels are indeed associated with an increased risk of stroke, more specifically, ischemic stroke. Their study had two components:

- Correlating blood plasma level of 25-hydroxyvitamin D (25[OH]D) with incidence of ischemic stroke in a group of 33,000 female nurses taking part in the Nurses' Health Study started in 1976.
- Performing a meta-analysis of 6 studies evaluating the association between 25(OH)D levels and the risk of stroke.

Nurses' Health Study

The researchers prospectively identified and confirmed 464 cases of ischemic stroke. These cases were matched with 464 stroke-free controls of similar age, menopausal status, hormone replacement therapy status, race, and smoking status. After adjusting for a large number of nutritional, disease-related and lifestyle factors, the researchers concluded that women with an average plasma level of 25(OH)D of 35 nmol/L (range of 9.2 to 45.7) had a significantly increased risk of suffering an ischemic stroke (<u>relative</u> risk of 1.53) when compared to those with an average 25(OH)D level of 77.6 nmol/L (range of 65.5 to 264.3). More specifically, a woman with a 25(OH)D level of 55 nmol/L had twice the risk of suffering an ischemic stroke than did a woman with a 25(OH)D level of 95 nmol/L. They also noted that more than 40% of the study participants were deficient in vitamin D as defined as a plasma level of 25(OH)D below 50 nmol/L.

Meta-analysis
Analysis of 6 studies involving 1214 stroke cases found a relative risk of 1.52 when comparing men and women with low vitamin D status with those with high levels of 25(OH)D. One study only considered ischemic stroke and when its results were combined with the results of the Nurses' Health Study, the relative risk of suffering an ischemic stroke associated with a low vitamin D level was 1.59. [6]

This study clearly links a high plasma level of 25(OH)D with a significantly reduced risk of suffering an ischemic stroke. Although the Nurses' Health Study involved women only, there is no reason to suspect that the results would not be applicable to men. Unfortunately, the diet provides relatively little vitamin D. In the Nurses' Health Study the average vitamin D intake was 350 IU/day resulting in an average 25(OH)D level of 56 nmol/L. To reach a level of 95 nmol/L would require supplementation with about 4000 IU/day.

Gamma-tocopherol in stroke prevention
Natural vitamin E is not a single compound but a complex of at least four tocopherols (alpha, beta, delta, and gamma) and four tocotrienols (alpha, beta, delta, and gamma). *Alpha*-tocopherol is the predominant form found in human blood, while *gamma*-tocopherol is the predominant form found in food. Based on the finding that *alpha*-tocopherol is the most abundant form in blood, scientists concluded that it was also the most active and beneficial form. This led to the formulation of vitamin supplements based solely on *alpha*-tocopherol, and later to the synthesis and marketing of synthetic (dl-) *alpha*-tocopheryl acetate. Dl-*alpha*-tocopheryl acetate also quickly became the preferred form used in clinical trials aimed at evaluating the benefits of vitamin E, particularly in regard to cardiovascular disease.

A team of *Australian and Chinese* researchers suggests that *gamma*-tocopherol may be significantly more effective than *alpha*-tocopherol and may be particularly beneficial in stroke prevention. Their clinical trial included 39 healthy volunteers (19 men and 20 women) between the ages of 20 and 40 years. The participants were randomly assigned to supplement with a placebo, or 100 mg/day or 200 mg/day of pure *gamma*-tocopherol. Blood samples were drawn for analysis at the beginning and end of the 5-week trial. Supplementation clearly increased *gamma*-tocopherol concentrations in blood serum from 5.3 to 16.8 mg/mL in the case of the 100-mg/day dose, and from 5.4 to 30.1 mg/mL in the case of the 200-mg/day dose. The serum concentration of *alpha*-tocopherol did not change significantly during the trial.

The researchers also noted a significant decrease in platelet activation, LDL cholesterol level, platelet aggregation, and mean platelet volume. They also made the following interesting observations:

- "Several independent investigations have demonstrated that the blood concentration of *gamma*-tocopherol, not *alpha*- tocopherol, is negatively correlated to the incidence of coronary heart disease."

- "Supplementation with large amounts of *alpha*-tocopherol was shown to increase the breakdown and decrease blood concentrations of *gamma*-tocopherol."
- Both natural and synthetic *alpha*-tocopherol suppresses serum *gamma*-tocopherol. The resulting imbalance between *alpha*- and *gamma*-tocopherol may have significant health consequences.

The researchers conclude that the results of their study suggest that, "the daily consumption of small amounts of gamma-tocopherol, in conjunction with usual dietary intake from mixed food sources may provide protection from oxidative damage and prevent thrombosis."[7]

The results of this study support my own long-held belief that supplements, especially vitamins and antioxidants, should always be taken in a formulation that mimics, as close as possible, the way the vitamin/antioxidant is found in nature. Thus, vitamin C should always be taken with the bioflavonoids with which it is associated in nature. B vitamins should always be taken as the whole complex, as should vitamin E with emphasis on natural gamma-tocopherol. The finding that gamma-tocopherol helps prevent thrombosis logically leads to the conclusion that it may also be effective in preventing transient ischemic attacks (TIAs) and ischemic stroke.

LYCOPENE

The carotenoid lycopene is a powerful antioxidant, particularly abundant in tomatoes. It owes its stroke preventing properties to its ability to prevent and reduce endothelial dysfunction and oxidative stress and its ability to prevent nitric oxide deficiency.

Lycopene decreases risk of stroke in men

Medical researchers associated with *University of Eastern Finland* provide convincing proof that high serum concentrations of lycopene is associated with a substantially decreased risk of ischemic stroke and any stroke.

Their study involved 1031 Finnish men aged 46-65 years at entry to the study. A total of 67 strokes (0.54%/year) of which 50 (0.40%/year) were ischemic occurred during the 12 year follow-up period. Serum concentrations of alpha-carotene, beta-carotene, retinol, alpha-tocopherol, and lycopene were measured at entry to the study and periodically during a 7-year period. No correlations were found between stroke risk and blood (serum) levels of alpha-carotene, beta-carotene, retinol, and alpha-tocopherol.

However, study participants with lycopene levels above 0.22 micromol/L were found to have a 55% lower <u>relative</u> risk of suffering a stroke than participants having a level below 0.030 micromol L. This corresponds to an <u>absolute</u> reduction in the risk of stroke from 0.80%/year to 0.35%/year. The <u>relative</u> risk of ischemic stroke associated with a high lycopene level was 58% lower than the risk for study participants with low lycopene. This corresponds to an absolute reduction in the risk of ischemic stroke from 0.64%/year to 0.26%/year. [8]

Researchers associated with *Newcastle University* in The UK report that high intakes and high serum levels of lycopene are significantly associated with lower risk of stroke and overall mortality.

Their meta-analysis involved eight studies including 211,704 participants. Four of the studies evaluated dietary intake of lycopene versus stroke risk while the remaining four evaluated serum concentration of lycopene versus stroke risk. A significant association between stroke risk and serum level of lycopene was found with study participants with high levels (mean serum concentration: 0.41 micromol/L) having a 39% lower relative risk of suffering a stroke than did participants with low levels (mean serum concentration: 0.15 micromol/L). Participants with a high dietary intake (mean daily intake: 9.81 mg)) of lycopene were found to have a 21% lower relative risk of experiencing a stroke than participants with lower intakes (mean daily intake: 1.85 mg).

The reduction in stroke risk associated with high dietary intakes or high serum levels of lycopene was more pronounced for men, participants over the age of 55 years, and participants with a BMI above 26. Studies carried out in the US reported a statistically non-significant relative risk reduction of only 12% while studies carried out in Finland and Japan reported a highly significant average relative risk reduction of 37%.

A separate analysis of five studies involving 6249 participants found a strong, statistically significant association between serum concentration of lycopene and overall mortality. Participants with high lycopene levels had a 37% lower relative risk of premature death than did participants with lower levels. [9]

NOTE: The data presented in the report did not make it possible to calculate absolute stroke and mortality risks.

MAGNESIUM AND POTASSIUM

Magnesium is of key importance to human health. It participates in over 300 enzymatic reactions in the body. A deficiency has been linked to conditions such as irregular heartbeat, asthma, emphysema, cardiovascular disease, high blood pressure, mitral valve prolapse, stroke and heart attack, diabetes, fibromyalgia, glaucoma, migraine, kidney stones, osteoporosis, and probably many more. Magnesium is helpful in reducing endothelial dysfunction and in inhibiting platelet aggregation; it also helps prevent stroke indirectly by reducing blood pressure. There is also evidence that magnesium injections given within 6 hours of suffering an ischemic stroke can remarkably reduce stroke damage.

Potassium has been found to materially reduce the risk of both ischemic and hemorrhagic stroke. It is likely that this is an indirect effect associated with the proven ability of potassium to lower blood pressure.

Magnesium in stroke prevention

A group of nutritional researchers at *Karolinska Institute* in Sweden has found that higher magnesium intakes are associated with a significantly reduced risk of suffering an ischemic stroke. Their meta-analysis covered 7 prospective studies involving 241,378 participants and 6477 cases of stroke, about 5100 of which were ischemic (caused by a blockage in an artery). The remaining strokes were hemorrhagic (caused by rupture of an artery), or of unknown origin. All studies compared stroke risk with at least 3 different levels of magnesium intake ranging from less than 186 mg/day to 575 mg/day and included adjustments for potential confounders such as age, sex, smoking, hypertension and diabetes; most also corrected for body mass index, physical activity and alcohol consumption. The conclusion of the meta-analysis was that the risk of ischemic stroke decreases by 9% for each 100 mg/day of additional magnesium intake. Thus, if a person with a daily intake of 200 mg (typical intake in North America) were to increase their intake by 400 mg/day they would decrease their risk of suffering an ischemic stroke by 36%.

In an accompanying editorial, Drs. Song and Liu of *Harvard Medical School* point out that researchers have been studying the role of magnesium in cardiovascular health for nearly 80 years, ever since Zwillinger in 1935 reported that intravenous injection of magnesium sulfate suppressed digitalis-induced cardiac arrhythmia in humans. They suggest that the time has come to perform a large, double-blind and placebo-controlled randomized trial of magnesium for the primary prevention of cardiovascular disease. They conclude with the following comment:

"Without a large trial that directly defines cardiovascular disease as a primary outcome, it is safe to predict that another 8 decades will go by while generations of nutritional scientists continue to debate magnesium's efficacy for the primary prevention of cardiovascular disease."[10, 11]

Many afibbers are already supplementing with 400 to 600 mg/day of elemental magnesium thus potentially reducing their risk of ischemic stroke by 36 to 54%. This is clearly highly significant and using magnesium supplementation to achieve it avoids the many adverse effects of aspirin and warfarin, and would have the added benefit of potentially preventing or reversing osteoporosis by increasing whole-body bone mass by about 8%.

Magnesium and potassium help prevent stroke in men

Researchers at *Harvard School of Public Health* report that a diet rich in magnesium, potassium and calcium is associated with a reduced risk of stroke in men. Their study included 42,669 male health professionals aged 40 to 75 years at enrollment in 1986. The participants were followed for 24 years during which time 1547 strokes occurred (895 ischemic, 179 hemorrhagic, and 473 of unknown type).

The researchers found a strong association between overall stroke risk and total magnesium intake (from diet and supplements) with an even stronger association with intake from supplements. Study participants with a high average magnesium intake (467 mg/day) had a 17% lower underline{relative }risk of suffering any stroke than did participants with a low average daily intake (267 mg/day). When considering only intake from supplements a high intake was associated with a 26% lower risk of any stroke and a 28% lower risk of ischemic stroke. There was no correlation between magnesium intake and risk of hemorrhagic stroke.

A high potassium intake was also associated with a reduced risk of stroke. Participants with a high average daily intake (4438 mg/day) had a 12% lower risk of any stroke than did participants with a low intake (2600 mg/day). When considering only intake from supplements a high intake was associated with a 34% lower risk of any stroke and a 41% lower risk of ischemic stroke. There was no correlation between potassium intake and risk of hemorrhagic stroke.

There was no statistically significant association between calcium intake and overall stroke risk. However, participants with a high combined intake of magnesium, potassium, and calcium were found to have a 21% reduced risk of any stroke. [12]

The article detailing the findings of the study unfortunately does not provide the data necessary to calculate the absolute incidence of stroke. However, assuming that all original enrollees completed the study (1,024 million person-years) the overall absolute rate of stroke would have been 0.15%/year. Even if only half the original enrollees completed the study (512,000 person-years) the rate of any stroke would have been only 0.30%/year. Corresponding rates for ischemic stroke alone would be 0.09%/year and 0.17%/year.

Magnesium, potassium, and calcium and stroke risk in women

Medical researchers at *Brigham and Women's Hospital* in Boston report that a diet rich in magnesium, potassium and calcium is associated with a reduced risk of stroke in women. Their study included 86,149 female registered nurses aged 30 to 55 years at enrollment in 1976 (NHS I) and 94,715 nurses aged 25 to 42 years at enrollment in 1989 (NHS 2). The nurses were followed for 30 years (until 2010) and 22 years (until 2011) years respectively. During the follow-up period a total of 3780 strokes (1850 ischemic, 636 hemorrhagic, and 1294 of unknown origin) were documented.

The researchers found a strong association between overall stroke risk and total magnesium intake (from diet and supplements). Nurses with a high average magnesium intake (383 mg/day) had a 13% lower underline{relative }risk of suffering any stroke than did participants with a low average daily intake (249 mg/day). Supplementing with magnesium was associated with a 19% lower risk of suffering an ischemic stroke. There was no statistically significant correlation between magnesium intake and risk of hemorrhagic stroke.

A high potassium intake was also associated with a reduced risk of stroke. Participants with a high average daily intake (3385 mg/day) had an 11% lower <u>relative</u> risk of any stroke than did participants with a low intake (2442 mg/day).

Supplementing with potassium was associated with a 29% lower risk of suffering an ischemic stroke. There was no statistically significant correlation between potassium intake and risk of hemorrhagic stroke.

There was no statistically significant association between total calcium intake and overall stroke risk. However, participants with a high combined intake of magnesium, potassium, and calcium were found to have a 28% reduced risk of any stroke and a 22% reduced risk of ischemic stroke.

The authors of the study also reviewed and updated meta-analyses of prospective studies of dietary magnesium, potassium, and calcium intakes and risk of stroke. They conclude that overall stroke risk (relative) decreases by 13% for every 100 mg/day increase in magnesium intake and by 9% for every 1000 mg/day increase in potassium intake. [13]

The article detailing the findings of the study, unfortunately, does not provide the data necessary to calculate the <u>absolute</u> incidence of stroke. However, assuming that all original enrollees completed the study (4,667 million person-years) the overall absolute rate of stroke would have been 0.08%/year. Even if only half the original enrollees completed the study (2,334 million person-years) the overall rate of any stroke would still be remarkably low at 0.16%/year. Corresponding rates for ischemic stroke alone would be 0.04%/year and 0.08%/year.

Magnesium and stroke risk in men and women

A team of medical researchers from *Norwich Medical School* and *Cambridge University* reports that a high dietary intake of magnesium is associated with a substantial decrease in the risk of suffering a stroke (ischemic, hemorrhagic or of unknown type). Their study included 2000 men and 2443 women (between the ages of 39 and 78 years) who were randomly selected from the EPIC-Norfolk cohort of 25,639 men and women believed to be representative of the UK population. All participants completed 7-day food diaries and were then followed for 10 years (till 2008).

During the follow-up period (42,556 person-years) a total of 928 strokes occurred (2.1%/ person-year). Annual stroke rate among men with a daily magnesium intake less than 214 mg (average 181 mg/day) was 3.27%/year as compared to 1.72% among men with an intake of more than 354 mg/day (average 427 mg/day). This equates to a <u>relative</u> reduction in stroke risk of 41% after multivariate adjustment.

Annual stroke rate among women with a daily intake less than 180 mg (average 156 mg/day) was 3.15%/year as compared to 1.58%/year among women with an intake of more than 295 mg (average 352 mg/day). This difference however, proved to be not statistically significant after multivariate adjustment.

The researchers also observed a significantly lower (by 7 mm Hg) systolic blood pressure among men with a magnesium intake above 386 mg/day (average 456 mg/day) when compared to men with a daily intake of less than 242 mg (average 206 mg/day). A similar reduction was observed in women but this reduction became statistically non-significant after multivariate adjustment.

Both men and women with the highest magnesium intake were found to have lower total cholesterol levels than did study participants with the lowest intake. [14]

The multivariate adjustment for stroke risk corrected for possible confounding by age, BMI, education status, physical activity, smoking status, alcohol intake, serum total cholesterol, baseline MI or diabetes, family history of stroke, systolic blood pressure, diastolic blood pressure, aspirin use, antihypertensive medication, calcium:magnesium ratio, and use of magnesium and calcium supplements. The authors of the study offer no explanation for the lack of post-multivariate adjustment statistical significance of the effect of magnesium on blood pressure and stroke incidence in women.

Mortality in stroke patients with low magnesium
Medical doctors at the *universities of Soochow (Suzhou) and Nanjing* in China report that patients admitted with acute ischemic stroke are more likely to die while in hospital if their magnesium level upon admission was low.

Their study included 2485 patients admitted with acute ischemic stroke to 22 hospitals in Suzhou (a city of 10 million people) during the period December 2013 to May 2014. During hospitalization 92 patients (3.7%) died from all causes. The number of deaths (43) was substantially higher among patients admitted with a serum magnesium level below 0.82 mmol/L than among patients with a level of 0.98 mmol/L or higher. NOTE: The normal range for serum potassium is 0.85 to 1.10 mmol/L (1.7 to 2.2 mg/dL).

After adjusting for confounding variables the authors of the study conclude that stroke patients admitted with low magnesium levels are twice as likely to die in hospital than are patients with higher levels. They surmise that lower magnesium level at admission might reflect high blood pressure, elevated blood sugar, or severe renal disease; factors that have all been implicated in poor outcome and mortality in stroke patients. They also point out that magnesium has been found to improve endothelial function and inhibit platelet aggregation. [15]

A team of researchers from *five American and a Chinese university* have just completed a study examining the association of serum magnesium concentrations and all-cause, cardiovascular and cancer mortality in a nationally representative sample of 14,353 US adults aged 25-74 years. During the 29 year follow-up 708 study participants died from a stroke.

Participants with a magnesium serum level below 0.70 mmol/L had a 2.5 times greater risk of dying from a stroke than did participants with levels of 0.8 mmol/L or higher. [16]

This is further evidence that low magnesium levels are associated not only with a substantially increased risk of suffering a stroke but also with a significantly increased risk of dying from one. It is a sobering thought that between 50 and 80% of adults in the United States do not consume the recommended daily allowance (RDA) of magnesium which is 420 mg/day for men and 320 mg/day for women.

Potassium and stroke risk

A team of scientists from *Boston University School of Public Health, Karolinska Institute* in Sweden, and *University of Modena and Reggio Emilia* in Italy reports that higher intakes of potassium are associated with a reduced risk of stroke. The scientists base their conclusion on a meta-analysis of 16 studies involving 639,440 participants.

When adjusted for blood pressure study participants with a daily potassium intake of 90 mmol/day (3500 mg/day) had a 22% lower relative risk of suffering a stroke than did participants with a daily intake (referent value) of 25 mmol/day (1000 mg/day). The unadjusted relative risk reduction with a 90 mmol/day vs. a 25 mmol/day intake was 33% indicating that patients with hypertension benefit more from a high potassium intake than do people with blood pressure within the optimal range.

The added benefit of increasing potassium intake to the current RDA (Recommended Daily Allowance) of 120 mmol/day (4700 mg/day) was nonsignificant in the adjusted model and slightly negative in the non-adjusted model indicating that an intake of 3500 mg/day is optimal for stroke prevention.

In the case of ischemic stroke the decrease in relative stroke risk when going from a daily intake of 25 mmol/day to 90 mmol/day was 29% in both the adjusted and unadjusted models.

In the case of hemorrhagic stroke the decrease in relative stroke risk was 27% in the adjusted model and 35% in the unadjusted model again indicating that a substantial part of potassium's protective effect is due to its ability to lower blood pressure.

The authors conclude that their meta-analysis supports an inverse association between potassium intake and the risk of total, hemorrhagic, and ischemic stroke, with the lowest risk occurring at a potassium intake of around 90 mmol/day (3500 mg/day). [17]

The average potassium intake by adult men and women in the United States is 2790 mg/day (71 mmol/day). [18]. Increasing this intake by 750 mg/day to reach the value recommended above would result in an overall 4% reduction in relative stroke risk (unadjusted model). While this may not seem impressive on its own, it would have a very significant impact if applied to the entire adult U.S. population.

FRUIT and TEA

An apple a day keeps stroke away!

There is ample evidence that a high consumption of fruits and vegetables lowers the risk of stroke. What is not known is whether some fruits and vegetables are more effective in stroke prevention than others. A group of researchers from *Wageningen University* in The Netherlands now answers this question.

Their study included 20,069 men and women between the ages of 20 and 65 years who were free of cardiovascular disease at baseline. During 10 years of follow-up, 226 nonfatal and 19 fatal strokes were recorded (0.11%/year). It is worth noting that 12 of the patients who suffered a fatal stroke had previously had a nonfatal stroke. The majority (60%) of the strokes was ischemic, 19% were hemorrhagic, and the remaining 21% were of unknown origin. All participants completed a validated, self-administered food-frequency questionnaire at enrolment between 1993 and 1997.

Fruit and vegetable intake was grouped according to the predominant colour of the produce. Thus, the green colour group consisted of broccoli, brussel sprouts, cabbage, kale, spinach, endive, and lettuce. The orange/yellow group included citrus fruit, cantaloupe, carrot, carrot juice, and peach. The red/purple group contained red beets, red cabbage, cherries, grapes, strawberries, red sweet pepper, tomato, and tomato juice. The white group consisted of garlic, leeks, onion, apples (including apple sauce and apple juice), pears, banana, cauliflower, chicory, cucumber, and mushrooms.

The average daily fruit and vegetable intake was 378 grams/day with white fruits and vegetables contributing 36%, and orange/yellow fruits and vegetables contributing 29% of total intake. Apples and pears constituted 55% of the white fruit and vegetable intake, while citrus fruits accounted for 78% of the orange/yellow group. After adjustment for lifestyle and other dietary factors, the researchers concluded that study participants whose intake of white fruits and vegetables exceeded 171 grams/day had halved their stroke risk as compared to those whose intake was 78 grams/day or less. Thus, a 25-gram/day increase in the intake of white fruits and vegetables corresponds to a 9% (relative) reduction in the risk of stroke. NOTE: In this study apples and pears constituted 55% of the total daily intake of white fruits and vegetables.

Consumption of green, orange/yellow and red/purple fruits was not associated with a decreased stroke incidence. The Dutch researchers point out that apples are a rich source of quercetin (3.6 mg/100 grams) and dietary fiber (2.3 grams/100 grams) and that other researchers have found that a high intake of flavonoids like quercetin is associated with a 20% reduction in stroke risk. [19]

Tea may help prevent stroke

Several studies have shown that habitual consumption of green tea is protective against cardiovascular disease, breast cancer, and prostate cancer. Now researchers at the *UCLA School of Medicine* report that habitual tea (green or black) drinking is also associated with a reduced risk of stroke.

The researchers performed a meta-analysis of 10 studies from 6 different countries (China, Japan, Finland, the Netherlands, Australia and the USA). Mortality from stroke (ischemic and hemorrhagic) among 35- to 74-year-old men in these countries ranged from 3 per 10,000 in Australia to 24 per 10,000 in rural China. The 10 studies covered 4378 strokes (fatal and non-fatal) that occurred in a total population of 194,965 men and women. The annual incidence of stroke in a subgroup of 162,700 individuals was 0.7% a year.

The researchers pooled the results of the 10 studies and arrived at the conclusion that individuals drinking 3 or more cups of green or black tea every day had a 21% lower risk of stroke than did those consuming less than one cup a day. They speculate that the protective effect of tea may be due to its ability to improve endothelial function and thereby increase blood flow to the brain, or to the ability of one of its components (theanine) to reduce the size of the area impacted by a stroke. They also point out that the protective effect of tea is primarily evident in the case of ischemic stroke and is likely to be considerably less important in the prevention of hemorrhagic stroke. [20]

Researchers at *Seoul National University College of Medicine* in South Korea provide evidence that while black tea is not effective in the prevention of hemorrhagic stroke green tea clearly is. Their study included 940 patients aged 20 to 84 years who had experienced a first, acute hemorrhagic stroke (non-traumatic) as well as 940 community controls and 940 hospital controls matched by age and gender. Study participants were asked to indicate the number of cups of tea (green, black, and oolong tea) consumed per day or week during the preceding year.

Analysis of the collected data showed that consumption of green tea was associated with a 29% reduction in relative risk of suffering a hemorrhagic stroke. Black tea and oolong tea exhibited no protective effect and there was no significant association between the amount of green tea consumed and degree of protection. [21]

Although there is, as yet, no conclusive evidence that green tea extract in capsule form provides the same benefits as green tea itself, it may be advisable for those who do not drink tea to supplement with a green tea extract containing its two most important components epigallocatechin and gallate (EGCG) and theanine.

Citrus fruits help prevent ischemic stroke

Citrus fruits are a rich source of flavanones such as hesperidin and naringenin. Flavanones are strong antioxidants and scavengers of free radicals, and they exhibit antiviral, antimicrobial, and anti-inflammatory properties. There is also evidence that flavanones inhibit platelet aggregation.

Researchers at *Emory University and University of Alabama* have found that a diet rich in flavanones is associated with a significantly reduced risk of ischemic stroke. Their study included 20,024 participants (56% women) in the REGARDS (**RE**asons for **G**eographic and **R**acial **D**ifferences in **S**troke) study. All study participants completed a 107-item food intake questionnaire and were then followed for 6.5 years. During this period 524 ischemic strokes were observed, 250 in women and 274 in men. Analysis of the collected data showed that a high intake (48 mg or more per day) of flavanones is associated with a 28% lower *relative* risk of ischemic stroke. More specifically, a high intake (average 267 g/day) of citrus fruit was associated with a 31% relative reduction in stroke risk. [22]

NOTE: One large orange without the skin weighs about 200 g and a large grapefruit (peeled) weighs about 280 g.

NATTOKINASE

An ischemic stroke is caused by a blood clot or plaque fragment obstructing the flow of blood through the small arteries in the brain. A heart attack (myocardial infarction) is caused by a blood clot or plaque fragment obstructing the flow of blood through the small arteries feeding the heart. Venous thromboembolism, also known as deep vein thrombosis (DVT), is caused by a blood clot forming in the veins, most often in the lower legs.

Thus, inhibiting blood clot (thrombus) formation is of primary importance in the prevention of all the above conditions. The drug warfarin (Coumadin) is the most commonly used anticoagulant and works by inhibiting the activation of the vitamin K-dependent coagulation factors V, VII and X in the extrinsic and common pathways of the coagulation cascade. The level of other important coagulation promoters, such as fibrinogen and factor VIII, are not affected by warfarin.

Nattokinase helps prevent blood clots

Nattokinase, an extract from fermented soybeans (natto), is known to inhibit blood clot formation (thrombosis), but does so by dissolving already formed fibrin-rich clots and by inactivating plasminogen activator inhibitor-1. Researchers at the *Changhua Christian Hospital* in Taiwan report that nattokinase also inhibits the synthesis of fibrinogen and coagulation factors VII and VIII. Elevated fibrinogen levels are associated with increased blood viscosity and an increased risk of cardiovascular disease (CVD). There is also evidence that elevated levels of factors VII and VIII are associated with atherosclerosis and coronary heart disease.

The Changhua study involved 15 healthy controls, 15 patients with CVD or at least 2 risk factors for CVD, and 15 patients undergoing dialysis for chronic kidney disease (a known risk factor for CVD). At the beginning of the study (baseline) the levels of fibrinogen, factor VII and factor VIII in the three groups were as follows:

Clotting Factor	Controls	CVD Group	Dialysis Group
Fibrinogen - mg/dL	335.0	376.2	433.5
Factor VII – IU	122.5	139.7	154.8
Factor VIII – IU	106.1	156.7	236.3

All study participants ingested 2 nattokinase capsules a day (2000 fibrinolysis units per capsule) for 2 months. At the end of this period levels of fibrinogen had decreased by 9% in the healthy group, by 7% in the CVD group, and by 10% in the dialysis group. Corresponding declines in factor VII level in the 3 groups were 14%, 13% and 7% and for factor VIII 17%, 19% and 19% respectively. No adverse events or increases in uric acid level were observed during the trial.

As an added benefit   18% of participants noticed a drop in blood pressure and/or increased vitality. Thirteen percent noticed an improvement in bowel function and 11% reported a lessening of shoulder-neck ache. The Taiwanese researchers conclude that supplementation with nattokinase would have a beneficial effect on risk factors associated with CVD through its reduction in fibrinogen, factor VII and factor VIII levels.[23]

This study confirms that nattokinase is effective in preventing the formation of fibrin-rich blood clots such as those associated with venous thromboembolism and atrial fibrillation (blood stagnation in the left atrial appendage). Although nattokinase also reduces the level of factor VIII I am not aware of any evidence that it would also reduce the formation of platelet-rich clots (plaque). Additional evidence for the effectiveness of nattokinase in preventing DVT can be found in a study by a group of British and Italian researchers involving 204 airline passengers at high risk for venous thrombosis traveling between London and New York. [24]

EXERCISE

Moderate physical activity helps prevent stroke

Physicians from *University of Minnesota, Osaka University, University of Tsukuba*, and the *National Cancer Centre* in Tokyo report that moderate-intensity physical activities may be optimum for stroke prevention in Japanese people.

Their study included 74,913 Japanese men and women between the ages of 52 and 68 years. Study participants were asked to provide information about the average daily amount of time and frequency spent in work-related and leisure-time physical activities. Daily total physical activity level (MET-hours per day) was calculated as the sum of physical activity levels spent during work-related walking and strenuous work and leisure-time physical activities, such as brisk walking and jogging.

> **MET** (metabolic equivalent) is a measure expressing the energy consumption associated with various physical activities where 1 MET is equal to the energy expenditure of an average person seated at rest. Walking and bicycling are the most common moderate-intensity activities with brisk walking expending about 3.3 MET/hour and leisurely bicycling expending about 4 MET per hour. More vigorous activities are bicycling at 10-16 mph (16-26 km/hour) which expends 6-10 MET/hour, jogging at about 7 MET/hour and snow shoveling at 6 MET/hour.

During the 698,946 person-years of follow-up a total of 2738 incident strokes were recorded (0.4%/person-year). Of these 1721 (0.24%/person-year) were ischemic (0.07%/person-year were embolic) and 1007 (0.14%/person/year) were hemorrhagic. The average (median) total daily physical activity of the participants varied between 1 and 28 MET-hours. The researchers found that men and women who expended 5 to 10 MET-hours in physical activity during the day had a 17% lower risk of any stroke than did participants who expended only 1 MET-hour in physical activity during the day.

The greatest relative risk reduction for ischemic stroke (21%) were found among participants spending 8-19 MET-hours per day in physical activities while the greatest relative risk reduction for hemorrhagic stroke (21%) was associated with a daily energy expenditure of 3 to 8 MET-hours. Expenditures in excess of 15 MET-hours/day actually increased the risk the risk of hemorrhagic stroke. It is of interest that the greatest relative risk reduction (24%/person-year) for an embolic stroke (such as strokes associated with atrial fibrillation) was achieved at a daily energy expenditure of 16 to 68 MET-hours.

The researchers conclude that for Japanese people, moderate levels of total physical activity, particularly achieved by moderate-intensity activities, may be optimal for stroke prevention because excessive vigorous-intensity activities may not be beneficial for prevention of hemorrhagic stroke. [25]

REFERENCES

1. Choe, H. et al. Intake of antioxidants and B vitamins is inversely associated with ischemic stroke and cerebral atherosclerosis. Nutrition Research and Practice, Vol. 10 (5), October 2016, pp. 516-23
2. Saposnik, G et al. Homocysteine-lowering therapy and stroke risk, severity and disability: additional findings from the HOPE 2 trial. Stroke, Vol. 40 (4), April 2009, pp. 1365-72
3. Myint, PK, et al. Plasma vitamin C concentrations predict risk of incident stroke over 10 years in 20,649 participants of the European Prospective Investigation into Cancer. American Journal of Clinical Nutrition, Vol. 87, January 1, 2008, pp. 64-69

4. Uesugi, S, et al. Dietary intake of antioxidant vitamins and risk of stroke: the Japan Public Health Center-based Prospective Study. European Journal of Clinical Nutrition, Vol. 71, July 12, 2017, pp. 1179-1185

5. Wynne, H, et al. Dietary related plasma vitamin C concentration has no effect on anticoagulation response to warfarin. Thrombosis Research, Vol. 118, 2006, pp. 501-04

6. Sun, Q, et al. 25-hydroxyvitamin D levels and the risk of stroke. Stroke, Vol. 43, June 2012, pp. 1470-77

7. Singh, I, et al. Effects of gamma-tocopherol supplementation on thrombotic risk factors. Asia Pacific Journal of Clinical Nutrition, Vol. 16, No. 3, 2007, pp. 422-28

8. Karppi, J, et al. Serum lycopene decreases the risk of stroke in men: a population-based follow-up study. Neurology, Vol. 79 (15), October 9, 2012, pp. 1540-7

9. Cheng, HM, et al. Lycopene and tomato and risk of cardiovascular diseases: A systematic review and meta-analysis of epidemiological evidence. Critical Reviews in Food Science and Nutrition. August 11, 2017

10. Larsson, SC, et al. Dietary magnesium intake and risk of stroke: a meta-analysis of prospective studies. American Journal of Clinical Nutrition, Vol. 95, 2012, pp. 362-66

11. Song, Y and Liu, S. Magnesium for cardiovascular health: time for intervention. American Journal of Clinical Nutrition, Vol. 95, 2012, pp. 269-70

12. Adebamowo, SN, et al. Intakes of magnesium, potassium, and calcium and the risk of stroke among men. International Journal of Stroke, Vol. 10 (7), October 2015, pp. 1093-1100

13. Adebamowo, SN, et al. Association between intakes of magnesium, potassium, and calcium and risk of stroke: 2 cohorts of US women and updated meta-analyses. American Journal of Chemical Nutrition. Vol. 101 (6). June 2015, pp. 1269-77

14. Bain, LK, et al. The relationship between dietary magnesium intake, stroke and its major risk factors, blood pressure and cholesterol, in the EPIC-Norfolk cohort. International Journal of Cardiology. October 1, 2015, pp. 108-14

15. You, S, et al. Admission low magnesium level is associated with in-hospital mortality in acute ischemic stroke patients. Cerebrovascular Diseases, Vol. 44 (1-2), August 2017, pp. 35-42

16. Zhang, X, et al. Serum magnesium concentrations and all-cause, cardiovascular, and cancer mortality among U.S. adults: Results from the NHANES I Epidemiologic Follow-up Study. Clinical Nutrition, August 30, 2017

17. Vinceti, M, et al. Meta-analysis of potassium intake and the risk of stroke. Journal of the American Heart Association. Vol. 5 (10), October 6, 2016

18. Hoy, MK, et al. Potassium intake of the U.S. population. U.S Department of Agriculture, Food Surveys Research Group, Brief No. 10, September 2012.

19. Oude Griep, LM, Geleijnse, JM, et al. Colors of fruit and vegetables and 10-year incidence of stroke. Stroke, Vol. 42, November 2011, pp. 3190-95

20. Arab, L, et al. Green and black tea consumption and risk of stroke: a meta-analysis. Stroke, Vol. 40, May 2009, pp. 1786-92

21. Lee, SM, et al. The impact of green tea consumption on the prevention of hemorrhagic stroke. Neuroepidemiology, Vol 44 (4), July 2015, pp. 215-20

22. Goetz, ME, et al. Flavanone intake is inversely associated with risk of incident ischemic stroke in the REasons for Geographic and Racial Differences in Stroke (REGARDS) Study. The Journal of Nutrition, Vol. 146 (11), November 2016, pp. 2233-2243

23. Hsia, CH, et al. Nattokinase decreases plasma levels of fibrinogen, factor VII, and factor VIII in human subjects. Nutrition Research, Vol. 29, 2009, pp. 190-96

24. Cesarone, MR, et al. Prevention of venous thrombosis in long-haul flights with Flite Tabs. Angiology, Vol. 54, No. 5, Sept-Oct 2003, pp. 531-39

25. Kubota, Y, et al. Daily total physical activity and incident stroke: The Japan Public Health Center-Based Prospective Study. Stroke, Vol. 48 (7), July 2017, pp.1730-1736

Chapter 12

Stroke Prevention with Aspirin

The Food and Drug Administration (FDA) in the USA has not approved the use of aspirin for the prevention of a first cardiovascular event (heart attack, stroke and cardiovascular death). Nevertheless, it is estimated that 50 million Americans take a daily aspirin (acetylsalicylic acid) for the primary prevention of cardiovascular events. This translates into roughly 10 billion to 20 billion tablets consumed annually in the USA alone. [1]

There is no evidence that daily aspirin consumption protects against a first ischemic stroke. As a matter of fact, there is evidence that it may do more harm than good in low-risk patients with atrial fibrillation. In a 2005 study of 871 low-risk AF patients Japanese researchers at *Osaka School of Medicine* conclude that daily aspirin therapy (150-200 mg/day) in this group is neither effective nor safe. They actually observed more cardiovascular deaths, strokes and TIAs in the aspirin group than in the placebo group. In addition, fatal or major bleeding was found to be more frequent in the aspirin group than in the placebo group. Overall, the incidence of strokes, deaths and other adverse events was 42% greater in the aspirin group than in the placebo group. The trial was stopped early since the probability that aspirin would prove superior to placebo in stroke prevention, if it continued, was deemed to be vanishingly small. [2]

Researchers at *Intermountain Medical Center Heart Institute* in Salt Lake City recently confirmed that daily aspirin therapy is neither effective nor safe in low-risk atrial fibrillation patients. Their study involved over 56,000 patients with atrial fibrillation and $CHADS_2$ scores of 0-1 or $CHADS_2VASc$ score of 0-2. The average age of the study participants was 67 years and 56.6% were male. A total of 9,682 patients were prescribed aspirin within 6 months of their initial diagnosis in order to prevent ischemic stroke. During a 5-year follow-up 4.6% of study participants on aspirin suffered a stroke compared to an incident rate of 2.3% (0.5%/year) among patients not on aspirin or any other stroke prevention medicine. Patients on aspirin were not only more likely to suffer a stroke but also experience a significantly higher incidence (17.6%) of serious bleeding than did patients not on aspirin (11.5%). The authors of the study conclude that aspirin therapy does not lower stroke rates in low-risk atrial fibrillation patients, but does increase the risk of significant bleeding and death. [3,4]

PRIMARY STROKE PREVENTION

Researchers from the *University of Alabama* carried out a meta-analysis of 6 large trials aimed at evaluating the benefits of aspirin in primary prevention of cardiovascular events (heart attack and stroke) and coronary heart disease.

The trials involved a total of 47,293 aspirin users and 45,580 controls not on aspirin who had no prior indication of cardiovascular disease. The dosage of aspirin involved in the trials varied from 75 mg/day to 500 mg/day. The researchers conclude that regular aspirin use reduces the <u>relative risk</u> of experiencing a first non-fatal heart attack by 24%, that of developing coronary heart disease by 23%, and reduces the risk of any cardiovascular event by 15% (relative). No risk reduction was observed for stroke, cardiovascular mortality or all-cause mortality. The authors conclude that their analysis supports the current recommendation for the use of aspirin for primary prevention in patients with a high risk of cardiovascular disease (10-year risk of 6% or higher). Unfortunately, they completely ignore the downside of aspirin usage – a substantially increased risk of hemorrhagic stroke and major gastrointestinal bleeding. NOTE: This study was funded by Bayer, the major manufacturer of aspirin. [5]

It is noteworthy that long-term aspirin usage has no effect on the risk of stroke in patients without prior cardiovascular disease. A previous meta-analysis of 5 of the 6 trials discussed above clearly showed that long-term aspirin usage increases the relative risk of hemorrhagic stroke (stroke caused by a burst blood vessel) by about 40% and the risk of major gastrointestinal bleeding by 70%. [6]

Thus it would seem prudent to keep in mind the conclusion of the U.S. Federal Drug Administration, *"The FDA has reviewed the available data and does not believe the evidence supports the general use of aspirin for primary prevention of a heart attack or stroke. In fact, there are serious risks associated with the use of aspirin, including increased risk of bleeding in the stomach and brain, in situations where the benefit of aspirin for primary prevention has not been established."* [7]

A group of researchers at *Oxford University* has concluded that aspirin is of questionable value in <u>primary prevention</u> since the risk reduction it confers is small and, to a large extent, is counterbalanced by an increase in hemorrhagic stroke and internal bleeding.

Their study of the results of 6 primary prevention trials found that the yearly incidence of serious vascular events (heart attack, stroke, or vascular death) among 95,000 participants with low risk for cardiovascular disease was 0.54%/year. Among participants who took aspirin daily, the incidence was 0.51%/year as compared to 0.57%/year among those who did not. On the other hand, 0.10%/year of participants on aspirin experienced a major gastrointestinal or intracranial bleed as compared to only 0.07% doing so among non-aspirin users. Of particular interest is the finding that taking aspirin on a daily basis did not reduce the risk of an ischemic or hemorrhagic stroke in participants at low average risk for cardiovascular disease.

There was no indication that the small reduction in vascular events observed among aspirin users was related to age, gender, smoking history, blood pressure, cholesterol level, body mass index, history of diabetes, or predicted risk of coronary heart disease. In particular, there was no significant trend in the proportional effects of aspirin in people at very low, low, moderate, and high estimated risk of heart disease.

Evaluation of the results of 16 <u>secondary prevention</u> trials revealed that daily aspirin consumption reduced the risk of a serious vascular event from 8.2%/year to 6.7%/year with a statistically non-significant increase in the risk of hemorrhagic stroke and major extracranial bleeds.

The Oxford researchers conclude that their observations *"do not seem to justify general guidelines advocating the routine use of aspirin in all apparently healthy individuals above a moderate level of risk of coronary heart disease".* [8]

A group of researchers from the *University of Utrecht and Harvard Medical School* reports that aspirin therapy is ineffective, or even harmful, for most women without a history of cardiovascular disease. Their study (Women's Health Study) included 27,939 initially healthy women who were randomized to receive either placebos or 100 mg of aspirin every second day. During 10 years of follow-up, 340 major cardiovascular events (heart attack, stroke and cardiovascular death) were observed in the placebo group (0.24%/year) as compared to 312 events (0.22%/year) in the aspirin-treated group. However, aspirin therapy was of no net benefit when taking into account its associated increased risk of major bleeding, in particular, gastrointestinal bleeding. Especially noteworthy was the finding that aspirin treatment of women with a 10% or greater 10-year risk for coronary heart disease, as advocated by most guidelines, was not associated with a net benefit.[9]

Researchers from the *Department of Clinical Pharmacology and Epidemiology* in Puglia, Italy report that the daily use of low-dose aspirin (300 mg/day or less) is associated with a significantly increased risk of major gastrointestinal and cerebral bleeding episodes. Their study involved 186,425 individuals being treated with low-dose aspirin and 186,425 matched controls not on aspirin. During an average follow-up of 5.7 years (1.6 million person-years) the incidence of major bleeding events was found to be 0.56%/year in the aspirin group versus 0.36%/year in the control group. This corresponds to a 55% relative risk increase in the aspirin group. The risk increase was similar for major gastrointestinal bleeding and cerebral bleeding.

The following factors were associated with a higher than average incidence of major bleeding amongst aspirin users – female sex, age below 50 years, previous hospitalization for cardiovascular or gastrointestinal problems, and use of oral anticoagulants and other antiplatelet agents. Protective effects were observed from the use of proton pump inhibitors (PPIs) and anti-hypertensive drugs. Multivariate analysis of factors associated with hospitalization for major bleeding events indicated that men were more likely to be hospitalized than women. Other factors associated with an increased risk of hospitalization were the use of aspirin, oral anticoagulants (warfarin), other antiplatelet agents (clopidogrel), anti-hypertensive medications, and previous hospital admittances for cardiovascular or gastrointestinal problems. A reduced risk of admittance was observed for those on PPIs and statin drugs.

Included in the study group were 56,000 patients with type 2 diabetes of which 27,000 were on daily aspirin. Amongst diabetics not on aspirin the incidence of major bleeding was 0.54%/year as compared to 0.33%/year amongst non-diabetics not on aspirin. Thus, it is clear that diabetes, by itself, is a strong risk factor for major bleedings (61% relative risk increase). However, being on aspirin did not significantly increase the risk of bleeding (0.58%/year). The Italian researchers conclude that daily use of low-dose aspirin is associated with a significantly increased risk of major gastrointestinal or cerebral bleeding episodes in non-diabetics. The use of aspirin was not found to increase the already elevated bleeding risk amongst diabetics. [10]

NOTE: Discontinuing long-term use of aspirin may temporarily increase the risk of stroke and TIA. [11,12]

A group of physicians associated with 14 different *universities and hospitals in Japan* recently reached the conclusion that *"aspirin did not show any benefit for the primary prevention of stroke in elderly Japanese patients with risk factors for stroke"*.

Their 6-year clinical trial included 14,464 patients with one or more of the following risk factors: hypertension (85%), dyslipidemia (high cholesterol) (72%) and diabetes (34%). The average (mean) age of the patients was 71 years (60-85 years) and 42% were men. Patients with coronary artery disease, atrial fibrillation, a prior stroke or TIA, atherosclerotic disease requiring treatment or a history of peptic ulcer or bleeding were excluded from the trial.

Study participants were randomized to receive either 100 mg/day of enteric-coated aspirin in tablet form or no aspirin, in addition to any ongoing medication. During an average (mean) follow-up period of 5 years 275 strokes and TIAs (transient ischemic attacks) and 88 intracranial hemorrhages (ICHs) occurred in the group. Patients in the aspirin group experienced fewer ischemic strokes (85), but more hemorrhagic strokes (38) than patients in the no-aspirin group (102 ischemic strokes and 23 hemorrhagic strokes), but these differences were statistically non-significant. Overall, the annual rate of ischemic stroke was 0.2% in the aspirin group and 0.3% in the non-aspirin group. The rate of intracranial hemorrhage was 0.15%/year in the aspirin group and 0.10%/year in the non-aspirin group.

It is clear that in this elderly Japanese population overall stroke rate is extremely low and taking aspirin does not reduce it further. However, age of 70 years and above, smoking, and diabetes were found to be significant risk factors with age of 70 years and older associated with a doubling of stroke risk and smoking and diabetes associated with a 1.5-fold increase in risk. There was no indication that elevated cholesterol or triglyceride levels affected stroke risk nor was there any indication that aspirin was more successful in reducing stroke rate in high-risk patients than in low-risk patients – it was unsuccessful in doing so in both sub-groups. [13]

The *JPAD Trial Investigators* in Japan recently reported the results of a trial aimed at determining the benefits of aspirin therapy in patients with type 2 diabetes. Their conclusion: *"Low-dose aspirin did not affect the risk for cardiovascular events but increased risk for gastrointestinal bleeding in patients with type 2 diabetes mellitus in a primary prevention setting."*

Their 10-year clinical trial involved 2160 Japanese patients with type 2 diabetes and without pre-existing cardiovascular disease. The average age of the patients was 65 years and 55% were men. More than half the patients had hypertension and/or dyslipidemia (high cholesterol). The patients were randomized to a control group that received no aspirin (1168 patients) or to an aspirin group (992 patients) that received either 100 mg enteric-coated aspirin every day or 81 mg of unbuffered, uncoated aspirin daily.

During the 10-year follow-up 37 patients in the aspirin group experienced an ischemic stroke and 7 suffered a hemorrhagic stroke yielding annual event rates of 0.37% and 0.07% respectively. Corresponding numbers were 45 ischemic strokes and 9 hemorrhagic strokes in the control group yielding annual rates of 0.39% and 0.07%. Gastrointestinal bleeding occurred in 2% of patients in the aspirin group and in 0.9% of patients in the no-aspirin group.

The difference in incidence of ischemic stroke between the two groups was thus 0.02% which means that treating 10,000 patients with aspirin would avoid 2 ischemic strokes per year while causing 110 gastrointestinal bleeds more than experienced in the control group.

There was no significant difference in the incidence of heart attacks and angina between the aspirin and no-aspirin groups. [14]

SAFETY AND DOSAGE

Aspirin is not innocuous. It can cause serious bleeding in the gastrointestinal tract and can aggravate existing ulcers. The estimated death rate from gastrointestinal (GI) bleeding ranges from 8-12% of all cases. Researchers at *Oxford University* have released the results of a very large study aimed at establishing the magnitude of aspirin-related bleeding incidents. They carefully studied the results of 24 major randomized clinical trials involving almost 66,000 participants. They conclude that when treated for a year 2.47% of aspirin users develop GI bleeding as compared to 1.42% among placebo users. Put in terms of the 50 million Americans now taking aspirin this means that the excess incidence of GI bleeding attributable to aspirin would be 525,000 and the excess mortality would be 50,000 every year.

The researchers also investigated whether lower dosages of aspirin would be safer. They found that they were not. The incidence of GI bleeding among low-dose aspirin users was 2.30% compared with 1.45% for placebo users.

Somewhat surprisingly, the study also found that enterically-coated or otherwise modified formulations were no safer than standard aspirin. The increase in GI bleeding among users of modified formulations was 93% as compared to 68% for all aspirin users and 59% for low-dose users. The researchers conclude that patients and their physicians need to consider the trade-off between the benefits and harms of long-term aspirin use. Dr. Martin Tramer of the Geneva University Hospitals in Switzerland wholeheartedly agrees with this conclusion and adds, *"It may be more appropriate for some people to eat an apple rather than an aspirin a day."*[15,16]

A study of 1225 patients with indications of adverse drug reactions admitted to two large *British hospitals* found that 18% of these reactions was associated with aspirin usage and most frequently involved gastrointestinal bleeding or peptic ulceration. The mortality among patients admitted with aspirin-related adverse events was 8% [17].

A team of *American and French physicians* reviewed 11 clinical trials involving over 10,000 patients in order to determine the efficacy of various doses of aspirin on the prevention of cardiovascular disease including stroke. Their conclusion: *"Currently available clinical data do not support the routine, long-term use of aspirin dosages greater than 75 to 81 mg/day in the setting of cardiovascular disease prevention. Higher dosages, which may be commonly prescribed, do not better prevent events but are associated with increased risks of gastrointestinal bleeding"*[1].

The *Oxford study* discussed above also noted that neither enteric-coated nor buffered aspirin formulations decreased bleeding risk. This outcome was also reported in a study carried out by researchers at *Boston University School of Medicine*. The researchers conclude that the increase in risk (comparing aspirin and non-aspirin users) of major upper gastrointestinal bleeding was 2.6-fold for plain aspirin, 2.7-fold for enteric-coated aspirin, and 3.1-fold for buffered aspirin. They did not observe any significant differences in risk attributable to the three aspirin forms according to bleeding site (gastric vs. duodenal). Their conclusion was, *"Use of low doses of enteric-coated or buffered aspirin carries a three-fold increase in the risk of major upper gastrointestinal bleeding. The assumption that these formulations are less harmful than plain aspirin may be mistaken."*[18]

Although people with low risk for future coronary heart disease events would not benefit from a daily aspirin, there are groups of patients who would indeed do so, especially patients who have already suffered a thrombotic stroke or a heart attack. An obvious question is how much aspirin is required on a daily basis to achieve optimum protection?

One 162 mg dose of aspirin irreversibly destroys the ability of platelets to form the aggregates that are involved in a thrombotic, ischemic stroke. The platelets recover their ability to aggregate at a rate of about 10% a day. Thus, a prophylactic regimen of a one-time, 325-mg dose (standard dosage) followed by a daily dose of 81 mg (baby aspirin) or even half a baby aspirin would provide the full beneficial effect of aspirin as far as prevention of secondary cardiovascular events is concerned. [1]

Limited data suggest that 100 mg of aspirin every other day is also effective in suppressing platelet function. [19]

The 325-mg loading dose, if taken in oral form, is effective within about an hour of ingestion. However, absorption and complete destruction of platelet activity can be achieved in 15 minutes by chewing and then swallowing the tablet, or by taking the aspirin in the form of Alka-Seltzer [1].

COMBINATIONS WITH CLOPIDOGREL OR WARFARIN

Clopidogrel + aspirin versus warfarin alone

Current medical practice specifies treatment with warfarin (Coumadin) for 3 weeks prior to and for 4 weeks after electrical cardioversion of AF. Warfarin has many drawbacks such as a high risk of internal bleeding and hemorrhagic stroke and the need to undergo frequent testing in order to determine the correct dosage for maintaining the desired INR. Italian physicians at *Campo di Marte Hospital* in Lucca have discovered that a combination of aspirin and clopidogrel (Plavix) may be just as effective as warfarin in preventing thrombosis and stroke related to cardioversion.

Their clinical trial involved 30 patients (11 women), 18 of whom had persistent AF and 12 of whom had low-risk permanent AF. Patients with a prior stroke or TIA, left ventricular dysfunction (ejection fraction less than 50%), mitral valve disease, prosthetic heart valves, coronary artery disease or untreated diabetes or hypertension were not included in the trial. After a thorough medical examination, including measurement of bleeding time, INR and thromboxane B2 (an important indicator of platelet aggregability), the patients underwent transesophageal echocardiography (TEE) to check for blood clots in the atrium and left atrial appendage (LAA). No clots or dense spontaneous echo-contrast (SEC) were observed in any of the patients. The study participants were then randomly assigned to receive warfarin (to an INR of 2.0-3.0) for 3 weeks or a 1-week course of 100 mg/day of aspirin followed by a 3-week course of 100 mg/day of aspirin plus 75 mg/day of clopidogrel.

At the end of the treatment period, the TEE and blood tests were repeated. The INR had not changed in the aspirin/clopidogrel group, but had increased in the warfarin group. However, aspirin by itself decreased thromboxane B2 levels by 98% (no further change with clopidogrel) and the aspirin/clopidogrel combination increased bleeding time by an astonishing 144%. The repeat TEE showed no clots or dense SEC and there were no strokes, TIAs or bleeding incidents in either group during the treatment period nor in the 4-week period following attempted cardioversion. The researchers conclude that aspirin + clopidogrel may be a safe alternative to warfarin in the pre and post electrical cardioversion period. NOTE: This study was funded by Bristol-Myers Squibb, Italy. [20]

Safety of clopidogrel + aspirin

While there is evidence that stroke prevention therapy with a combination of clopidogrel (Plavix) and aspirin is effective and safe in the short term there is concern that prolonged use of this combination may result in an unacceptable increase in intracranial bleeding (hemorrhagic stroke).

A group of researchers from *Sun Yat-Sen University in China* evaluated the results of fourteen clinical trials designed to evaluate the relative effectiveness and safety of aspirin alone versus aspirin + clopidogrel therapy in the prevention of ischemic and hemorrhagic stroke.

Six of the trials were short-term (1 month or less) and involved a total of 54,800 patients at high risk for ischemic stroke. Patients were randomized to dual antiplatelet therapy with clopidogrel + aspirin or to monotherapy with aspirin alone. The incidence of stroke (ischemic + hemorrhagic) in the dual antiplatelet group was 1.6% vs 2.2% in the aspirin group for a relative risk reduction of 24%. Major bleeding incidence was 0.74% in the dual antiplatelet group versus 0.66% in the aspirin group for a relative risk increase of 11%. The incidence of intracranial bleeding was 0.25% in the dual antiplatelet group versus 0.23% in the aspirin group for a relative risk increase of 8%. The researchers conclude that dual antiplatelet therapy for less than one month is safe and effective in high vascular risk patients.

The remaining eight trials were long-term (3 months or longer) and involved a total of 42,000 patients at high risk for ischemic stroke. Patients were randomized to dual antiplatelet therapy with clopidogrel + aspirin or to monotherapy with aspirin alone. The incidence of stroke (ischemic + hemorrhagic) in the dual antiplatelet group was 3.4% vs 4.3% in the aspirin group for a relative risk reduction of 19%. Major bleeding incidence was 4.6% in the dual antiplatelet group versus 0.3.0% in the aspirin group for a relative risk increase of 52%. The incidence of intracranial bleeding was 1.4% in the dual antiplatelet group versus 0.8% in the aspirin group for a relative risk increase of 76%. The researchers conclude that dual antiplatelet therapy for more than three months substantially increases the risk of major bleeding and intracranial bleeding in high vascular risk patients. [21]

Aspirin and warfarin: Should they be used together?

It is well established that combining aspirin and warfarin therapy in AF patients increases the risk of major bleeding. Thus, it is surprising that a study carried out by *Duke University* researchers found that 35% of AF patients prescribed warfarin for stroke prevention had also been prescribed aspirin. The study was part of the ORBIT-AF study and involved 7347 AF patients on oral anticoagulation with warfarin. Of the 35% of study participants prescribed both warfarin and aspirin, 39% had no atherosclerosis or other condition that would warrant prescribing aspirin in addition to warfarin. Conversely, 37% of patients with known cardiovascular disease who might benefit from added aspirin were only prescribed warfarin. Furthermore, a significant proportion of patients prescribed both warfarin and aspirin was known to have elevated bleeding risk. Not surprisingly, patients prescribed both warfarin and aspirin had a relative

50% greater risk of being hospitalized for major bleeding and a 3-fold increased risk of suffering a hemorrhagic stroke when compared to patients on warfarin only. These findings confirm earlier results from a Danish study which concluded that combining warfarin and aspirin doubles the risk of bleeding events when compared to warfarin alone.

The authors of the *Duke University* study conclude that physicians prescribing warfarin or one of the newer anticoagulants to AF patients need to carefully consider the benefit/risk ratio of adding aspirin.

This study adds to the proof that aspirin, whether used on its own or in combination with warfarin, is not innocuous and should be used with caution in AF patients. One of the authors of the study, Dr. Eric Peterson put it this way, *"In general, if I see a patient in my clinic who has only atrial fibrillation and no other risk factors, they should not be on aspirin because I know for sure their risk of bleeding is going to be one and a half times what it was before."* [22,23]

NOTE: Discontinuing long-term use of aspirin may temporarily increase risk of stroke and TIA. [11,12]

OTHER OBSERVATIONS

Preventive properties of aspirin decline over time

Aspirin (acetylsalicylic acid) is widely used in the prevention of heart attacks and stroke. It works by preventing platelet aggregation in the blood, specifically that induced by collagen and adenosine diphosphate (ADP). Researchers at Rome's *La Sapienza University* now report that aspirin's antiplatelet effect decreases markedly with continued use. Their clinical trial involved 64 men and 86 women who were treated with aspirin (100 or 330 mg/day) and a matched control group of 80 patients who received 250 mg/day of ticlopidine (Ticlid), another antiplatelet agent. The researchers measured the degree of platelet aggregation induced by collagen and ADP at baseline and after 2, 6, 12 and 24 months. They also measured the delay (lag phase) between the addition of collagen and the beginning of aggregation. Their results were:

- Collagen-induced platelet aggregation declined from 88.2% to 37.9% after 2 months of treatment with aspirin. However, after 1 year it had risen to 58.5% and after 2 years to 61.9% indicating that most patients lost their sensitivity to aspirin with time. After 2 years 43% of all aspirin-treated patients had the same degree of collagen-induced platelet aggregation as they had prior to their treatment with aspirin.

- The collagen-induced lag phase was significantly prolonged after 2 months of treatment when compared to baseline (76.6 seconds versus 36.1 seconds). However, after 2 years the lag time had fallen to 42.5 seconds. After 2 years 42% of aspirin-treated patients had the same lag phase as before they began aspirin therapy.

- Aspirin inhibited ADP-induced platelet aggregation to a significantly lesser degree than that observed in regard to collagen-induced aggregation. The baseline value was 85.1% with a decline to 68.3% at 12 months and a subsequent gradual return towards baseline after 2 years of treatment.

- Ticlopidine did not affect collagen-induced aggregation or lag phase significantly, but did result in a substantial and sustained drop in ADP-induced aggregation from 86.1% at baseline to 37.2% after 2 years.

The aspirin results were not affected by dosage (100 mg or 330 mg/day). The finding that aspirin loses its platelet aggregation preventive effects with continued use, thus making patients insensitive to it over time, is a serious concern. Other research has shown that patients who are not sensitive to aspirin therapy have more than twice (24% versus 10%) the rate of cardiovascular events than do those who are sensitive to aspirin. The researchers urge further studies to determine if a combination of clopidogrel (Plavix) and aspirin may maintain antiplatelet aggregation benefits over time. [24]

Perils of aspirin discontinuation

It is estimated that more than 50 million Americans now take a daily aspirin for the prevention of cardiovascular disease. While there is evidence that this practice may help prevent heart attacks in high-risk populations, there is no evidence that it may help prevent a first stroke or TIA (transient ischemic attack) in low-risk patients such as lone afibbers. Nevertheless, the ritual of the daily aspirin is clearly very popular and it is therefore of concern that interrupting this ritual may result in an increased risk of stroke.

Researchers at the *University Hospital in Lausanne* report a 3-fold increased risk of ischemic stroke in a group of high-risk patients who discontinued their aspirin therapy prior to scheduled surgery, because they experienced bleeding complications or interactions with other drugs, or because they or their physician decided that they no longer needed the aspirin. The study included 309 patients with an average age of 72 years who had suffered a recent stroke or TIA, and a control group of 309 patients who had a history of stroke or TIA, but had not suffered an event in the last 6 months. Neither group was particularly healthy with about 70% having hypertension, and 36% and 18% (control group) respectively having coronary heart disease. Thirteen participants in the patient group and 4 in the control group had discontinued aspirin at least 4 weeks prior to their TIA or stroke (patient group) or 4 weeks prior to being interviewed (control group).

The researchers found (after correcting for possible confounding variables such as coronary heart disease) that those who discontinued aspirin were 3.4 times more likely to experience a TIA or ischemic stroke than were patients who remained on the aspirin. Seventy percent of the strokes occurred within 10 days after discontinuation (mean: 9 days). The researchers conclude that the discontinuation of aspirin therapy could increase the risk of ischemic stroke in patients with multiple cardiovascular risk factors, mainly in those with coronary heart disease. [11,12]

The patient groups evaluated in this study had multiple cardiovascular risk factors including hypertension, coronary heart disease, and diabetes. Thus, it is not at all clear whether the increased stroke risk accompanying aspirin withdrawal applies to afibbers with no underlying heart disease or other stroke risk factors. My guess would be that it probably does not. Nevertheless, if an afibber wishes to wean off the daily aspirin it may be prudent to replace it, at least for a couple of months, with one or more natural antiplatelet aggregation agents such as vitamin C, vitamin E, vitamin B6, niacin, fish oil, ginkgo biloba, or garlic.

Gender differences in aspirin effectiveness

Aspirin has been found effective in the prevention of heart attack (myocardial infarction), ischemic stroke, and cardiovascular death in patients who have already experienced a heart attack or stroke. Its benefits in <u>primary prevention</u>, that is in the prevention of a first heart attack or stroke, are much less clear. Researchers at the *University Medical Center in Utrecht* have published a major study aimed at determining the benefits and risks of taking a daily aspirin for primary prevention of cardiovascular events. Taking into account all major studies on the subject as well as discharge statistics from Dutch hospitals, the researchers developed a computer model for predicting the risk of a first heart attack, ischemic stroke, hemorrhagic stroke, major gastrointestinal bleeding, and death in four specific age groups of men and women who were, or were not, taking aspirin on a daily basis.

Using a 55-year-old man with no cardiovascular risk factors as an example, they found an annual incidence of a first heart attack to be 0.40%/year with no aspirin and 0.28%/year with daily aspirin, or a relative risk decrease of 30%. There was no decrease in risk of a first ischemic stroke, but the relative risk increase of a first hemorrhagic stroke was 42%, and that of major gastrointestinal bleeding 42%. The daily aspirin did not prevent a first heart attack in 55-year-old women, but did reduce the risk of ischemic stroke from 0.07%/year to 0.05%/year, or a relative risk reduction of 24%. However, this benefit was offset by a relative risk increase of hemorrhagic stroke of 5% and of major gastrointestinal bleeding of 70%.

Overall, the researchers concluded that the risk involved in the daily aspirin ritual outweighs the benefit in healthy 55-year-old women. A healthy 55-year-old man may gain 3 days of "Quality Adjusted Life Years" (QALY) over a 10-year period by taking aspirin on a daily basis.

The net benefits of daily aspirin usage increased with increasing age and the presence of cardiovascular risk factors. For healthy men, the gain in QALY over a 10-year period was 9 days at age 65 years and 15 days at age 75 years. Corresponding numbers for women were a loss of one day at age 65 years and a gain of 6 days at age 75. However, for men with 5 times normal cardiovascular risk the net gain in QALY over a 10-year period was 34 days at age 55, 68 days at age 65, and 108 days at age 75. Corresponding numbers for women were 2 days, 12 days, and 38 days.

The researchers conclude that for most women aspirin treatment results in increased health care costs and worse health outcomes. However, for women 65 years or older with 5-times-increased cardiovascular risk, aspirin may have a favourable benefit/risk ratio. The benefits for healthy men are not impressive until age 75, but daily aspirin would generally seem to be beneficial for men with moderate or high risk for cardiovascular disease. [25]

The major "take-home" message from this study is that one size definitely does not fit all when it comes to using aspirin for prevention of a first cardiovascular event. In general, aspirin may benefit men with a 10-year cardiovascular disease risk greater than 10% and women with a 10-year cardiovascular disease risk greater than 15%. [26]

REFERENCES

1. Campbell, CL, et al. Aspirin dose for the prevention of cardiovascular disease: A systematic review. JAMA, Vol. 297, May 9, 2007, pp. 2018-24
2. Sato, H, et al. Low-dose aspirin for prevention of stroke in low-risk patients with atrial fibrillation. Stroke, Vol. 37, February 2006, pp. 447-51
3. Intermountain Medical Center. "New study finds antithrombotic therapy has no benefit for low-risk atrial fibrillation patients." Science Daily, 17 March 2017
4. Golive, A, et al. The population-based long-term impact of anticoagulant and antiplatelet therapies in low-risk patients with atrial fibrillation. American Journal of Cardiology. Vol. 120, July 1, 2017, pp. 75-82.
5. Bartolucci, AA and Howard, G. Meta-analysis of data from the 6 primary prevention trials of cardiovascular events using aspirin. American Journal of Cardiology, Vol. 98, September 15, 2006, pp. 746-50
6. Hayden, M, et al. Aspirin for the primary prevention of cardiovascular events. Annals of Internal Medicine, Vol. 136, January 15, 2002, pp. 161-72
7. U.S. Food & Drug Administration. Use of Aspirin for Primary Prevention of Heart Attack and Stroke.
   https://www.fda.gov/drugs/resourcesforyou/consumers/ucm390574.htm
8. Baigent, C, et al. Aspirin in the primary and secondary prevention of vascular disease. The Lancet, Vol. 373, May 30, 2009, pp. 1849-60
9. Dorresteijn, JAN, et al. Aspirin for primary prevention of vascular events in women: individualized prediction of treatment effects. European Heart Journal, Vol. 32, 2011, pp. 2962-69
10. De Berardis, G, et al. Association of aspirin use with major bleeding in patients with and without diabetes. Journal of the American Medical Association (JAMA), Vol. 307, June 6, 2012, pp. 2286-94
11. Maulaz, AB, et al. Effect of discontinuing aspirin therapy on the risk of brain ischemic stroke. Archives of Neurology, Vol. 62, August 2005, pp. 1217-20
12. Llinas, RH. Could discontinuation of aspirin therapy be a trigger for stroke? Nature Clinical Practice Neurology, Vol. 2, June 2006, pp. 300-01

13. Uchiyama S, et al. Aspirin for stroke prevention in elderly patients with vascular risk factors: Japanese Primary Prevention Project. Stroke. Vol. 47 (6), June 2016, pp. 1605-11

14. Saito Y, et al. Low-dose aspirin for primary prevention of cardiovascular events in patients with type 2 diabetes mellitus. Circulation, Vol 135 (7), February 2017, pp. 659-670

15. Derry, S and Loke, YK. Risk of gastrointestinal haemorrhage with long term use of aspirin: Meta-analysis. BMJ, Vol. 321, November 11, 2000, 1183-87

16. Tramer, MR. Aspirin, like all other drugs, is a poison. BMJ, Vol. 321, November 11, 2000, 1170-71

17. Pirmohamed, M, et al. Adverse drug reactions as cause of admission to hospital: Prospective analysis of 18,820 patients. BMJ, Vol. 329, July 3, 2004, pp. 15-19

18. Kelly, JP, et al. Risk of aspirin-associated major upper-gastrointestinal bleeding with enteric-coated or buffered product. Lancet, Vol. 348, November 23, 1996, pp. 1413-16

19. Ridker, PM, et al. Anti-platelet effects of 100 mg alternate day oral aspirin: a randomized, double-blind, placebo-controlled trial of regular and enteric-coated formulations in men and women. Journal of Cardiovascular Risk 1996; 3:209-212

20. Lorenzoni, R, et al. Short-term prevention of thromboembolic complications in patients with atrial fibrillation with aspirin plus clopidogrel. American Heart Journal, Vol. 148, July 2004, pp. 11-18

21. Chen S, et al. Efficacy and safety of adding clopidogrel to aspirin on stroke prevention among high vascular risk patients: a meta-analysis of randomized controlled trials. PLoS One, Vol 9 (8), August 2014, pp. 1-10

22. Steinberg, BA, et al. Use and associated risks of concomitant aspirin therapy with oral anticoagulation in patients with atrial fibrillation. Circulation, Vol. 128, August 13, 2013, pp. 721-28

23. Patrono, C and Andreotti, F. Antithrombotic therapy for patients with atrial fibrillation and atherothrombotic vascular disease. Circulation, Vol. 128, August 13, 2013, pp. 684-86 (editorial)

24. Pulcinelli, FM, et al. Inhibition of platelet aggregation by aspirin progressively decreases in long-term treated patients. Journal of the American College of Cardiology, Vol. 43, March 17, 2004, pp. 979-84

25. Greving, JP, et al. Cost-effectiveness of aspirin treatment in the primary prevention of cardiovascular disease events in subgroups based on age, gender, and varying cardiovascular risk. Circulation, Vol. 117, June 3, 2008, pp. 2875-83

26. Mosca, L. Aspirin chemoprevention – one size does not fit all [Editorial]. Circulation, Vol. 117, June 3, 2008, pp. 2844-46

Chapter 13

Stroke Prevention with Warfarin

Despite several studies unequivocally showing that anticoagulation therapy does not benefit but may actually harm lone afibbers who have no or, at the most, one risk factor for ischemic stroke, warfarin is still widely prescribed for this patient population. A study carried out by a team from *Massachusetts General Hospital, University of California, and Kaiser Permanente of Northern California* will, hopefully, go a long way towards banishing the excessive prescription of warfarin (Coumadin) for lone afibbers. The California study involved 13,559 patients with nonvalvular atrial fibrillation who were followed for 6 years, accumulating a total of over 66,000 person-years of actual experience on warfarin usage in AF. At entry to the study about 53% of the patients were on warfarin.

In past studies aimed at proving the benefits of warfarin therapy among afibbers the focus has been entirely on the prevention of ischemic stroke with no, or very scant, attention paid to the harm done by the drug. The California study takes a bold step forward in this respect in that it introduces a new concept "net clinical benefit". In other words, it considers both the benefit (reduction in ischemic stroke) and harm (increase in hemorrhagic stroke) in administering the drug. **Net Clinical Benefit** (NCB) is defined as:

NCB = (TE rate off warfarin – TE rate on warfarin) – W x (ICH rate on warfarin – ICH rate off warfarin)

- TE rate is the annualized rate of thromboembolic events (ischemic stroke and systemic emboli)
- W is a weighting factor designed to reflect the fact that the consequences of a hemorrhagic stroke (intracranial bleeding) are far more serious than that of an ischemic stroke. The authors used a W equal to 1.5.
- ICH rate is the annualized rate of intracranial bleeding (incl. hemorrhagic stroke).

During the 6-year follow-up there were 407 thromboembolic events, 93% of which were ischemic strokes, in the total group treated with warfarin vs. 685 in patients not receiving warfarin, resulting in annualized TE rates of 1.25% and 2.29% respectively. ICH rates were 0.33% and 0.57% respectively. Not surprisingly, the net clinical benefit of warfarin therapy was highest for patients with a serious risk of stroke and negligible to negative in other cases. Thus, afibbers with a $CHADS_2$ score (this score assigns 1 point each for congestive heart failure, hypertension, age 75 years or older and diabetes, and 2 points for previous stroke or TIA) of 0 (no risk factors for stroke) had a NCB of –0.11% indicating that for this group, which includes most lone afibbers, warfarin therapy is actually more likely to be harmful than beneficial. The likelihood of harm was particularly strong among those aged 65 years or less where the NCB was –0.25%. On the other hand, for patients over the age of 85 years, NCB was a positive 2.34% and for those who had already suffered a stroke it was 2.48%.

The researchers conclude that the net benefit of warfarin therapy is essentially zero in atrial fibrillation patients with a CHADS$_2$ score of 0 or 1, i.e. with, at the most, one risk factor for ischemic stroke. [1]

In an accompanying editorial Drs. Robert Hart and Jonathan Halperin (*University of Texas Health Sciences Center*) make the following salient statements:

- "The authors failed to include major gastrointestinal bleeding as a negative impact of warfarin therapy. Had they done so the NCB would likely have been even less favourable.
- The annual rate of ischemic stroke among afibbers with one stroke risk factor was only 1.2% even without warfarin therapy." Editor's note: *This number is far lower than the 4 to 5% per year reported in the original studies aimed at proving the benefits of warfarin in stroke prevention.*
- "Participants with CHADS$_2$ scores of 0 and 1, about half of the afibbers in the study, gained no benefit from warfarin therapy." [2]

Ever since I first began researching the role of warfarin in stroke prevention among lone afibbers, I invariably arrived at the conclusion that for a lone afibber with none or, at most, one risk factor for ischemic stroke warfarin therapy is contra-indicated. Not only is warfarin not beneficial in this patient group, but considering its many potential adverse effects (hemorrhagic stroke, major gastrointestinal bleeding, serious interactions with foods and herbs, arterial calcification, osteoporosis, skin necrosis, and serious eye damage in patients with age-related macular degeneration) and the difficulty in maintaining INR within the prescribed range, it is likely to cause more harm than good. It is indeed rewarding to see this conclusion confirmed by such a large and well-designed study.

It is estimated that about 90% of afib-related blood clots (thrombi) form in the left atrial appendage (small sac attached to the left atrium). The thrombi can escape into the blood stream and cause a stroke (cerebral infarction). Researchers at *University of Bonn in Germany* have found that anticoagulants are not very effective in eliminating left atrial appendage (LAA) thrombi or in preventing stroke. Their study involved 43 patients who had been admitted to hospital with permanent AF and who had been found to have thrombi in the LAA. Twenty-three (53%) of the patients were effectively anticoagulated before admission to hospital (they still had atrial thrombi) and the remaining 47% were put on phenprocoumon (a cousin of warfarin) before being released from hospital. The patients were re-examined at 1, 3, 6 and 12 months after discharge using transesophageal echocardiography (TEE) to check for LAA thrombi and magnetic resonance imaging (MRI) to check for embolisms (blood clots) in the brain.

The researchers found that 16% of the LAA thrombi disappeared after 1 month, 42% after 3 months, 49% after 6 months, and 56% after 12 months. Patients whose thrombi disappeared had smaller initial thrombi and smaller left atrial size. Six patients (14%) developed clinically apparent neurologic deficits and cerebral infarctions (stroke) as documented by cranial MRI. The researchers conclude that, "continued effective anticoagulation does not prevent thromboembolic events in patients with permanent AF and prevalent LA thrombi". [3]

This study clearly shows that coumarin derivatives (warfarin and phenprocoumon) are not very effective in preventing strokes caused by blood clots in the left atrial appendage, nor are they very effective in eliminating (dissolving) existing blood clots. That this is so should not come as a surprise. Coumarins work by destroying vitamin K and thus reducing the production of vitamin K-dependent clotting factors. In other words, they work to prevent the formation of blood clots. There is, as far as I know, no evidence that they have any effect on fibrinolysis (the digestion and removal of existing blood clots). The body does produce fibrinolytic enzymes that, over time, remove blood clots, so it is likely that any reduction in the number and size of thrombi observed during the study was due to the body's own natural blood clot removing capabilities rather than to anticoagulation.

The study also underscores the relative futility of placing prospective ablation candidates on warfarin for 1 or 2 months prior to the procedure. More than half the patients admitted to the study had LAA thrombi even though they had been effectively anticoagulated prior to admission – only a small percentage of the clots disappeared during 1 month of anticoagulation. Fortunately, there are highly effective alternatives. Nattokinase has proven ability to prevent the formation of blood clots and is also effective in dissolving existing clots. Vitamin C inhibits plasminogen activator inhibitor PAI-1 and thereby allows the beneficial plasminogen activators to accelerate fibrinolysis. It should also be noted that, while blood clot formation in the LAA is a real and serious problem in patients with permanent AF and underlying heart problems, there is no evidence that it is a problem in otherwise healthy lone paroxysmal afibbers.

A group of Italian researchers (*GISSI-AF investigators*) has concluded that the risk of a thromboembolic (TE) event is low in both paroxysmal and persistent AF with moderate stroke risk. Their study involved 1234 participants in the GISSI-AF trial originally designed to evaluate the efficacy of the angiotensin II receptor blocker valsartan (Diovan) in preventing AF recurrence in patients with hypertension.

The average age of the participants was 67 years, 40% were women (46% in the paroxysmal group), 62% had paroxysmal and 38% had persistent AF. The majority (85%) had hypertension, 4% had coronary artery disease, 8% had heart failure or reduced left ventricular ejection fraction, and 6% had suffered a prior TE event. Heart failure was significantly more common among persistent afibbers than among paroxysmal ones (14% vs 4%). The average CHADS$_2$ score for the total patient population was 1.41.

During a 1-year intensive follow-up period, 12 patients (0.97%) died, 12 patients (0.97%) suffered a TE event, and 10 patients (0.81%) suffered a major bleeding event (intracranial hemorrhage or major bleed requiring blood transfusion or hospitalization). There was no statistically significant difference in the incidence of TE events, major bleeding events or mortality between the paroxysmal group and the persistent group. However, the rate of TE events was significantly higher in women than in men. The incidence of TE and major bleeding events in untreated patients and in those treated with warfarin or antiplatelet agents is shown below.

Thromboembolic and Bleeding Events, %/year

Type of Treatment	% of total group	TE event	Bleeding event
No treatment	16%	0.5%	0%
Warfarin	48%	0.84%	0.84%
Antiplatelet	34%	1.47%	0.98%
Warfarin + antiplatelet	2%	-	-

Warfarin therapy was significantly more common among persistent afibbers (87% were treated with warfarin) than among paroxysmal afibbers (25% were treated with warfarin). Warfarin therapy was under-prescribed in patients with a $CHADS_2$ score of 2 or greater and overprescribed for those with a $CHADS_2$ score of 0. Thirty-five percent of patients with a zero score were still on warfarin at the end of the study period.

The GISSI investigators conclude that the incidence of TE and bleeding events were remarkably low in both paroxysmal and persistent AF despite a significant degree of over- or under-treatment with warfarin. [4]

This study adds to accumulating evidence that warfarin is often overprescribed and is not terribly effective except in the case of patients having suffered a previous stroke or TIA. It is also clear that the net benefit of warfarin therapy leaves much to be desired and that it is inappropriate in the case of lone afibbers with no risk factors for stroke.

Researchers at the *University of Toronto* carried out an investigation aimed at determining if patients (aged 66 years and older) are at increased risk of stroke if they discontinue warfarin therapy after suffering major trauma. Their study involved 8450 warfarin-taking individuals who had sustained major traumas (82% due to falls) during a 10-year period. During the 6 months following the trauma, 78% of the study participants resumed anticoagulation with warfarin, while the remaining 22% did not. During an average 3.3 years of follow-up a total of 592 patients (2.2% a year) sustained an ischemic stroke and 399 (1.5% a year) experienced a heart attack (myocardial infarction). There was no difference in the incidence of ischemic stroke and heart attacks between the patients on warfarin and those who had discontinued anticoagulation therapy. The long-term risk of major hemorrhage (hemorrhagic stroke and internal bleeding requiring blood transfusion) was significantly higher among patients on warfarin (1.9% a year) than among those who had discontinued the drug

(1.3% a year). The incidence of deep vein thrombosis was, however, almost twice as high among patients not on warfarin, but was fairly low overall (0.4% a year). There was no difference in the incidence of pulmonary embolism in the two groups. The researchers conclude that discontinuing warfarin in patients prone to falls will not increase their risk of stroke and heart attack, but will materially reduce the risk of major hemorrhage at the expense of a fairly small increase in the risk of deep vein thrombosis. [5]

This study certainly casts considerable doubt on the wisdom of routinely anticoagulating elderly patients at risk for ischemic stroke, particularly if they are prone to falls. The slight increase in deep vein thrombosis could easily be counteracted by giving nattokinase to patients not on warfarin. At least one clinical trial has found nattokinase to provide very effective protection against deep vein thrombosis. [6]

BLEEDING RISK WITH WARFARIN THERAPY

Cardiologists at *University Hospital in Groningen, The Netherlands* involved in trials to determine the relative merits of rate control versus rhythm control in AF have studied the results in a subgroup of lone afibbers. They define lone atrial fibrillation as AF not associated with hypertension or any underlying heart disease. Their study group included 522 patients with AF of which 89 had the lone variety (persistent). The lone afibbers were more likely to be men, tended to be younger (average of 65 years versus 69 years), and had fewer complaints of fatigue and breathing difficulties. During a mean follow-up of 2.3 years three lone afibbers (3%) died from internal bleeding or hemorrhagic stroke. They were all on warfarin at the time of their death with an INR in excess of 3.5. Two patients suffered non-fatal bleeding (also on anticoagulants) and 2 experienced an ischemic stroke or TIA. The two lone afibbers having a stroke or TIA were not taking anticoagulants at the time even though they had one or more additional risk factors for stroke. Among non-lone afibbers, 6 (1%) died from bleeding, while another 16 (4%) suffered serious bleeding. Thirty-three (8%) had a stroke or TIA even though 70% of them were on anticoagulation at the time of their stroke.

None of the lone afibbers suffered severe adverse effects from their antiarrhythmic drugs, while 3% of the non-lone afibbers did. None of the lone afibbers died from heart disease or heart failure, while 5% of the non-lone afibbers did. Overall, death or serious adverse effects were significantly more common among lone afibbers using rate control than among those using rhythm control, but due to the small sample size the researchers could not conclude whether rate control is an acceptable alternative for patients with persistent lone AF. They do conclude though that lone AF is a far more benign disorder than is AF with underlying heart disease. [7]

Although the sample size was small, it is clear that the most serious complication facing lone afibbers is death or serious bleeding from inadequately controlled anticoagulation (warfarin) therapy. The study provided no evidence that lone afibbers with no additional risk factors for stroke would benefit from warfarin therapy – actually quite the opposite.

Clinical trials carried out in 1994 concluded that the use of warfarin in atrial fibrillation (AF) patients was relatively safe with an annual rate of major hemorrhage of 1.3%. Major hemorrhage is defined as a fatal bleeding incident, a bleeding incident requiring hospitalization with transfusion of 2 or more units of packed red blood cells, or a bleeding incident involving a critical site (intracranial, intraspinal, pericardial, intraocular, etc). The average annual reduction in ischemic stroke rate in the five 1994 trials was 1.8% for patients over the age of 75 years with no risk factors for stroke, and 6.9% for those with one or more risk factors. Thus, it was concluded that treating older patients with warfarin had a favourable benefit/risk ratio.

Elaine Hylek and colleagues at the *Boston University School of Medicine* have questioned this conclusion. Their clinical trial involved 472 AF patients with an average age of 77 years (32% were 80 years or older). Forty-seven percent of the patients were women and 91% had one or more risk factors for ischemic stroke (75% had hypertension and 35% had coronary artery disease). After being admitted with a first AF episode (59%), a recurrent episode (35%), or permanent AF (6%) all study participants were prescribed warfarin with an INR target of 2.0 – 3.0. Management of warfarin dosage was carried out by the hospital's own anti-coagulation clinic. More than 10,000 INR measurements were made during the 1-year follow-up period. The time spent within the prescribed INR range (2.0 – 3.0) was only 58% with 29% being spent below 2.0 and 13% above 3.0.

The overall incidence of major hemorrhage was 7.2% and that of intracranial hemorrhage (hemorrhagic stroke) was 2.5%. A third of the hemorrhagic strokes were fatal and 89% of them occurred in patients 75 years or older. The incidence of major hemorrhage was particularly high (13.1%) among patients 80 years or older. Age and an INR greater than 4 were strong risk factors and 58% of the major hemorrhages occurred within the first 90 days after initiation of warfarin therapy. Concomitant use of aspirin was also a significant risk factor for major bleeding and there was no indication that taking 81 mg/day was any safer than taking the standard 325 mg/day.

During the study 26% of participants aged 80 years or older were taken off warfarin – 81% because of safety concerns and 19% because they regained normal sinus rhythm. The Boston researchers conclude that the risk of major bleeding among older AF patients on warfarin has been significantly underestimated in previous trials. They also point out that the rate of bleeding observed in their closely controlled clinical trial would likely be significantly lower than that experienced in the "real world". [8]

In an accompanying editorial Dr. George Wyse of the *Health Sciences Center* in Calgary, Canada states, "there is reason to be sceptical about net benefit when warfarin is used in some elderly patients with AF." Dr. Wyse also points out that warfarin therapy would appear to be over-utilized in patients with low to moderate risk of ischemic stroke. A recent European study found that 50% of AF patients with no risk factors for stroke were being treated with warfarin or similar anticoagulants. [9]

This study adds to the growing evidence that warfarin therapy is far from ideal for AF patients. It would appear to be over-prescribed for patients who don't need it and of no overall benefit for older patients with one or more risk factors for ischemic stroke.

Surgeons have long been aware that trauma patients on warfarin (Coumadin) have significantly poorer survival than do those who are not anticoagulated at the time of their accident. In order to determine more precisely exactly how dangerous being on warfarin is, Dr. Lesly Dossett and colleagues at *Vanderbilt University Medical Center* reviewed the records of 1,230,422 trauma patients listed in the National Trauma Databank maintained by the American College of Surgeons. They found that 36,270 of the patients were on warfarin when their trauma occurred. After adjusting for comorbidities associated with warfarin, they found that its use increased trauma-related mortality by 30%. The Vanderbilt team also noted that the use of warfarin had almost doubled in the period 2002 to 2006. Overall, 2.3% of the patient population was on warfarin in 2002 as compared to 4.0% in 2006. Among patients over the age of 65 years warfarin usage increased from 7.3% in 2002 to 12.8% in 2006. [10]

The finding that trauma victims on warfarin therapy experienced a substantially increased rate of mortality is disturbing indeed, particularly in view of the fact that an approved and effective antidote to warfarin poisoning is readily available. This, unfortunately, is not the case when it comes to the new oral anticoagulants like Pradaxa and Eliquis.

Although the bleeding risk involved in warfarin therapy has been evaluated in several clinical trials, there is very little data on the actual incidence of hemorrhage amongst patients not participating in clinical trials. It is conceivable that there could be a significant difference between clinical trial incidence and the incidence found in the real world, since time spent in the usually recommended INR range of 2.0 to 3.0 is often as low as 50% in community surveys, but much higher in closely controlled clinical trials.

A group of *Canadian researchers* sponsored by the *Ontario Drug Policy Research Network* reports the results of a study aimed at determining the actual incidence of hemorrhage in a population of 125,195 atrial fibrillation (AF) patients who were prescribed warfarin during the period April 1, 1997 to March 31, 2008. The average age of the study participants (evenly split between men and women) was 77 years with 57.5% being 76 years or older. The majority had one or more comorbid conditions such as hypertension (75%), congestive heart failure (35%), and diabetes (24%), which would increase their risk of ischemic stroke. Only 7% had a $CHADS_2$ score of 0 and 69% had a score of 2 or higher. Patients were followed until one of the following events occurred:

- Visit to hospital for hemorrhage
- End of warfarin therapy
- Death
- Five years of follow-up
- End of study period (March 31, 2010)

If a patient had multiple hospital admissions during warfarin therapy, only the first admission was counted.

The overall rate of hemorrhage (major bleeding) was 3.8%/year. However, during the first 30 days of treatment it was 11.8% (16.7% for patients with a $CHADS_2$ score of 4 or greater). Over the 5-year follow-up, 10,840 patients were hospitalized for major bleeding and, of these, 1963 (18.1%) died in hospital or within 7 days of being discharged. The mortality was highest (42%) for patients admitted with intracranial hemorrhage (hemorrhagic stroke). The risk of major bleeding was significantly lower for patients with a $CHADS_2$ score of 0 or 1 (1.8% and 2.5% respectively), but was higher among patients aged 76 years or older (4.6%) than among those younger (2.9%). The most common bleeding sites were lower gastrointestinal at 36.5%, upper gastrointestinal at 26.1%, and intracranial (hemorrhagic stroke) at 5.1%. Eighteen percent of patients admitted to hospital with warfarin-related bleeding died in hospital or within 7 days of discharge. Mortality was particularly high (42%) amongst patients admitted for intracranial bleeding.

The researchers conclude that warfarin-related hospital admissions of AF patients is substantially higher than that reported in clinical trials designed to evaluate the safety and efficacy of warfarin therapy. [11]

It seems to me that this study is somewhat misleading in that patients were no longer followed-up once they had experienced a first bleeding event after starting on warfarin therapy. If all warfarin-related hemorrhages had been recorded, I would be very surprised if the annual incidence of bleeding would not have overshadowed any protective effect against ischemic stroke, except in cases where the patient had already suffered a previous stroke.

DANGEROUS WARFARIN COMBINATIONS

Painkillers and warfarin – A lethal combination?

Warfarin (Coumadin) is effective in the prevention of blood clots (thromboembolism) and is frequently prescribed for atrial fibrillation and other conditions requiring anticoagulation. It is a highly toxic drug and its actual level in patients must be monitored frequently. The level is measured with the prothrombin time test and expressed in terms of International Normalized Ratio (INR). An INR of 2.0 to 3.0 is deemed optimum in most patients while an INR of 4.0 or greater markedly increases the risk of internal hemorrhage particularly in the brain. Now researchers at *Harvard Medical School* report that people who take both warfarin and acetaminophen (Tylenol, Paracetamol) vastly increase the risk of elevating their INR above 4.0 and thereby multiply their chances of suffering internal bleeding. Acetaminophen is the most frequently used medication in the United States and many patients on warfarin routinely take it.

The Harvard study involved 93 patients whose routine prothrombin test had produced results above 6.0 and 196 controls whose results were in the target range of 2.0 to 3.0. Patient interviews were conducted within 24 hours of the test results becoming available and covered the use of medications and alcohol and the intake of foods rich in vitamin K during the previous week. The correlation between acetaminophen use and INR was quite astonishing. Patients who had taken four or more regular strength (325 mg) tablets per day for a week were 10 times more likely to have an INR of 6.0 or greater than were the controls. Even just taking two to three tablets a day for a week increased the risk of a dangerously high INR by a factor of almost seven. In general, the use of acetaminophen was much higher among cases (56 %) than among controls (36 %) and the average amount consumed per week was approximately 21 tablets among cases and only 9 tablets among controls.

Several other medications were also found to increase INR as was advanced cancer. Patients with advanced malignancy taking standard dosages of warfarin were found to have a 16-fold increase in their risk of having an INR of 6.0 or higher. On the other hand, patients who regularly consumed alcohol lowered their risk of developing high INRs as did people eating a diet rich in vitamin K-containing foods. The researchers conclude that acetaminophen usage is an important risk factor and recommend increased monitoring of INR values to reduce the frequency of dangerously high levels of anticoagulation. Dr. William Bell, MD of the *Johns Hopkins University School of Medicine* suggests in an accompanying editorial that patients on warfarin who also take acetaminophen need to have their prothrombin time checked once or twice a week to ensure that their INR does not exceed 4.0. [12,13]

Warfarin + aspirin – Not a good idea
Patients at high risk for cardiovascular events are sometimes prescribed a combination of warfarin and aspirin in an attempt to provide added protection. A team of medical doctors from *Canada, Finland, France, and the United States* reports that the combination does not confer added stroke protection among patients with atrial fibrillation, but does increase the incidence of major and minor bleeding events.

The study involved 7300 patients who participated in the SPORTIF III and V trials comparing the efficacy and safety of warfarin and ximelagatran for stroke prevention in AF patients. (NOTE: The trial participants were not lone afibbers, but afibbers with a high risk of ischemic stroke). The trial protocol discouraged the concomitant use of aspirin, but doses up to 100 mg/day were allowed at the discretion of participating physicians. Those prescribed aspirin were significantly more likely to have diabetes, coronary artery disease, and left ventricular dysfunction.

Trial participants were followed for an average of 16.5 months during which time INR was closely controlled between 2.0 and 3.0 and all strokes (ischemic or hemorrhagic), transient ischemic attacks (TIAs), and major and minor bleeding events were recorded. Bleeding events were defined as major if fatal, involving a critical anatomical site, or requiring transfusion of 2 units of blood or more.

The researchers found no significant difference in the incidence of stroke between patients taking warfarin and those taking warfarin + aspirin nor was there any difference between patients taking ximelagatran and those taking ximelagatran + aspirin. Overall, annual ischemic stroke rates ranged from 1.2% to 1.7%. The incidence of major bleeding events was, however, significantly higher for patients taking warfarin + aspirin (3.9%/year) than for those taking warfarin alone (2.3%/year). The rate of minor bleeds was also significantly higher when aspirin was added with a rate from warfarin alone of 37% vs. 63% with warfarin + aspirin. The most common site for major bleeds was the gastrointestinal tract.

The researchers conclude that the results suggest the risks associated with addition of aspirin to anticoagulation in patients with atrial fibrillation outweigh the benefits. [14]

Anticoagulation – Dangerous combinations

Cardiologists at *Copenhagen University Hospital* in Denmark warn that the practice of combining antiplatelet and anticoagulation therapy in the same patients is associated with a substantially higher risk of fatal and non-fatal internal bleeding.

Their study included 118,606 patients who were discharged from hospital between January 1, 1997 and December 31, 2006 with a diagnosis of atrial fibrillation (AF). The mean age of the patients was 74 years and 52% were male. Many had comorbidities such as hypertension (16%), heart failure (18%) or ischemic heart disease (16%), while 7% had suffered a previous ischemic stroke. About 77% were taking antiarrhythmic drugs and 27% were being treated with angiotensin-converting-enzyme (ACE) inhibitors or angiotensin II receptor antagonists. About 70% of the patients were discharged with a prescription for antiplatelet agents and/or warfarin. The pattern of prescriptions was as follows:

- Warfarin – 42.9%
- Aspirin – 40.1%
- Clopidogrel – 3.1%
- Clopidogrel + aspirin – 2.4%
- Warfarin + aspirin – 15.5%
- Warfarin + clopidogrel – 1.2%
- Warfarin + aspirin + clopidogrel – 1.1%

Patients treated only with aspirin were older and more often female than were those in the other treatment groups. During the 10-year follow-up period, 1381 patients (1.2%) experienced a fatal bleeding, while 12,191 (10.3%) were hospitalized as the result of a non-fatal internal bleeding. Using warfarin as a reference point, aspirin-treated patients had a 4% reduced risk of experiencing a bleeding event but all combination treatments were associated with a substantial increase in risk.

- Clopidogrel monotherapy – 45% increased risk
- Aspirin + clopidogrel – 91% increased risk
- Aspirin + warfarin – 75% increased risk
- Clopidogrel + warfarin – 257% increased risk
- Clopidogrel + aspirin + warfarin – 303% increased risk

The use of clopidogrel either alone or in combination was primarily associated with an increased risk of gastrointestinal bleeding. Patients who had experienced a non-fatal bleeding event during therapy had a 145% increased risk of dying during the follow-up period. It is also worth noting that the 3.9% annual bleeding incidence observed in this "real world" study is substantially higher than that found in closely controlled clinical trials. Also, the bleeding incidence during the first year of warfarin therapy is 7% among elderly patients. Perhaps most surprising, there was no indication that combining warfarin with an antiplatelet agent (aspirin, clopidogrel or both) reduced the risk of ischemic stroke.

The article concludes with the following note from the editor, *"They [the Danish researchers] find that adding clopidogrel or aspirin to warfarin monotherapy greatly increases the fatal and non-fatal bleeding risk while showing no benefit to prevention of ischemic stroke."* [15]

This study clearly shows that there is no advantage and much potential risk in using combined antiplatelet/anticoagulation therapy in atrial fibrillation patients needing stroke prevention therapy. It is unfortunate that the authors did not include actual data on the incidence of stroke in the different treatment groups and compared it to a group receiving no treatment.

AGE-RELATED RISK OF WARFARIN THERAPY

The risk of a thromboembolic event [ischemic stroke (cerebral infarction), heart attack (myocardial infarction), or peripheral arterial embolism] increases sharply with age, especially in patients with mechanical heart valve prostheses, atrial fibrillation, or a prior heart attack. These patients, especially older ones, are commonly prescribed warfarin in order to reduce the risk of a thromboembolic event. Unfortunately, warfarin therapy is associated with an increased risk of major hemorrhage (mainly gastrointestinal) and hemorrhagic stroke.

Researchers at *Leiden University Medical Center* in Holland carried out a study to determine the relative risks of thromboembolic and bleeding events in older patients treated with warfarin. The study included 4202 patients treated at a regional anticoagulation clinic. Half of these patients were on warfarin because of atrial fibrillation and their target INR was 2.5 to 3.5. The remaining patients were on warfarin because they had experienced a heart attack or had a mechanical heart valve. At baseline about 13% of patients in the entire study group was under the age of 60 years, 24% were between the ages of 60 and 70 years, 40% between 71 and 80 years, and the remaining 23% were over the age of 80 years.

Overall, the warfarin-treated patients were within their INR target range 61-68% of the time. The incidence (%/year) of ischemic stroke (fatal and non-fatal), heart attack (fatal and non-fatal), hemorrhagic stroke, and major bleeding were as follows:

Stroke and Bleeding Events, %/year

AGE, years EVENT	< 60	61-70	71-80	> 80
Fatal ischemic stroke	0%	0%	0%	0%
Non-fatal ischemic stroke	0.1%	0.4%	0.2%	0.5%
Fatal heart attack	0.3%	0.3%	0.3%	0.5%
Non-fatal heart attack	0.6%	0.7%	1.0%	1.3%
Total thromboembolic events	**1.0%**	**1.4%**	**1.6%**	**2.4%**
Fatal hemorrhagic stroke	0.1%	0.3%	0.3%	0.2%
Non-fatal hemorrhagic stroke	0%	0.2%	0.4%	0.4%
Fatal major bleeding	0%	0.04%	0.07%	0.09%
Non-fatal major bleeding	0%	1.5%	1.8%	3.6%
Total bleeding events	**1.5%**	**2.1%**	**2.5%**	**4.2%**

The researchers conclude that anticoagulant treatment in elderly patients presents a major clinical dilemma and state that, *"The question is whether an overall benefit remains for elderly patients who are treated with oral anticoagulants."*[16]

WARFARIN: THE GENE CONNECTION

The risks of bleeding complications and stroke are highest during the first 3 months of warfarin (Coumadin) therapy. It is also clear that the dosage necessary to achieve an INR of 2.0 to 3.0 varies considerably between patients. Studies have shown that patients who require relatively low daily doses have a considerably higher risk of major bleeding events than do people who need higher doses. Researchers at *Chinese University of Hong Kong* have found that patients requiring lower doses are 6 times more likely to have a genetic abnormality (polymorphism) in the cytochrome P450 enzyme system involved in the metabolism of pharmaceutical drugs and herbs.

The researchers found that determining if patients had the abnormal gene prior to initiating warfarin therapy could reduce the risk of major bleeding from about 8% to about 7% per year. Inasmuch as the cost of genotyping (determining if variant genes are present) is about $100 US and the average cost of treating a major bleeding event is $15,000 US, genotyping would appear to be a worthwhile investment, not only from the patient's point of view, but also from the point of overall cost to the health care system. The researchers emphasize, however, that patients with the variant gene may require closer INR monitoring. [17]

The FDA recently approved a new genetic test designed to determine the presence or absence of three genes affecting warfarin metabolism [CYP2C9 *2, CYP2C9 *3, and VKORC1(C1173T)].

Researchers at *University Of Utah School Of Medicine* report on the first trial of genotype-guided warfarin dosing. Two hundred patients starting on warfarin were randomized into a standard treatment arm and the genotype-guided arm. Patients in the standard arm were given 10 mg/day of warfarin for the first two days, 5 mg/day for the third day, and then an adjusted dosage based on their day 3 INR value. Patients in the genotype-guided arm were given an initial dose of from 2 to 16 mg/day for two days as determined by an algorithm taking into account age, weight, gender, and the presence or absence of the variant genotypes. Dosage was halved on day 3 and then adjusted according to INR. The adjustment was calculated as the ratio of the estimated individual weekly maintenance dose determined with the algorithm to the standard weekly dose. INR measurements were made on days 0, 3, 5, 8, 21, 60, and 90.

Somewhat surprisingly, the use of the genotype algorithm did not reduce the time patients had an INR outside the therapeutic range. In both cases, patients were outside the range about 30% of the time pretty evenly split between being too high and too low. It should be pointed out that the study participants were hospitalized, so likely received better care and follow-up than if they had been outpatients. The researchers did notice that patients in the genotype arm required slightly fewer dose adjustments than did those in the standard arm. They also observed that patients who carried both the CYP2C9 and the VKORC1 variants had a greater risk of experiencing an INR greater than 4 than did those without these two gene variants. They recommend further, much larger (at least 2000 patients) trials to further evaluate their findings. [18]

This study clearly shows that genotype-guided warfarin therapy does not reduce the time spent outside the recommended INR range of 2.0 to 3.0. It is possible that identifying carriers of both the gene variants may avoid some cases of overdosing, but this particular study did not have the statistical power to prove this. Says the lead investigator of the study, Dr. Jeffrey Anderson, *"I think this approach has a lot of promise for the future, but it's maybe not ready for right now."* Dr. Raymond Gibbons of the Mayo Clinic shares this view, *"I definitely do not think doctors should rush out there and start giving genetic tests to all the patients they want to put on warfarin at the moment. Maybe one day this will happen, and yes, it does make sense, but we need evidence that it will have a real benefit, and that's not there yet."*

WARFARIN: THE GENDER CONNECTION

A team of researchers from *University of California, Massachusetts General Hospital and Boston University School of Medicine* has completed a study aimed at determining whether women with afib have a higher risk of ischemic stroke than do men. The study included 13,559 adults with atrial fibrillation. The majority of the study participants had one or more recognized risk factors for stroke, such as hypertension (57.7%), congestive heart failure (26.7%), coronary artery disease (23.9%), or diabetes (14.2%). Only 15.8% of women and 23.8% of men could be classified as non-hypertensive lone afibbers.

The overall incidence of ischemic stroke during 15,494 person years was 2.4%. The annual average rate on warfarin was 1.5% for women and 1.2% for men as compared to 3.5% and 1.8% when not on warfarin. However, the rate among lone afibbers (not on warfarin) with no additional risk factors for stroke was only 0.6% for women and 0.5% for men – in other words, no higher than would be expected in the general population.

The incidence of major hemorrhage (fatal bleeding, blood transfusion requiring two units or more of packed blood cells, or bleeding into a critical anatomical site) was 1.0% a year among warfarin-treated women and 1.1% among men. Of the major hemorrhages 0.36% among women and 0.55% among men were intracranial (hemorrhagic stroke). The authors of the study point out that, *"the health consequences of intracranial hemorrhage are worse than those resulting from the ischemic strokes we seek to prevent through anticoagulation."*[19]

These recent findings confirm earlier ones that neither men nor women with LONE atrial fibrillation and no other risk factors for stroke benefit from warfarin therapy. As a matter of fact, for this group the risk of major hemorrhage is almost twice as high as the risk of ischemic stroke and the risk of hemorrhagic stroke for men on warfarin is actually higher than the risk of ischemic stroke when not on warfarin. Even for lone afibbers with one additional minor risk factor such as hypertension, diabetes or age over 75 years, the benefits of warfarin therapy are not at all clear-cut. Women with one additional risk factor would have an annual ischemic stroke risk of 1.8% if not on warfarin. On warfarin this risk would be reduced to 0.7%, but would be accompanied by a 1.0% risk of major hemorrhage of which 0.36% would be associated with hemorrhagic stroke. For men the ischemic stroke risk when not on warfarin would be 1.2%. On warfarin this would be reduced to 0.7%, but would be accompanied by a 1.1% risk of major hemorrhage of which 0.55% would involve hemorrhagic stroke – in other words, pretty well a toss-up.

WARFARIN: THE VITAMIN K CONNECTION

Warfarin implicated in osteoporosis

Vitamin K is a crucial element in the process of bone formation. As warfarin (Coumadin) is known to inhibit this action of vitamin K, it is relevant to ask the question, "Is long-term use of warfarin associated with an increased risk of osteoporotic fractures?" A team of researchers from *Washington University School of Medicine and the NYU Medical Center* provides the answer. The researchers investigated the association between osteoporotic fractures and warfarin usage in over 14,000 Medicare beneficiaries who were hospitalized with atrial fibrillation. Most of the study participants (70%) had hypertension, 48% had heart failure, and 35% had a history of stroke. A total of 1005 of the study participants (6.9%) experienced an osteoporotic fracture during the 3-year study period. The researchers found that men who had been taking warfarin for a year or more had a 63% higher relative risk of experiencing an osteoporotic fracture when compared to men not taking warfarin. Hip fractures were most common (65% of all fractures) and were associated with a 30-day mortality of 39%. Women and men using warfarin for less than a year did not have an increased risk of osteoporotic fractures.

Other prominent risk factors for osteoporotic fractures were increasing age (63% increased risk per decade), frequent falls (78% increased risk), hyperthyroidism (77% increased risk), dementia, Parkinson's disease or schizophrenia (51% increased risk), and alcoholism (50% increased risk). On the other hand, the use of beta-blockers was associated with a 16% lower risk of osteoporotic fractures.

The researchers point out that patients taking warfarin are often advised to limit their intake of vitamin K-rich green vegetables. They believe this may be poor advice and that ensuring an adequate intake of vitamin K-1 (found especially in green vegetables) and vitamin K-2 (present in fermented dairy and soy products, fish, meat, liver and eggs) would be more appropriate. They also caution that avoiding green vegetables may lead to a folic acid deficiency and subsequent high levels of homocysteine, a known promoter of atherosclerosis. [20]

The results of this study support the findings of other studies that an adequate, but consistent, intake of vitamin K containing foods is advisable for patients taking warfarin. It would also be advisable to undertake an active osteoporosis-prevention program including regular exercise and supplementation with vitamin D and calcium.

Vitamin K stabilizes INR in warfarin therapy

Maintaining an INR (International Normalized Ratio) in the therapeutic range (usually 2.0-3.0) when on warfarin (Coumadin) therapy can be problematical. Some studies have concluded that patients on warfarin are out of range at least a third of the time. Too low an INR increases the risk of an ischemic stroke, while too high a reading increases the risk of a hemorrhagic stroke or a major internal bleeding event. Warfarin works by reducing the amount of vitamin K available for the synthesis of clotting factors II, VII, IX and X. Patients on warfarin are therefore often counseled to avoid dark green leafy vegetables (the major dietary source of vitamin K) and to strictly avoid vitamin K-containing supplements.

Medical doctors at *University of Newcastle upon Tyne in the* UK report that minimizing vitamin K intake while on warfarin might be precisely the wrong thing to do. Their study involved 26 patients (stable) whose INR had remained within the therapeutic range for at least 6 months without a change in warfarin dosage. The daily vitamin K intake of these patients was compared to that of 26 patients (unstable) whose INR had been varying considerably (standard deviation of INR values greater than 0.5) over a 6-month period and thus requiring continuous adjustment of warfarin dosage. All participants carefully weighed their food intake for two 7-day periods and completed detailed food diaries. Analysis of the data showed that the unstable patients had a significantly lower average daily intake of vitamin K (K_1) than did stable patients (29 versus 76 micrograms/day). As a matter of fact, the daily vitamin K intake of the unstable patients was significantly lower than the daily intake of 60-80 micrograms estimated for the general UK population.

The researchers conclude that INR levels can be stabilized by increasing daily vitamin K intake. They point out that even a daily increase in vitamin K intake of 100 micrograms has comparatively little effect on INR (reduction of about 0.2). While it would be theoretically possible to improve the consistency of daily vitamin K intake through a strictly controlled diet, it is unlikely that this would be a viable solution. The researchers conclude their report with the statement, "Daily supplementation with vitamin K could be an alternative method in stabilizing anticoagulation control, lessening the impact of variable dietary vitamin K intake. We are currently evaluating this possibility." [21]

Johannes Oldenburg, a German medical researcher at *University Clinics in Bonn, Germany*, concurs and suggests that a continuous low-dose intake of vitamin K may stabilize the INR and subsequently reduce risk of bleeding complications. [22]

This is indeed a revolutionary study. The idea of avoiding vitamin K when taking warfarin is firmly entrenched in the medical community. So firmly in fact that vitamin K supplements and multivitamins containing vitamin K used to be banned in Canada, so as to "protect" the small minority of the Canadian population who are on warfarin therapy. Seemingly no thought had been given to the thousands upon thousands of Canadians who may develop osteoporosis due to a lack of vitamin K. Hopefully, this will all change now! The immediate practical implication of the study is for anyone who has trouble controlling their INR to supplement with 50-75 micrograms/day of vitamin K – with their doctor's approval, of course.

REFERENCES

1. Singer, DE, et al. The net clinical benefit of warfarin anticoagulation in atrial fibrillation. Annals of Internal Medicine, Vol. 151, September 1, 2009, pp. 297-305

2. Hart, RG and Halperin, JL. Do current guidelines result in overuse of warfarin anticoagulation in patients with atrial fibrillation? Annals of Internal Medicine, Vol. 151, September 1, 2009, pp. 355-56

3. Bernhardt, P, et al. Fate of left atrial thrombi in patients with atrial fibrillation determined by transesophageal echocardiography and cerebral magnetic resonance imaging. American Journal of Cardiology, Vol. 94, September 15, 2004, pp. 801-04

4. Disertori, M, et al. Thromboembolic event rate in paroxysmal and persistent atrial fibrillation. BMC Cardiovascular Disorders, Vol. 13, 2013, pp. 28-37

5. Hackam, DG, et al. Prognostic implications of warfarin cessation after major trauma. Circulation, Vol. 111, May 3, 2005, pp. 2250-56

6. Cesarone, MR, et al. Prevention of venous thrombosis in long-haul flights with Flite Tabs. Angiology, Vol. 54, No. 5, Sept-Oct, 2003, pp. 531-39

7. Rienstra, M, et al. Clinical characteristics of persistent lone atrial fibrillation in the RACE Study. American Journal of Cardiology, Vol. 94, December 15, 2004, pp. 1486-90

8. Hylek, EM, et al. Major hemorrhage and tolerability of warfarin in the first year of therapy among elderly patients with atrial fibrillation. Circulation, Vol. 115, May 29, 2007, pp. 2689-96

9. Wyse, DG. Bleeding while starting anticoagulation for thromboembolism prophylaxis in elderly patients with atrial fibrillation. Circulation, Vol. 115, May 29, 2007, pp. 2684-86

10. Dossett, LA, et al. Prevalence and outcomes associated with warfarin use in injured adults. Journal of the American College of Surgeons, Vol. 209, 2009, p. S46

11. Gomes, T, et al. Rates of hemorrhage during warfarin therapy for atrial fibrillation. Canadian Medical Association Journal, Vol. 185, No. 2, February 5, 2013, pp. E121-E127

12. Hylek, Elaine M., et al. Acetaminophen and other risk factors for excessive warfarin anticoagulation. Journal of the American Medical Association, Vol. 279, March 4, 1998, pp. 657-62

13. Bell, William R. Acetaminophen and warfarin: undesirable synergy. Journal of the American Medical Association, Vol. 279, March 4, 1998, p. 702-03 (editorial)

14. Flaker, GC, et al. Risks and benefits of combining aspirin with anticoagulation therapy in patients with atrial fibrillation: An exploratory analysis of stroke prevention using an oral thrombin inhibitor in atrial fibrillation (SPORTIF) trials. American Heart Journal, Vol. 152, November 2006, pp. 967-73

15. Hansen, ML, et al. Risk of bleeding with single, dual, or triple therapy with warfarin, aspirin, and clopidogrel in patients with atrial fibrillation. Archives of Internal Medicine, Vol. 170, No. 16, September 13, 2010, pp. 1433-41

16. Torn, M, et al. Risks of oral anticoagulant therapy with increasing age. Archives of Internal Medicine, Vol. 165, July 11, 2005, pp. 1527-32

17. You, JHS, et al. The potential clinical and economic outcomes of pharmacogenetics-oriented management of warfarin therapy – a decision

analysis. Thrombosis & Haemostasis, Vol. 92, September 2004, pp. 590-97

18. Anderson, JL, et al. Randomized trial of genotype-guided versus standard warfarin dosing in patients initiating oral anticoagulation. Circulation, Vol. 116, November 27, 2007, pp. 2563-70

19. Fang, MC, et al. Gender differences in the risk of ischemic stroke and peripheral embolism in atrial fibrillation. Circulation, Vol. 112, September 20, 2005, pp.1687-91

20. Gage, BF, et al. Risk of osteoporotic fracture in elderly patients taking warfarin: results from the National Registry of Atrial Fibrillation 2. Archives of Internal Medicine, Vol. 166, January 23, 2006, pp. 241-46

21. Sconce, E, et al. Patients with unstable control have a poorer dietary intake of vitamin K compared to patients with stable control of anticoagulation. Thrombosis and Haemostasis, Vol. 93, May 2005, pp. 872-75

22. Oldenburg, J. Vitamin K intake and stability of oral anticoagulant treatment. Thrombosis and Haemostasis, Vol. 93, May 2005, pp. 799-800

Design and Analysis of Clinical Trials

The gold standard of clinical trials involving drugs and medical devices is the *superiority* trial. In this type of trial the outcome of an active intervention is compared to the outcome of no treatment or "treatment" with a placebo. The conclusion of such a trial is unequivocal. Either the active treatment confers a benefit or it does not.

However, with the growth of look-alike pharmaceuticals and medical devices it is now considered unethical to compare results of treatment with a new drug/device with results of no treatment or treatment with a placebo. Hence the now almost exclusive use of *noninferiority* trials. The goal of this type of trial is to establish that the outcome of a new treatment is not (much) worse than the outcome of an existing, accepted treatment for the same condition.

The two most common protocols for analyzing clinical trial data are the intention-to-treat (ITT) method and the per-protocol (PP) approach. In the ITT method patient population is defined as all patients randomized to receive treatment irrespective of whether they actually received the treatment, dropped out of the trial, or switched to another treatment. The PP approach, on the other hand, limits the population to patients that actually received the specified treatment for the specified period of time.

Using the ITT approach in superiority trials tends to increase the certainty that a result showing superiority is actually valid, while using the ITT method in the analysis of a noninferiority trial tends to favour the novel treatment being evaluated. An example:

400 patients (ITT population) are randomized to receive a treatment. After randomization 50 patients are deemed ineligible to receive the treatment leaving 350 patients who actually received it (PP population). At the 1-year follow-up 10 patients had suffered a stroke. Using the ITT approach one would conclude that the annual stroke rate was 2.5% while using the PP approach one would conclude that it was 2.9%. It is clear that a difference such as this could result in a treatment being declared non-inferior when in fact it was not non-inferior, or in layman's term "inferior" or "not as good as".

For this reason most experts in the field of medical statistics recommend that trial results only be classified as non-inferior if both ITT and PP analyses show that the new treatment is indeed non-inferior to current, accepted treatment.

- Lesaffre, Emmanuel. Superiority, Equivalence, and Non-inferiority Trials. Bulletin of the NYU Hospital for Joint Diseases. Vol. 66 (2), 2008, pp.150-4
- Christensen, Erik. Methodology of superiority vs. equivalence trials and non-inferiority trials. Journal of Hepatology. Vol. 46 (5), May 2007, pp. 947-54
- Mauri, Laura, and D'Agostino, Ralph B. Challenges in the Design and Interpretation of Noninferiority Trials. New England Journal of Medicine. Vol. 377 (14), October 5, 2017, pp. 1357-1367

Chapter 14

Novel Oral Anticoagulants

Oral anticoagulation with vitamin K antagonists such as warfarin (Coumadin) is still the most commonly prescribed preventive therapy for atrial fibrillation patients at risk for stroke. Unfortunately, warfarin interacts with many foods and drugs and treatment requires constant, costly monitoring. Its use also substantially increases the risk of hemorrhagic stroke and major internal bleeding, particularly in older people, a group that, ironically, is also most at risk for an ischemic stroke. Effective warfarin therapy is based on maintaining an INR (international normalized ratio) between 2.0 and 3.0. In real life this ratio is only achieved on a continuous basis in about 50 to 60% of patients. Too low a ratio increases the risk of ischemic stroke, while too high a ratio increases the risk of hemorrhagic stroke and major bleeding.

The uncertain efficacy in preventing thromboembolism, the increased risk of major bleeding, the cost and inconvenience of regular INR monitoring, and the potential for interactions with many common foods and pharmaceutical drugs thus makes warfarin a less than perfect drug and it is not surprising that substantial effort has been expended on finding a replacement. Warfarin acts by inhibiting the activation of the vitamin K-dependent coagulation factors V, VII and X in the extrinsic and common pathways of the coagulation cascade. Research aimed at replacing warfarin has focused on developing new pharmaceutical drugs that inhibit specific coagulation factors. Currently the four favorites are:

- Dabigatran (*Pradaxa*) developed by Boehringer Ingelheim
- Rivaroxaban (*Xarelto*) developed by Bayer and Johnson & Johnson
- Apixaban (*Eliquis*) developed by Pfizer and Bristol-Myers Squibb.
- Edoxaban (*Lixiana, Savaysa*) developed by Daiichi Sankyo.

Dabigatran

Research aimed at replacing warfarin has essentially focused on developing new pharmaceutical drugs which will inhibit specific coagulation factors. A new direct thrombin inhibitor dabigatran etexilate (*Pradaxa*) has successfully undergone 3 large-scale phase III trials for the treatment of deep vein thrombosis (DVT). Dabigatran works by inhibiting thrombin's ability to form fibrin and thus prevents the formation of blood clots.

In September 2009 a large group of researchers from 41 countries reported on the RE-LY trial involving over 18,000 atrial fibrillation patients who had one or more risk factors for stroke (average $CHADS_2$ score was 2.1). NOTE: 79% of the participants had hypertension, 32% had heart failure, 20% had experienced a prior heart attack or stroke, and 23% had diabetes. The study participants were randomly allocated to receive 110 or 150 mg of dabigatran twice daily or standard warfarin therapy (INR range aim of 2.0 to 3.0). The patients were re-examined 2 weeks and 1 and 2 months after randomization, every 3 months thereafter in the first year, and then every 4 months until the end of the 2-year follow-up period. The INR of warfarin users was checked monthly, but no monitoring of blood levels of dabigatran was required. Warfarin users were within INR range 64% of the time.

A comparison of the incidence of ischemic stroke and systemic embolism, hemorrhagic stroke, major bleeding, heart attack, and overall mortality is shown below:

Incidence of Events, %/year

Event	Warfarin	Dabigatran	Dabigatran
	INR 2.0-3.0	110 mg twice daily	150 mg twice daily
Ischemic stroke and embolism	1.69	1.53	1.11
Hemorrhagic stroke	0.38	0.12	0.10
Heart attack	0.53	0.72	0.74
Major bleeding	3.36	2.71	3.11
Overall mortality	4.13	3.75	3.64

It is clear that dabigatran, either at 110 mg or 150 mg twice daily, gives better protection against strokes (ischemic and hemorrhagic) and bleeding than does warfarin, although an increased risk of heart attack (myocardial infarction) was noted at both levels of dabigatran. There was a significantly higher rate of gastrointestinal bleeding with dabigatran at the 150 mg dose than with warfarin (1.51%/year vs. 1.02%/year).

Adverse events were similar in the 3 groups except in the case of indigestion (dyspepsia) which was experienced by about 11.5% of dabigatran users versus only 5.8% among warfarin users. Several other direct thrombin inhibitors, most prominent among them, ximelagatran, proved to cause liver toxicity and, for this reason, has not been approved by the FDA for stroke prevention in atrial fibrillation patients. The RE-LY trial specifically excluded participants with compromised liver function but there was no indication that liver function was affected by dabigatran. Nevertheless, dabigatran is not recommended for patients with impaired liver function.

The RE-LY investigators concluded that low-dose dabigatran (110 mg twice daily) is associated with an ischemic stroke rate similar to that experienced with warfarin, but results in a lower incidence of hemorrhagic stroke and major bleeding. High-dose dabigatran (150 mg twice daily) is superior to warfarin when it comes to preventing ischemic and hemorrhagic stroke, but has a similar rate of major hemorrhage.

NOTE: The description of the financial ties between the authors of this report and the pharmaceutical industry takes up half a page of fine print! [1]

In September 2010 a FDA advisory panel recommended that dabigatran be approved for stroke prevention in atrial fibrillation patients. This was followed by full approval by the FDA on October 20, 2010. The approval covered two doses – a twice daily 150-mg dose for patients with normal kidney function, and a twice daily 75-mg dose for elderly patients and those with impaired kidney function. It was assumed that 75 mg twice a day would be effective in preventing ischemic stroke without increasing bleeding risk in this patient group. However, there is no long-term clinical data to prove that this assumption is correct.

One of the major disadvantages of warfarin is that it is metabolized by CYP 450 enzymes. These enzymes are also involved in the metabolism of numerous pharmaceutical drugs, common foods, and supplements thus setting the stage for many interactions that may increase or decrease the blood level of warfarin. CYP 450 enzymes are not involved in the metabolism of dabigatran so the potential for interactions is substantially less. Another major advantage of dabigatran is that its use does not involve the constant monitoring of INR levels required when using warfarin. Dabigatran was approved in Europe in 2008 for anticoagulation after knee-and-hip replacement surgery and in August 2011 for stroke prevention in atrial fibrillation patients. The approved doses were 150 mg twice daily for general use and 110 mg twice daily for patients over the age of 80 and for patients with known bleeding problems.

A follow-up study specifically aimed at quantifying bleeding risk associated with dabigatran was reported in May 2011. The researchers looked at the effect of age and kidney impairment on intracranial (intracerebral, hemorrhagic stroke) and extracranial (mainly gastrointestinal) bleeding. They conclude that low-dose dabigatran therapy (110 mg twice daily) compared with warfarin is associated with a 20% lower relative risk of major bleeding and a 70% reduced risk of intracranial bleeding (0.23%/year vs. 0.76%/year) with no significant difference in extracranial bleeding. There was no significant difference in the incidence of ischemic stroke between low-dose dabigatran and warfarin. The incidence of major bleeding in patients under the age of 75 years was significantly lower in the dabigatran group, but no difference was observed in the 75 years or older group. The incidence of intracranial bleeding was substantially lower in the dabigatran group irrespective of age, whereas the incidence of gastrointestinal bleeding was substantially higher among patients aged 75 years or older (2.19%/year for dabigatran vs. 1.59%/year for warfarin).

High-dose dabigatran therapy (150 mg twice daily) was associated with a major bleeding risk similar to that of warfarin and a 58% reduced risk of intracranial bleeding (0.32%/year vs. 0.76%/year) with no difference in extracranial bleeding. The incidence of ischemic stroke in the high-dose dabigatran group was significantly lower than in the warfarin group (1.69%/year vs. 1.10%/year) irrespective of age.

However, the incidence of gastrointestinal bleeding was substantially higher among patients aged 75 years or older (2.80%/year for dabigatran vs. 1.59%/year for warfarin). The researchers observed that the risk of major bleeding increased with the concomitant use of aspirin. They also found that renal impairment (kidney dysfunction) was a strong risk factor for bleeding with a creatinine clearance of less than 50 mL/min associated with a 2-fold higher risk of major bleeding than if creatinine clearance was more than 80 mL/min. The researchers speculate that renal impairment may be a major cause of the increased tendency for gastrointestinal bleeding observed with dabigatran therapy in elderly patients (dabigatran is renally excreted so a kidney dysfunction may result in higher blood concentrations of the drug). [2]

During the RE-LY trial 1270 participants underwent cardioversion (84% electrical). The number of cardioversions performed in the three study groups – dabigatran, 110 mg twice daily (D110), dabigatran, 150 mg twice daily (D150), and warfarin to achieve an INR of 2.0 to 3.0 were similar at 647, 672, and 664.

Transesophageal echocardiography (TEE) was performed in 21% of patients and left atrial appendage thrombi were found in 1.8% of patients in the D110 group, 1.2% in the D150 group, and 1.1% in the warfarin group. The differences in the incidence of stroke and systemic embolism within 30 days of cardioversion in the three groups were not statistically significant and neither were the differences in the incidence of major bleeding.

Events related to cardioversion, %

Event	D110	D150	Warfarin
Stroke and systemic embolism	0.77	0.30	0.60
Major bleeding	1.70	0.60	0.60

NOTE: The reason that the differences in the incidence of stroke and bleeding events are not statistically significant relates to the fact that the total number of patients affected was very small (only 11 cardioversions were followed by a stroke or thromboembolism and only 19 were followed by major bleeding).

There was no difference in the incidence of stroke and systemic embolism between patients who had a TEE prior to cardioversion and those who had not, likely indicating that TEE may not be necessary in patients who have been adequately anticoagulated for at least 3 weeks prior to cardioversion. NOTE: This study was funded by Boehringer Ingelheim, the manufacturer of dabigatran, and all the authors had received grants or consulting fees from the company. [3]

In August 2011 the Japanese Ministry of Health, Labor, and Welfare issued a safety advisory noting that there had been 81 cases of serious side effects from dabigatran use including gastrointestinal bleeding.

In October 2011 the Therapeutic Goods Administration in Australia issued a safety advisory prompted by an increase in the number of bleeding-related adverse events reported since more people began taking dabigatran. Some of the bleeding events occurred during the transition from warfarin to dabigatran and the most common site of serious bleeding was the gastrointestinal tract.

Apart from the bleeding concerns, especially among patients with kidney impairment, emergency room physicians also expressed concern about the fact that there was no approved antidote to stop dabigatran-induced bleeding. [4]

In early January 2012 the association between dabigatran use and an increased risk of heart attack (myocardial infarction) and acute coronary syndrome (unstable angina, heart attack and cardiac death) was confirmed. A meta-analysis of 7 studies comparing dabigatran (150 mg twice daily) to warfarin, enoxaparin or placebo found that dabigatran use was associated with a relative 33% (absolute 0.27%) increased risk of heart attack or acute coronary syndrome. [5]

As of January 2012 the recommended dosage in the USA for dabigatran is 150 mg twice daily for patients under the age of 75 years with normal kidney function and 75 mg twice daily for older patients and those with impaired kidney function. The drug is not recommended for patients with impaired liver function. It should be noted that there is no clinical data supporting the use of the 75-mg dose and that only the 110- and 150-mg doses have been approved in Europe.

NOTE: In May 2014 Boehringer Ingelheim agreed to pay $650 million to settle 4000 lawsuits claiming harm or death from the use of dabigatran (Pradaxa). According to the Institute for Safe Medication Practices more than 1000 deaths have been linked to the use of the drug. [6]

Rivaroxaban

Rivaroxaban (*Xarelto*) is a direct inhibitor of factor Xa and works by reducing thrombin production which in turn reduces the conversion of fibrinogen to fibrin, thus preventing the formation of blood clots. Like dabigatran it was initially approved for temporary use following knee and hip operations. After lengthy deliberations and some controversy, the drug was approved by the FDA in November 2011 for stroke prevention in AF patients.

The FDA approval was based on the results of a large clinical trial (ROCKET AF) involving 14,000 patients with non-valvular AF treated at 1178 participating sites in 45 countries. The average (median) age of the patients was 73 years and 40% were female. Most of the study participants had persistent (probably including permanent) AF and had a CHADS$_2$ score of at least 2 (mean score of 3.5). All in all, the trial involved a group of very sick people – in no way comparable to a group of otherwise healthy afibbers. Over 90% of the group had hypertension, 63% had heart failure, and 55% had experienced a prior stroke or transient ischemic attack (TIA).

The study participants were randomized to receive standard therapy with oral warfarin (INR range of 2.0 – 3.0) or 20 mg/day of rivaroxaban (15 mg/day for patients with kidney impairment). All patients also received a placebo pill and regular INR checks to blind them to the treatment received. The warfarin-treated patients were within INR target range 55% of the time and average follow-up period was 2 years. A comparison of the incidence of ischemic stroke and systemic embolism, major bleeding, hemorrhagic stroke, gastrointestinal bleeding, and overall mortality (from any cause) is shown below:

Incidence of Events, %/year

Event	Warfarin	Rivaroxaban
Ischemic stroke or embolism	2.2	1.7
Major bleeding**	14.5	14.9
Hemorrhagic stroke	0.7	0.5
Gastrointestinal bleeding	2.2	3.2
Fatal bleeding	0.5	0.2

** Major and non-major clinically relevant bleeding

About 23% of participants dropped out of the study before its completion. The rate of ischemic stroke, TIA and systemic embolism during a median 117 days of follow-up was 4.7% in the rivaroxaban drop-out group and 4.3% in the warfarin drop-out group. The ROCKET AF investigators conclude that rivaroxaban is non-inferior to warfarin in the treatment of AF patients at moderate to high risk of stroke.

NOTE: This study was funded by Johnson & Johnson and Bayer, and all the investigators had substantial financial ties to the pharmaceutical industry. [7]

Rivaroxaban and its metabolites are partially (66%) excreted through the kidneys thus raising concerns that poor kidney function may result in an increase in drug concentration and commensurate increase in bleeding risk. The ROCKET AF trial included 2950 patients with moderately impaired kidney function (creatinine clearance between 30 and 49 mL/min) who were randomized to receive warfarin or 15 mg/day of rivaroxaban. The average age of these patients was 79 years and their average $CHADS_2$ score was 3.7, 82% had persistent AF (probably including permanent AF), 50% had suffered a prior stroke or TIA, 92% had hypertension, and 66% had congestive heart failure.

Incidence of Events, %/year

Event	Warfarin	Rivaroxaban
Ischemic stroke or embolism	2.77	2.32
Ischemic stroke	1.78	1.98

Incidence of Events, %/year [continued]

Event	Warfarin	Rivaroxaban
Major Bleeding	4.70	4.49
Intracranial Bleeding	0.88	0.71

None of the differences in outcome were statistically significant indicating that rivaroxaban is non-inferior to warfarin in patients with moderate renal impairment. However, it should be kept in mind that that the average time (TTR) that patients on warfarin were in the specified INR range (2.0-3.0) was only 58%. This means that patients on warfarin would be more likely to suffer a stroke (if INR <2.0) or a bleeding event (if INR >3.0) than if their anticoagulation protocol had been more rigorously enforced. NOTE: This study was funded by Johnson & Johnson and Bayer Healthcare. [8, 9]

An independent evaluation of rivaroxaban was carried out by FDA's Center for Drug Evaluation and Research and reported in October 2016. The study involved 52,240 elderly atrial fibrillation patients treated with dabigatran (150 mg twice daily) and 66,651 elderly atrial fibrillation patients treated with rivaroxaban (20 mg once daily). During follow-up there were 306 thromboembolic strokes, 176 intracranial bleeding events, 1209 major extracranial bleeding events of which 1018 were gastrointestinal, and 846 deaths. Incidence rates for the two groups are presented below:

Incidence of Events, %/year

Event	Dabigatran	Rivaroxaban	Difference	Difference
	Unadjusted	Unadjusted	Unadjusted	Adjusted
Thromboembolic stroke	0.97	0.77	-0.20	-0.18
Intracranial hemorrhage	0.37	0.58	0.21	0.23
Extracranial bleeding*	2.66	3.94	1.28	1.30
Gastrointestinal bleeding	2.33	3.25	0.92	0.94
Mortality	2.22	2.47	0.25	0.31

*Including gastrointestinal bleeding

The statistically significant greater incidence of bleeding events with rivaroxaban was even more pronounced in patients over the age of 75 and in patients with a $CHADS_2$ score greater than 2. The FDA researchers suggest that the once-a-day dosing of rivaroxaban (half-life 9-13 hours in the elderly) would lead to higher peak and lower through serum concentrations and that this may at least partly explain the greater incidence of bleeding in the rivaroxaban group. [10]

NOTE: On December 5, 2017 a Philadelphia state court jury ordered Bayer AG and Johnson & Johnson to pay $27.8 million to an Indiana couple where the wife had been hospitalized with severe gastrointestinal bleeding attributed to Xarelto. More than 18,500 other lawsuits against the makers of Xarelto are pending in U.S. federal court. [11]

Apixaban

Apixaban (*Eliquis*) is a direct inhibitor of factor Xa and works by reducing thrombin production which in turn reduces the conversion of fibrinogen to fibrin, thus preventing the formation of blood clots.

A study comparing apixaban (5 mg twice daily) with aspirin (81 – 324 mg/day) in a group of 5600 AF patients found that apixaban reduced the relative risk of stroke and systemic embolism by about 50% when compared to aspirin (yearly event rates 1.6% with apixaban and 3.7% with aspirin) without significantly increasing the risk of major bleeding. [12]

A large-scale study (ARISTOTLE) comparing apixaban to warfarin was recently completed. It involved 18,200 atrial fibrillation patients recruited at 1000 sites in 40 countries (3,000 patients in Russia and 4,000 patients in China). The average (median) age of the patients was 70 years and 35% were female. Most of the participants (85%) had persistent or permanent AF and had a $CHADS_2$ score of at least 1 (mean score of 2.1). All in all, the trial involved a group of very sick people, in no way comparable to a group of otherwise healthy afibbers. Almost 90% were being treated for hypertension, 35% had heart failure or abnormally low left ventricular ejection fraction, over 30% had experienced a prior heart attack, stroke, TIA (transient ischemic attack) or systemic embolism, and 25% had diabetes. None of the study participants had a $CHADS_2$ score of zero.

The participants were randomized to receive standard therapy with oral warfarin (INR range of 2.0 to 3.0) or 5 mg twice daily of apixaban (2.5 mg twice daily for elderly or frail persons and those with impaired kidney function). The warfarin-treated patients were within INR target range 66% of the time (median value). The average (median) follow-up was 1.8 years. A comparison of the incidence of ischemic stroke and systemic embolism, major bleeding, hemorrhagic stroke, gastrointestinal bleeding, and overall mortality (from any cause) follows:

Incidence of Events, %/year

Event	Warfarin	Apixaban
Ischemic stroke or embolism	1.60	1.27
Major bleeding	3.09	2.13
Intracranial bleeding	0.80	0.33

Incidence of Events, %/year [continued]

Event	Warfarin	Apixaban
Hemorrhagic Stroke	0.47	0.24
Gastrointestinal bleeding	0.86	0.76
Mortality (from any cause)	3.94	3.52

The ARISTOTLE AF investigators conclude that apixaban is superior to warfarin in regard to preventing stroke and systemic embolism and non-inferior in all other aspects where a comparison was made. NOTE: This study was funded by Bristol-Myers Squibb and Pfizer and all the investigators have substantial financial ties to the pharmaceutical industry. [12-14]

Apixaban was approved for sale to atrial fibrillation patients in the USA in 2012. The approval by the Federal Drug Administration (FDA) was delayed for nine months due to numerous problems with the conduct of the clinical trial (ARISTOTLE) used to support the approval of the drug.

The most significant problems were [15, 16]:

- Missing data for more than 300 patients – primarily involving presumed deaths.
- Dispensing errors – a substantial fraction of patients might have been given the wrong treatment (active drug instead of placebo or vice versa). The vast majority of medication errors occurred at Russian trial sites.
- Cover-up of the extent of dispensing errors.
- Deliberate falsification of records.
- Fraudulent behaviour by BMS employees at a test site in China.

The FDA employees reviewing the data from the ARISTOTLE trial expressed serious reservations about the conduct of the trial but had no other data on which to base the decision as to whether the drug should be approved or not. Nevertheless, on December 28, 2012 apixaban, under the tradename Eliquis, was approved by FDA for the prevention of stroke in atrial fibrillation patients. [17]

Bleeding risk with apixaban

Anticoagulants are designed to prevent the formation of blood clots which, if carried to the brain, can cause an ischemic stroke, and if ending up in the heart's capillaries, can cause a heart attack (myocardial infarction). Unfortunately, as part of the process involved in preventing blood clots, anticoagulants such as warfarin also tend to destroy the collagen fibers forming the backbone of the walls of capillaries. This enables blood cells to leak through the capillaries and possibly cause a hemorrhagic stroke or severe gastrointestinal bleeding. In general, the risk of serious (major) bleeding is significantly greater than the risk of an ischemic stroke in anticoagulated patients.

In the ARISTOTLE trial the annual risk of stroke was 1.3% for patients on apixaban vs. 1.6% for patients on warfarin. The risk of major bleeding was 2.1% on apixaban and 3.1% on warfarin. The most serious adverse effect of anticoagulation is intracranial hemorrhage (including hemorrhagic stroke) which occurred at a rate of 0.33%/year in apixaban-treated patients vs. a rate of 0.80%/year in the warfarin group. The overall incidence of any treatment-related bleeding was 18%/year in the apixaban arm and 26%/year in the warfarin arm [13].

A detailed analysis of intracranial hemorrhage (ICH) cases revealed that the median time to ICH (from start of anticoagulation) was 348 days in patients randomized to apixaban vs. 279 days among patients randomized to warfarin. In most patients ICH was identified through a CT scan. Almost a third of all ICH patients were on aspirin the day before their ICH and about half of them had no medical reason to be on aspirin. Patients with ICH were older, weighed less, and had more history of prior embolic events than patients without ICH. They were also more likely to have renal dysfunction at enrollment. [18]

Mortality rates after ICH were substantial with 43.3% of ICH patients dying within 30 days of the event, 45.3% within 90 days and 47.6% at 6 months. Among survivors, disability was at least of moderate degree in 37.8% of patients. [18]

Unfortunately the design of the ARISTOTLE trial had at least one major flaw. The incidence of stroke and bleeding was not evaluated in subgroups of patients grouped according to their stroke risk as graded by their $CHADS_2$ score (a measure of the risk of ischemic stroke). It is well established that warfarin has a substantially higher benefit/risk ratio at higher $CHADS_2$ scores (especially if the patient has experienced a previous ischemic stroke) than at low scores where the ratio may even be negative. Is the same the case for apixaban? All that is known about inherent stroke risk in the ARISTOTLE population is that the average $CHADS_2$ score was 2.1 in both arms. The question as to whether apixaban is as effective as warfarin in preventing a second stroke is thus not answered.

The fact that anticoagulants are associated with an increased risk of serious bleeding raises the obvious question: "Is anticoagulation safe in patients who are already at elevated risk for intracranial or gastrointestinal bleeding?"

Unfortunately the ARISTOTLE trial cannot answer this question as patients with elevated bleeding risk were specifically excluded from participating in the trial (NOTE: This applies to both the apixaban arm and the warfarin arm of the trial). One would have to assume that this was due to the fairly obvious assumption that it would be unsafe, even unethical, to expose patients with elevated bleeding risk to an agent known to further increase bleeding risk. [19]

The fact that patients with elevated bleeding risk were excluded from participating in the trial means that the FDA reviewers had no data on which to base a decision as to the safety of apixaban in this patient group. The obvious conclusion therefore must be that the FDA approval of apixaban does not apply to patients with elevated bleeding risk and that the drug therefore cannot safely be prescribed to this patient group.

It is indeed unfortunate that the main report on the ARISTOTLE trial published in the *New England Journal of Medicine* failed to disclose that elevated bleeding risk was an absolute contraindication to enrollment in the trial [13]. It is also unfortunate that the official prescribing information for apixaban (Eliquis) lists only pregnancy, nursing, severe hepatic impairment and the presence of prosthetic heart valves as contraindications for prescribing Eliquis. Since apixaban was never tested in patients with elevated bleeding risk there is presumably no legal requirement to even advise caution in its use in this patient group.

Stroke risk upon discontinuation of apixaban

The prescribing information for Eliquis states:

An increased rate of stroke was observed following discontinuation of Eliquis in clinical trials in patients with nonvalvular atrial fibrillation. If anticoagulation with Eliquis must be discontinued for reasons other than pathological bleeding, coverage with another anticoagulant should be strongly considered.

A review of data from the ARISTOTLE trial comparing apixaban (Eliquis) with warfarin concluded that transitioning from apixaban to warfarin is associated with a stroke incidence of 4%/year and an incidence of major bleeding of 5%/year. This compares to a stroke incidence of 1%/year and a major bleeding incidence of 2%/year for patients who remained on warfarin during and after the trial. It is however, not clear whether a short interruption of Eliquis therapy would be as detrimental as complete discontinuation. It is also not clear whether the increased risks associated with switching from Eliquis to warfarin can be blamed on Eliquis or on warfarin (not that this really matters to the patient – the elevated stroke risk remains the same) [20].

Edoxaban

Edoxaban (*Lixiana, Savaysa)* is a direct inhibitor of factor Xa and works by reducing thrombin production which in turn reduces the conversion of fibrinogen to fibrin, thus preventing the formation of blood clots.

The results of a large-scale study (ENGAGE AF-TIMI 48) comparing edoxaban to warfarin was reported in 2013. It involved 21,105 atrial fibrillation patients with moderate to high stroke risk. The average (median) age of the patients was 72 years and 38% were female. Most of the participants (75%) had persistent or permanent AF and had a CHADS$_2$ score of at least 2. All in all, the trial involved a group of very sick people, in no way comparable to a group of otherwise healthy afibbers. Over 90% were being treated for hypertension, 58% had heart failure, 28% had experienced a prior stroke or TIA (transient ischemic attack), and 36% had diabetes. More than 60% of study participants were from regions other than North America and Western Europe.

The participants were randomized to receive standard therapy with oral warfarin (INR range of 2.0 to 3.0) or 60 mg/day of edoxaban (high-dose) or 30 mg/day of edoxaban (low-dose). The dose of edoxaban were halved at randomization or whenever indicated for patients (32% of total) who had an estimated creatinine clearance of 30 to 50 mL/min, a body weight of 60 kg or less, or were using verapamil, quinidine or dronedarone. Full doses were resumed if any of these limitations were no longer applicable. Premature permanent discontinuation of the study drugs occurred in 7141 patients evenly split between the three groups.

The median duration of drug treatment was 907 days and the median follow-up was 1022 days (2.8 years). The warfarin-treated patients were within INR target range 68.4% of the time (median value). A comparison of the incidence of ischemic stroke and systemic embolism, major bleeding, gastrointestinal bleeding, and overall treatment-related mortality is shown below.

Incidence of Events, %/year

Event	Warfarin	High Edoxaban	Low Edoxaban
Ischemic stroke or embolism	1.50	1.18	1.61
Ischemic stroke	1.25	1.25	1.77
Hemorrhagic stroke	0.47	0.26	0.16
Major bleeding	3.43	2.75	1.61
Gastrointestinal bleeding	1.23	2.47	0.84

The ENGAGE AF-TIMI 48 investigators conclude that both doses of edoxaban are non-inferior to warfarin in regard to preventing stroke and systemic embolism with the high-dose edoxaban tending to be more effective than warfarin. They also conclude that both edoxaban doses were associated with a lower incidence of major bleeding and hemorrhagic stroke. Edoxaban was approved by the FDA for sale to atrial fibrillation patients in the US in January 2015.

NOTE: The ENGAGE AF-TIMI 48 study was funded by Daiichi Sankyo, the manufacturer of edoxaban, and 15 of the 21 investigators involved with and reporting on the study were either employees of Daiichi Sankyo or had substantial financial ties to Daiichi Sankyo or other members of the pharmaceutical industry. [21]

Summary

Preventing the coagulation of blood on a permanent basis clearly increases the risk of prolonged and serious bleeding and there is no such thing as an entirely safe pharmaceutical-based anticoagulant. Thus, it is best to avoid anticoagulation unless one has definite specific risk factors for ischemic stroke. If, however, anticoagulation is required, then individual circumstances should be taken into account when selecting one's anticoagulant.

A direct comparison of the efficacy and safety of the four novel anticoagulants is not possible due to the heterogeneity of the patient populations involved in the clinical trials. Average (mean) CHADS$_2$ scores varied from 2.1 in the dabigatran and apixaban trials to 2.8 in the edoxaban trial and 3.5 in the rivaroxaban trial. Furthermore, average time spent in the therapeutic range for warfarin therapy (TTR) differed significantly with TTR being 55% in the rivaroxaban trial, 62% in the apixaban trial, 64% in the dabigatran trial, and 68% in the edoxaban trial (ENGAGE AF-TIMI 48). Being outside the specified INR limits (2.0-3.0) would be detrimental to warfarin performance with an INR below 2.0 increasing the risk of ischemic stroke and an INR above 3.0 increasing the risk of bleeding. [22]

Nevertheless, if one has a tendency to bleeding, especially gastrointestinal bleeding, then apixaban would likely be the best choice. If one is prone to falls or is involved in contact sports, downhill skiing, mountain biking or similar activities, then warfarin would probably be the preferred option as its anticoagulant effect can be reversed by a vitamin K infusion. A second choice would be apixaban. Dabigatran, apixaban, and edoxaban all significantly reduce the risk of hemorrhagic stroke compared to warfarin, while dabigatran (150 twice daily) may be the best choice if one wishes to focus solely on avoiding an ischemic stroke.

However, dabigatran (150 mg twice daily) is not recommended for patients with impaired kidney or liver function and should be used with caution in patients over the age of 75 years as it materially increases gastrointestinal bleeding in this patient group. It is now also clear that dabigatran is associated with a small but significant increased risk of heart attack and acute coronary syndrome.

Apixaban is primarily excreted through the liver and is probably the best choice for patients with renal impairment. Apixaban and edoxaban are probably the best choices for patients with a high risk of gastrointestinal bleeding and apixaban may also be the best choice for patients who are at high risk for ischemic stroke or who have already suffered a stroke or TIA. [22, 23]

Guidelines for the use of the novel oral anticoagulants

Warfarin (Coumadin) has a long history and much experience has been gained over the past 30 years to ensure safe and effective use of this drug. Recently four new oral anticoagulants – dabigatran (*Pradaxa*), rivaroxaban (*Xarelto*), apixaban (*Eliquis*), and edoxaban (*Lixiana, Savaysa*) – have entered the market as replacements for warfarin. A major advantage of the new anticoagulants is that, unlike warfarin, they do not require regular monitoring to ensure that their anticoagulation effect is optimal. Several clinical trials have been done to establish their benefit in preventing ischemic stroke and the risks (major bleeding and hemorrhagic stroke) associated with their use.

However, while guidelines for the use of warfarin are well established, this is not the case for the newer anticoagulants. A group of European cardiologists/electrophysiologists has now released a set of guidelines for the use of the new anticoagulants in patients with non-valvular atrial fibrillation (AF). Highlights are: [24]

- It is recommended that patients on the new anticoagulants carry a card giving details about their treatment and other medications they may be taking. It is also recommended that patients undergo testing for liver and kidney function at least once a year and more frequently if they have reduced kidney function or have been prescribed dabigatran. Finally, patients should see their doctor at regular intervals, preferably every 3 months, for on-going review of their treatment.

- The new anticoagulants do not require routine monitoring of coagulation efficacy. The value of measuring activated partial thromboplastin time (aPTT) to provide a qualitative assessment of the presence of dabigatran, or prothrombin time (PT) to provide an assessment of the presence of rivaroxaban and apixaban is questionable, and INR monitoring is not applicable to patients on the new anticoagulants.

- It is expected that the new anticoagulants will have less interactions with foods, but interactions with other drugs will still be a problem. Not surprisingly, bleeding risk increases significantly if the new anticoagulants are taken in conjunction with other anticoagulants, platelet inhibitors or NSAIDs. Combining them with aspirin increases bleeding risk by at least 60%. Several drugs strongly potentiate the effect of the new anticoagulants and should be used with extreme caution or not at all. Among these drugs are dronedarone (Multaq), antifungal drugs such as ketoconazole and itraconazole, and HIV protease inhibitors (ritonavir). Other drugs weaken the anticoagulation effect. Most important among these are rifampicin, carbamazepine, phenytoin, phenobarbital, and the herb St. John's Wort. Some drugs potentiate the coagulation effect to a lesser extent, and this may be countered by reducing the dose of anticoagulant. Among these drugs are verapamil and quinidine.

- Finally, some drugs potentiate the anticoagulant effect, but unless two or more of these drugs are taken in combination with other potentiating drugs, anticoagulant dose does not need to be changed. Among this category of drugs are diltiazem, amiodarone, and certain antibiotics (cyclosporine, clarithromycin, and erythromycin). NOTE: For a more complete list of drug interactions see the complete article. [25]

- Special precautions need to be taken when switching between different anticoagulant therapies, especially when switching from one of the new anticoagulants to warfarin. [25]

- In Europe the standard dose for dabigatran is 110 or 150 mg twice a day, for rivaroxaban it is 15-20 mg once a day, for apixaban 5 mg twice a day, and for edoxaban 30 or 60 mg/day. NOTE: Dosages are reduced for patients with impaired kidney function. It is very important to follow the dosing schedule and to follow instructions regarding missed doses. [25].

- Chronic kidney disease is a risk factor for both thromboembolic events (ischemic strokes) and bleeding in AF patients. Use of the new anticoagulants is not recommended in patients with a creatinine clearance of less than 30 mL/min or in dialysis patients.

- As of May 2013 there are no specific, FDA-approved antidotes for the new anticoagulants and no effective and readily available protocols for dealing with severe bleeding complications, although some success has been achieved with the use of dialysis and blood transfusions. The effect of an accidental overdose can sometimes be mitigated by the prompt use of activated charcoal.

- Some forms of surgery require discontinuation of anticoagulation. The last dose should generally be taken 24 to 48 hours prior to surgery depending on the extent of the surgery and the patient's creatinine clearance level. Anticoagulation can generally be restarted 6 to 8 hours after the completion of surgery, but in some cases a wait period of 72 hours or more is required. For AF patients undergoing catheter ablation, anticoagulation with warfarin (INR between 2.0 and 3.0) would still seem to be the safest option. Patients with both AF and coronary artery disease require special consideration and different protocols may be needed depending on whether the patient has suffered a heart attack or not. [25].

- In the case of AF patients whose episode has lasted more than 48 hours (or is of unknown duration), anticoagulation is required for 3 weeks before and 4 weeks after cardioversion. If there is doubt about the patient's compliance with their anticoagulation protocol, transesophageal echocardiography should be performed prior to cardioversion.

- Patients suffering an ischemic stroke should not receive thrombolytic therapy with recombinant tissue plasminogen activator or should wait for this therapy for at least 48 hours after taking the last dose of the new anticoagulants. NOTE: Thrombolytic therapy is not effective if given more than 3 hours after stroke occurred. There is no established protocol for dealing with a hemorrhagic stroke (intracranial bleeding) occurring in a patient taking one of the new anticoagulants.

- Patients with cancer are at an increased risk for thromboembolic events and some cancer therapies may increase bleeding tendency. Because of the wealth of experience in using heparin and warfarin in cancer patients and the complete lack of experience using the new anticoagulants, they are not recommended for cancer patients. [24, 25]

Drug Interactions

It is well known that warfarin interacts with numerous prescription drugs, over-the-counter medications, herbs, and some foods. One of the major selling points of the novel anticoagulants (NOACs) is that they would be much less likely to interact with drugs, foods, and herbs. Although there is still next to no actual data about possible interactions between NOACs and herbs and foods the general consensus seems to be that the chance of any such interactions would be minor except in the case of St. John's Wort. However, there is clear evidence that NOACs do interact with several common drugs and over-the-counter medications. In some cases the drugs potentiate the effect of the NOAC and may thereby increase the risk of bleeding and hemorrhagic stroke, while in other cases they inhibit the effect and thereby increase the risk of thrombosis and ischemic stroke.

Because dabigatran (a direct thrombin inhibitor) and the direct inhibitors of factor Xa (rivaroxaban, apixaban, and edoxaban) work by different mechanisms, are metabolized by different enzymes, and are excreted via different pathways (liver or kidneys) there are some significant differences in interactions with pharmaceutical drugs.

NOACs – General Observations

Characteristic	Dabigatran	Rivaroxaban	Apixaban	Edoxaban
Elimination half-life	12-17 h	5-13 h **	12 h	10-14 h
Renal clearance*	80%	66%	27%	50%
Need to take with food	no	mandatory	no	no
May cause indigestion	yes	no	no	no

* Of drug and its metabolites
** 5-9 h for young patients, 11-13 h for elderly

NOACs – Drug Interactions

Drug	Dabigatran	Rivaroxaban	Apixaban	Edoxaban
Antiarrhythmics				
Amiodarone	up 12-60%	Minor effect	No data	up 40%
Dronedarone	Avoid	Avoid	No data	up 85%
Digoxin	No effect	No effect	No data	No effect
Diltiazem	No effect	Minor effect	Up 40%	No data
Quinidine	Up 53%	Effect unknown	No data	Up 77%
Verapamil	Up 12-180%	Minor effect	No data	Up 53%
Other Drugs				
Rimfampicin	Avoid	Avoid	Avoid	Avoid
Ritonavir	Avoid	Avoid	Avoid	Avoid
Fluconazole	No data	Use w/caution	No data	No data
Itraconazole	Avoid	Avoid	Avoid	Up 87-95%
Ketoconazole	Avoid	Avoid	Avoid	Up 87-95%
Voriconazole	Avoid	Avoid	Avoid	Up 87-95%
Cyclosporin	Avoid	Use w/caution	No data	Up 73%
Carbamazepine	Avoid	Avoid	Avoid	Down 35%
Phenobarbital	Avoid	Avoid	Avoid	Down 35%
Phenytoin	Avoid	Avoid	Avoid	Down 35%
Clarithromycin	Up 15-20%	Up 30-54%	No data	Up 90%
Erythromycin	Up 15-20%	Up 30-54%	No data	Up 90%
Naproxen	No data	No data	Up 55%	No effect
St. John's wort	Avoid	Avoid	Avoid	Down 35%
H2-blockers	Use caution	No effect	No effect	No effect
PPIs	Use caution	No effect	No effect	No effect

Up xx% means that the drug increases plasma concentration of the NOAC by xx%.

In the case of edoxaban it is recommended to reduce dose by 50% if plasma level increase exceeds 84%.

Down xx% means that the drug decreases plasma concentration of the NOAC by xx%.

Data on interaction between apixaban and other pharmaceutical drugs is scarce, but there is no reason to believe that apixaban has fewer interactions than the other two factor Xa inhibitors (rivaroxaban and edoxaban).

NOTE: The above table is based on the 2015 *Updated European Heart Rhythm Association Practical Guide on the use of non-vitamin K antagonist anticoagulants in patients with non-valvular atrial fibrillation* and is in general agreement with data presented in the 2017 *Old and new oral anticoagulants: Food, herbal medicines and drug interactions* . [26, 27]

Caution is advised when contemplating use of the NOACs in the following cases: [26]

- Concomitant use of antiplatelet agents, NSAIDs, or other anticoagulants*
- Concomitant use of systemic steroid therapy
- History of gastrointestinal bleeding or recent surgery on a critical organ
- Thrombocytopenia (e.g. chemotherapy)
- Patients having a HAS-BLED score of 3 or higher
- Patients being 75 years of age or older
- Patients weighing 60 kg (132 lbs.) or less
- Patients with impaired renal function.

* Apixaban can be safely combined with aspirin or clopidogrel in atrial fibrillation patients except in patients with acute coronary symptoms. [27]

Safely prescribing NOACs is clearly not a simple matter. A patient's age, weight, renal function, history and tendency to bleeding, and concomitant use of other medications must be taken into account. Furthermore, many drugs that interact with NOACs increase the plasma concentration of the NOAC, thus increasing the risk of major bleeding. Combine this with the lack of reliable and readily available methods for testing plasma concentration and anticoagulation effect with the lack of FDA-approved reversal agents for factor Xa inhibitors and it becomes clear that the decision to prescribe NOACs to a patient is not only technically challenging, but in many cases also presents a major moral dilemma.

Reversal Agents

In the period 2007-2009 adverse drug events accounted for more than 265,000 emergency department visits annually in the United States by adults aged 65 years or older. Almost 100,000 of these visits resulted in hospitalization and 21,000 of these were associated with hemorrhages caused by warfarin. Gastrointestinal hemorrhage was by far the most common type of hemorrhage and was associated with an 85% hospitalization rate. [28]

Intracranial hemorrhage, including hemorrhagic stroke, was much less common but far more likely to result in death or permanent disability. A study involving over 13,000 patients with nonvalvular atrial fibrillation found that of the 0.5% of patients who experienced intracranial bleeding 76% had severe disability or had died at hospital discharge. This despite the fact that there is a well-established protocol for monitoring anticoagulation with warfarin (INR test) and equally well-established protocols for reversing life-threatening warfarin-related bleeding. [29]

The first step in the reversal protocol involves the use of intravenous vitamin K and blood transfusion as needed. This may be followed by injection of a prothrombin complex concentrate or, if that is not available, injection of thawed, fresh frozen plasma. Plasma injection unfortunately is slow to act, is not very effective in lowering INR and its effectiveness in the treatment of intracranial hemorrhage is very low. A somewhat better approach, if prothrombin complex is not available, involves the injection of recombinant factor VIIa (rFVIIa). rFVIIa works very quickly to normalize INR, but carries a serious risk of thrombosis and associated ischemic stroke.

It is clear that although proven protocols exist for the reversal of warfarin-related hemorrhage their execution is, by no means, simple and a satisfactory outcome by no means assured. [30, 31]

A similar problem exists with NOACs, except in this case, there is currently no proven, quickly available method of measuring coagulation intensity (INR test is not applicable) nor are there effective, FDA-approved reversal agents for the factor Xa inhibitors (rivaroxaban, apixaban, edoxaban). A reversal agent for dabigatran (idarucizumab) was approved by FDA in October 2015.

The protocols for the reversal of warfarin-induced bleeding are based on restoring the concentration of vitamin-K-dependent coagulation factors, the formation of which is inhibited by warfarin. Unfortunately, these protocols do not work for NOACs as they do not work by inhibiting vitamin-K-dependent coagulation factors.

At present there are three reversal agents either approved (idarucizumab) or under development for reversing NOAC-associated bleeding.

- Idarucizumab (*Praxbind*) developed by Boehringer Ingelheim
- Andexanet alfa (*Annexa*) under development by Portola Biologics
- Ciraparantag (PER977) under development by Perosphere

Idarucizumab

Dabigatran binds to thrombin and works by inhibiting thrombin's ability to form fibrin and thus prolongs the time before blood clots are formed.

Idarucizumab (*Praxbind*) is a humanized mouse monoclonal antibody fragment that also binds to thrombin, but has no anticoagulation effect on its own. Idarucizumab has a 350 times greater affinity than dabigatran for binding to thrombin and thus rapidly replaces dabigatran at thrombin receptor sites resulting in almost immediate cessation of dabigatran's anticoagulant effect. The half-life of idarucizumab is about 45 minutes and its effect lasts for about 72 hours. [32, 33]

In an ideal world laboratory tests to rapidly determine a bleeding patient's blood level of dabigatran would be readily available to guide treatment with idarucizumab. Unfortunately, standard tests for anticoagulation level such as the INR test, thrombin clotting time (TCT), prothrombin time (PT), activated clotting time (ACT) and activated partial thromboplastin time (APTT) are poor predictors of dabigatran level although normal PT, ACT, and APTT results would tend to rule out very high dabigatran levels. [34, 35]

However, two specific tests, the ecarin clotting time (ECT) and the diluted thrombin time (dTT) can accurately measure the concentration and coagulation activity of dabigatran and other direct thrombin inhibitors, but they are not useful for use in emergency departments as they can only be performed in specially equipped laboratories. [36, 37]

Ecarin clotting time (ECT) is based on the ability of ecarin (an extract from the venom of the saw-scaled viper) to convert prothrombin to meizothrombin the concentration of which can be measured by recording prolongation of plasma clotting time. Dabigatran quenches meizothrombin and therefore the clotting time (ECT) will be proportional to the anticoagulation effect of dabigatran (linear correlation). A typical reference range for ECT in patients anticoagulated with dabigatran (150 mg twice daily) is 34.7 to 158 seconds with the higher value indicating maximum anticoagulation (maximum dabigatran concentration).

Dilute thrombin time (dTT) is based on measuring the clotting time for a mixture of the patient's plasma, pooled normal plasma (1:4 ratio), and a thrombin reagent. Dabigatran inhibits the activity of thrombin and therefore the prolongation of dTT is proportional to the inhibiting effect of dabigatran (linear correlation). A typical reference range for dTT in patients anticoagulated with dabigatran (150 mg twice daily) is 70.2 to 195.1 seconds with the higher value indicating maximum anticoagulation (maximum dabigatran concentration).

NOTE: Reference ranges vary from laboratory to laboratory.

The developer of idarucizumab, Boehringer Ingelheim, has carried out numerous animal experiments and human trials in order to establish the efficacy and safety of the drug. The results of a phase 1 trial involving 48 healthy men were reported in 2015. Idarucizumab in doses up to 5 g (administered intravenously) was found to be safe and well tolerated. A 5-minute infusion of 4 g idarucizumab in patients pretreated with dabigatran for 4 days (220 mg twice daily) immediately reversed dabigatran-induced anticoagulation (98% reduction). The effect was dose- dependent with a dose of 2 g producing a 94% reduction in anticoagulation effect as measured with the dTT test. [38]

Another phase 1 clinical trial treated 46 healthy elderly and middle-aged volunteers (18 with mild or moderate renal impairment) with 220 mg or 150 mg dabigatran twice daily for 4 days. On the fourth day (2 hours after the last dose) study participants were given 5-minute infusions of idarucizumab at dosages of 1 g, 2.5 g, 5 g, or 2x2.5 g 1 hour apart. Dabigatran-prolonged dTT,

APTT, and ECT were immediately reversed to baseline in the volunteers given doses of 2.5 g or 5 g. Idarucizumab was well tolerated regardless of age; however, study participants with impaired kidney function showed decreased dabigatran clearance and prolonged idarucizumab half-life. [39]

In June 2014 enrollment began for the RE-VERSE AD phase 3 trial of idarucizumab. The trial would investigate the outcome of treating patients with dabigatran-induced serious bleeding with idarucizumab. By February 2015 90 patients had been enrolled with 51 patients (96% with atrial fibrillation) experiencing life-threatening bleeding (Group A) and 39 patients (Group B) needing prompt anticoagulation reversal prior to urgent surgery. All patients received 5 g of idarucizumab administered as two 50-mL bolus infusions of 2.5 g each given no more than 15 minutes apart. Blood samples for measurement of ecarin clotting time (ECT) and diluted thrombin time (dTT) were collected at baseline, immediately after idarucizumab infusion, and periodically thereafter and sent to a central laboratory for special analysis. The analysis showed that 22 of the patients had normal dTT levels at baseline indicating ineffective anticoagulation. These patients were excluded from further analysis. The idarucizumab infusion normalized ECT and dTT in the remaining 68 patients within minutes and after 4 hours reversal was 100%. [40]

By July 2016 a total of 503 patients on dabigatran had been enrolled in the RE-VERSE AD trial and final results were reported in August 2017. Of the 503 patients, 301 had uncontrolled bleeding (Group A) and 95% of Group A patients had atrial fibrillation. The remaining 202 patients needed urgent surgery (Group B). Of the 301 patients in Group A 45.5% presented with gastrointestinal bleeding, 32.6% with intracranial hemorrhage and 25.9% had suffered trauma. Comorbidities were frequent in both groups with 78% having hypertension, 36% having congestive heart failure, and 35% having coronary artery disease.

Trial participants were evaluated and treated with idarucizumab as outlined in the interim study of 90 patients discussed above. At baseline 276 patients in Group A and 185 patients in Group B had prolonged ECT or dTT and were included in the primary efficacy analysis. Reversal of dabigatran's anticoagulation effect was 100% within 4 hours of idarucizumab administration as assessed by ECT or dTT. Among Group A patients who could be assessed for bleeding 67.7% had confirmed bleeding cessation within 24 hours.

The 30-day mortality rate (after idarucizumab infusion) was 16.4% among patients with intracranial hemorrhage, 11.1% among patients with gastrointestinal bleeding, and 12.7% among patients with bleeding at other sites.

NOTE: The four trials discussed above were funded by Boehringer Ingelheim, the manufacturer of dabigatran and idarucizumab, and the majority of investigators involved in the trials were either employees of Boehringer Ingelheim or have financial ties to the company. [41]

Andexanet alfa

Andexanet alfa (Annexa) is a genetically modified protein designed to serve as an antidote to direct factor Xa inhibitors such as rivaroxaban, apixaban, and edoxaban.

The direct factor Xa inhibitors bind to factor Xa and thereby inhibit its ability to participate in the reaction that forms blood clots by converting prothrombin to thrombin. Andexanet competes with factor Xa for binding to factor Xa inhibitors and thereby frees up factor Xa to do its job of promoting blood clotting (and stopping bleeding) by cleaving prothrombin to thrombin. Despite its similarity to factor Xa andexanet does not have the ability to promote thrombin formation. It acts very quickly (within 2 to 5 minutes) to stop anticoagulation and its half-life is between 30 and 60 minutes.

Andexanet is administered intravenously either as a 400 mg initial bolus and a 480 mg infusion over 2 hours or an 800 mg initial bolus and a 960 mg infusion over 2 hours. [42]

The developer of andexanet, Portola Pharmaceuticals, has carried out several animal experiments and human trials in order to establish the efficacy and safety of the drug. Outcomes of phase I and phase II trials involving healthy volunteers were reported in 2013 and 2014 with the conclusion that andexanet alfa is safe and effective in reversing the anticoagulant effect of rivaroxaban, apixaban, and edoxaban. [42]

In 2015 results of the ANNEXA-A and ANNEXA-R clinical trials were reported. The investigators concluded that andexanet safely reverses the anticoagulant activity of apixaban and rivaroxaban in older, healthy volunteers within minutes after administration of an intravenously administered bolus and for the duration of a subsequent infusion. [43]

In April 2015 enrollment began for the ANNEXA-4 study. This study would investigate the outcome of treating patients with serious bleeding induced by apixaban, rivaroxaban, or edoxaban with andexanet alfa. By June 2016 results were available for 67 patients (average age: 77 years, 52% male) of which 73% had atrial fibrillation, 30% had deep vein thrombosis, and 25% had suffered a prior stroke. Patients were eligible to participate in the study if they had received a dose of apixaban, rivaroxaban, or edoxaban less than 18 hours before presenting to an emergency department with potentially life-threatening bleeding. Gastrointestinal bleeding was substantially higher among patients taking rivaroxaban (61%) than among patients taking apixaban (33%) while intracranial bleeding was more common among patients taking apixaban (61%) than among patients taking rivaroxaban (36%). The mean time from arrival in the emergency department to administration of andexanet was 4.8 hours.

Andexanet was administered intravenously as a bolus of 400 mg followed by a 2-hour infusion of 480 mg in patients who had taken apixaban (mean daily dose 5 mg) or rivaroxaban (mean daily dose 20 mg) more than 7 hours before the administration of andexanet. For patients who had taken rivaroxaban or edoxaban 7 hours or less before or at an unknown time the initial bolus was 800 mg and the infusion dose was 960 mg.

The anticoagulant effect of apixaban was reduced by 93% from baseline immediately after administration of the initial bolus and by 92% at the end of the 2-hour infusion. Four hours later the reduction in anticoagulant effect was 39% from baseline. Corresponding anticoagulant activity decreases for rivaroxaban were 89%, 86%, and 39% respectively.

During a 30-day follow-up 10 study participants (15%) died (mostly from cardiovascular events). The investigators involved in the study suggest that a controlled study would be required in order to determine whether the incidence of serious adverse events and death observed in the ANNEXA-4 study was higher than expected for a group of patients with similar cardiovascular risk factors. [44]

FDA rejected Portola's initial licence application in August 2016 and a revised version was submitted in August 2017. A decision by FDA was expected by February 2018 but has now been postponed until May 2018.

NOTE: The ANNEXA trials discussed above were sponsored by Portola Pharmaceuticals, the manufacturer of andexanet alfa, and the majority of investigators involved in the trials were either employees of Portola or have financial ties to the pharmaceutical industry.

Ciraparantag

Ciraparantag (PER 977) is a small, synthetic, water-soluble, cationic molecule that was originally designed to bind to heparin and low-molecular-weight-heparin and thereby inhibit their anticoagulant activity. Recent research has shown that ciraparantag binds in a similar way to the new oral factor Xa inhibitors (apixaban, edoxaban, and rivaroxaban), and to the oral thrombin inhibitor, dabigatran. Animal experiments have shown that ciraparantag reverses the anticoagulant activity of the above mentioned NOACs. Ciraparantag does not bind to human coagulation factors or serum albumin and thus has no procoagulant effect. [45]

In November 2014 Perosphere, the developer of ciraparantag, reported the results of a trial carried out to determine if ciraparantag would reverse the anticoagulant effect of edoxaban. The trial involved 80 healthy volunteers who were given a single dose of 60 mg of edoxaban. Three hours later they were either given a placebo or a dose of ciraparantag (5, 15, 25, 50, 100, 200, or 300 mg). Edoxaban increased whole blood clotting time by 37% over baseline. Ciraparantag in the 100 and 300 mg doses reduced clotting time to within 10% of baseline within 10 minutes and this effect was maintained for 24 hours. In contrast, study participants given placebo required 12 to 15 hours to return to a clotting time within 10% of baseline. [46, 47]

Guidelines for Managing Anticoagulant-Induced Bleeding

Guidelines for the management of anticoagulant-induced bleeding was issued by the American College of Cardiology in December 2017. [48]

The first step in the decision pathway is to determine if the bleeding is major or non-major. Bleeding is considered to be <u>major</u> if one or more of the following factors apply:

- Bleeding in a critical site e.g. intracranial hemorrhage, central nervous system bleeds, intramuscular bleeds.
- Hemodynamic instability. An increased heart rate or a significant drop in blood pressure are usually the first signs of this.
- Overt bleeding with a drop in hemoglobin level of 2 g/dL or greater, or the requirement for transfusion of two or more units of red blood cells.

In cases of non-major bleeds local therapy/manual compression and, if applicable, discontinuation of antiplatelet therapy may suffice to stop the bleeding. In more severe bleeds anticoagulation should be stopped, but the use of NOAC reversal agents is not recommended.

In the case of major bleeding the first step is to stop anticoagulation. This should be followed by an injection of vitamin K (5-10 mg) if the patient is on warfarin. Next would be local therapy/manual compression and, if applicable, discontinuation of antiplatelet therapy. The patient should also be assessed and treated for comorbidities (especially renal and liver dysfunction) which may contribute to bleeding and, if necessary, surgery may be performed at the bleeding site to stop the hemorrhage. Blood transfusion and volume resuscitation should be administered as needed. Only in the case of life-threatening bleeding should NOAC reversal agents be administered.

The choice of reversal agent depends on which anticoagulant the patient is on.

Warfarin. Administer *four-factor prothrombin complex concentrate* (4F-PCC) in a dose depending on INR.

Dabigatran. Administer 5 g of idarucizumab intravenously. If idarucizumab is not available administer 4F-PCC or, if that is not available, *activated prothrombin complex concentrate* (aPCC) intravenously at 50 units/kg. If the last dose of dabigatran was taken within 2-4 hours oral administration of activated charcoal should be considered.

Apixaban, edoxaban, rivaroxaban. Administer 4F-PCC or, if that is not available, aPCC intravenously at 50 units/kg. If the last dose of the anticoagulant was taken within 2-4 hours oral administration of activated charcoal should be considered.

Depending on the risk of renewed bleeding and the risk of thrombosis if anticoagulation is withheld, anticoagulation may be restarted with the patient's informed consent when, as judged by the treating physician, it is safe to do so.

Summary

The novel anticoagulants were received with great anticipation and once approved were widely prescribed to patients with atrial fibrillation and venous thromboembolism. The main advantages of the NOACs were promoted as one size fits all, no monitoring required, decreased risk of stroke and bleeding, and less drug and food interactions. Unfortunately, reality has proven a little different.

One size fits all. Patients with kidney impairment cannot tolerate generally prescribed doses of NOACs and dabigatran is not recommended for patients with impaired liver function. In the case of dabigatran the minimum prescribed dose of 75 mg twice daily has not been tested in a clinical trial to establish whether it is actually effective in preventing ischemic stroke. NOTE: The minimum dose approved in Europe is 110 mg twice daily.

No monitoring required. This does not mean that the ability to measure blood concentration of the NOACs would not be highly desirable, particularly in emergencies, but simply that no accurate, reliable, readily available test procedures exist.

Decreased risk of stroke and bleeding
Dabigatran (150 mg twice daily) is superior to warfarin in preventing ischemic stroke, embolism and hemorrhagic stroke but is associated with a 40% (relative) increased risk of heart attack.

Rivaroxaban was deemed non-inferior to warfarin in the treatment of AF patients at moderate to high risk of stroke; however the rate of gastrointestinal bleeding was 45% (relative) higher in patients treated with rivaroxaban than in patients treated with warfarin.

Apixaban (5 mg twice daily) was found to be superior or at least non-inferior to warfarin in the large ARISTOTLE trial which formed the basis for its approval. However, the ARISTOTLE trial had several shortcomings and its conduct caused concern among FDA personnel involved in its evaluation. It remains to be seen if the favourable clinical trial results are replicated in real life.

Edoxaban (60 mg/day) is no more effective than warfarin in preventing ischemic stroke, but does have an advantage when it comes to protecting against hemorrhagic stroke. However, the risk of gastrointestinal bleeding is twice as high with edoxaban as with warfarin. Low dose edoxaban (30 mg/day) is inferior to warfarin when it comes to protecting against ischemic stroke but does have an advantage over warfarin and high-dose edoxaban in respect to the risk of hemorrhagic stroke and gastrointestinal bleeding.

Drug interactions. NOACs interact with many drugs including antiarrhythmics commonly prescribed for atrial fibrillation patients.

Of considerable concern is the fact that INR control was generally sub-optimal in the clinical trials performed to evaluate the efficacy and safety of the novel anticoagulants. This would translate into warfarin being cast in a more unfavourable light than if control had been optimized.

Finally, it is of perhaps greater concern that three of the NOACs (rivaroxaban, apixaban, and edoxaban) do not have an approved antidote which could be used to stem life-threatening bleeding in patients on these drugs.

REFERENCES

1. Connolly, SJ, et al. Dabigatran versus warfarin in patients with atrial fibrillation. New England Journal of Medicine, Vol. 361, September 17, 2009, pp. 1139-51
2. Eikelboom, JW, Yusuf, S, et al. Risk of bleeding with 2 doses of dabigatran compared with warfarin in older and younger patients with atrial fibrillation. Circulation, Vol. 123, May 31, 2011, pp. 2363-72
3. Nagarakanti, R, et al. Dabigatran versus warfarin in patients with atrial fibrillation: an analysis of patients undergoing cardioversion. Circulation, Vol. 123, January 18, 2011, pp. 131-36
4. Cotton, BA, et al. Acutely injured patients on dabigatran. New England Journal of Medicine, Vol. 365, November 24, 2011, pp. 2039-40
5. Uchino, K and Hernandez, AV. Dabigatran association with higher risk of acute coronary events. Archives of Internal Medicine, January 9, 2012 [Epub ahead of print]
6. New York Times, May 29, 2014, page B5
7. Patel, MR, Califf, RM, et al. Rivaroxaban versus warfarin in nonvalvular atrial fibrillation. New England Journal of Medicine, August 10, 2011 [Epub ahead of print]
8. Fox, KAA, et al. Prevention of stroke and systemic embolism with rivaroxaban compared with warfarin in patients with non-valvular atrial fibrillation and moderate renal impairment. European Heart Journal, Vol. 32, 2011, pp. 2387-94
9. Hohnloser SH and Connolly, SJ. Atrial fibrillation, moderate chronic kidney disease, and stroke prevention: new anticoagulants, new hope. European Heart Journal, Vol. 32, 2011, pp. 2347-49
10. Graham, DJ, et al. Stroke, Bleeding, and Mortality Risks in Elderly Medicare Beneficiaries Treated with Dabigatran or Rivaroxaban for Nonvalvular Atrial Fibrillation. JAMA Internal Medicine, Vol. 176 No. 11, November 1, 2016, pp. 1662-1671
11. https://uk.reuters.com/article/us-bayer-xarelto/jury-orders-bayer-jj-to-pay-28-million-in-xarelto-lawsuit-idUKKBN1DZ2NH
12. Connolly, SJ, et al. Apixaban in patients with atrial fibrillation. New England Journal of Medicine, Vol. 364, March 3, 2011, pp. 806-17
13. Granger, Christopher B. et al. Apixaban versus Warfarin in Patients with Atrial Fibrillation. The New England Journal of Medicine, September 15, 2011, pp. 981-992.
14. Mega, JL. A new era for anticoagulation in atrial fibrillation. New England Journal of Medicine, Vol. 365, 2011, pp. 1052-54

15. FDA Summary Review of Apixaban Application2021550rig1s000
    http://www.accessdata.fda.gov/drugsatfda_docs/nda/2012/2021550rig1s
    000SumR.pdf
16. FDA Medical Review of Apixaban Application 2021550rig1s000
    http://www.accessdata.fda.gov/drugsatfda_docs/nda/2012/2021550rig1s
    000MedR.pdf
17. FDA Medical Review of Apixaban Application 2021550rig1s000 page 309
    (182)
18. Lopes, RD, et al. Intracranial hemorrhage in patients with atrial fibrillation
    receiving anticoagulation therapy. Blood, Vol. 129 No.22, June 1, 2017, pp.
    2980-2987
19. FDA Medical Review of Apixaban Application 2021550rig1s000 pages 199-
    200 (72-73)
20. Granger, Christopher B et al. Clinical events after transitioning from apixaban
    versus warfarin to warfarin at the end of the Apixaban for reduction in Stroke
    and Other Thromboembolic Events in Atrial Fibrillation (ARISTOTLE) trial.
    American Heart Journal, January 2015, pp. 25-30.
21. Giugliano, RP, et al. Edoxaban versus warfarin in patients with atrial
    fibrillation. New England Journal of Medicine, November 28, 2013, pp. 2093-
    104
22. Umut Kocabas, et al. Novel oral anticoagulants in non-valvular atrial
    fibrillation: Pharmacological properties, clinical trials, guideline
    recommendations, new antidote drugs and real-world data. International
    Journal of the Cardiovascular Academy, Vol.2, 2016, pp. 167-173
23. Shields AM and Lip GY. Choosing the right drug to fit the patient when
    selecting oral anticoagulation for stroke prevention in atrial fibrillation.
    Journal of Internal Medicine, Vol. 278, July 2015, pp. 1-18
24. Heidbuchel, H, et al. EHRA practical guide on the use of new oral
    anticoagulants in patients with non-valvular atrial fibrillation: Executive
    summary. European Heart Journal, Vol. 34, July 2013, pp. 2094-2106
25. Heidbuchel, H, et al. European Heart Rhythm Association Practical Guide on
    the use of new oral anticoagulants in patients with non-valvular atrial
    fibrillation. Europace, Vol. 15 (5), May 2013, pp. 625-51.
26. Heidbuchel, H, et al. Updated European Heart Rhythm Association Practical
    Guide on the use of non-vitamin K antagonist anticoagulants in patients with
    non-valvular atrial fibrillation. Europace, Vol. 17 (10), October 2015, pp. 1467-
    507.
27. Di Minno, A, et al. Old and new oral anticoagulants: Food, herbal medicines
    and drug interactions. Blood Reviews, Vol. 31 (4), July 2017, pp. 193-203.
28. Budnitz, DS, et al. Emergency hospitalizations for adverse drug events in older
    Americans. New England Journal of Medicine, Vol. 365 (21), November 2011,
    pp. 2002-12.
29. Fang, MC, et al. Death and disability from warfarin-associated intracranial and
    extracranial hemorrhages. American Journal of Medicine, Vol. 120 (8), August
    2007, pp. 700-5.
30. Zareh, M, et al. Reversal of warfarin-induced hemorrhage in the emergency
    department. Western Journal of Emergency Medicine, Vol. 12 (4), November
    2011, pp. 386-92.
31. Frumkin, Kenneth. Rapid reversal of warfarin-associated hemorrhage in the
    emergency department by prothrombin complex concentrates. Annals of
    Emergency Medicine, Vol. 62 (6), December 2013, pp. 616-626.
32. Reilly, PA, et al. Idarucizumab, a specific reversal agent for dabigatran: Mode
    of action, pharmacokinetics and pharmacodynamics, and safety and efficacy

in phase 1 subjects. American Journal of Medicine, Vol. 129 (11S), November 2016, pp. S64-S72.

33. Hu, TY, et al. Reversing anticoagulant effects of novel anticoagulants: Role of ciraparantag, andexanet alpha, and idarucizumab. Vascular Health and Risk Management, Vol. 12, February 2016, pp. 35-44.

34. Hawes, EM, et al. Performance of coagulation tests in patients on therapeutic doses of dabigatran: A cross-sectional pharmacodynamics study based on peak and trough plasma levels. Journal of Thrombosis and Haemostasis, Vol. 11 (8), August 2013, pp.1493-502.

35. Tripodi, Armando. Results expression for tests used to measure the anticoagulant effect of new oral anticoagulants. Thrombosis Journal, Vol. 11 (1), 2013.

36. Nowak, G. The ecarin clotting time, a universal method to quantify direct thrombin inhibitors. Pathophysiology of Haemostasis and Thrombosis, Vol. 33 (4), July 2003-August 2004, pp. 173-183

37. Avecilla, ST, et al. Plasma-diluted thrombin time to measure dabigatran concentrations during dabigatran etexilate therapy. American Journal of Clinical Pathology, Vol. 137 (4), April 2012, pp. 572-4.

38. Glund, S, et al. Safety, tolerability, and efficacy of idarucizumab for the reversal of the anticoagulant effect of dabigatran in healthy male volunteers: a randomized, placebo-controlled, double-blind phase 1 trial. Lancet, Vol. 386 (9994), August 15, 2015, pp. 680-90.

39. Glund, S, et al. Effect of age and renal function on idarucizumab pharmacokinetics and idarucizumab-mediated reversal of dabigatran anticoagulant activity in a randomized, double-blind, crossover phase 1b study. Clinical Pharmacokinetics, Vol. 56 (1), January 2017, pp. 41-54.

40. Pollack, CV Jr, et al. Idarucizumab for dabigatran reversal. New England Journal of Medicine, Vol. 373 (6), August 2015, pp. 511-20.

41. Pollack, CV Jr, et al. Idarucizumab for dabigatran reversal – Full cohort analysis. New England Journal of Medicine, Vol. 377 (5), August 3, 2017, pp. 431-441.

42. Kaatz, S, et al. Reversing factor Xa inhibitors – clinical utility of andexanet alfa. Journal of Blood Medicine, Vol. 8, September 13, 2017, pp. 141-149.

43. Siegal, DW, et al. Andexanet alfa for the reversal of factor Xa inhibitor activity. New England Journal of Medicine, Vol. 373 (25), December 17, 2015, pp. 2413-24.

44. Connolly, SJ, et al. Andexanet alfa for acute major bleeding associated with factor Xa inhibitors. New England Journal of Medicine, Vol. 375 (12), September 22, 2016, pp. 1131-41.

45. Summers, Richard L and Sterling, Sarah A. Emergent bleeding in patients receiving direct oral anticoagulants. Air Medical Journal, Vol. 35, 2016, pp. 148-155.

46. Ansell, JE, et al. Use of PER977 to reverse the anticoagulant effect of edoxaban. New England Journal of Medicine, Vol. 371 (22), November 27, 2014, pp.2141-2.

47. Ansell, JE, et al. Single-dose ciraparantag safely and completely reverses anticoagulant effects of edoxaban. Thrombosis and Haemostasis, Vol. 117 (2), January 26, 2017, pp. 238-245.

48. Tomaselli, GF, et al. 2017 ACC Expert Consensus Decision Pathway on Management of Bleeding in Patients on Oral Anticoagulants; A Report of the American College of Cardiology Task Force on Expert Consensus Decision Pathways. Journal of American College of Cardiology, Vol. 70 (24), December 19, 2017, pp. 3042-3067.

Chapter 15

LAA Occlusion

The left atrial appendage (LAA) is a small pouch-like sac protruding from the left atrium of the heart. It is a remnant of the original embryonic left atrium formed during the third week of gestation. The LAA lies within the pericardium in close contact with the free wall of the left ventricle. It is therefore likely that blood flow in and out of the LAA depends, to a significant degree, on a properly functioning left ventricle. The LAA empties into the left atrium through an orifice located between the left upper pulmonary vein and the left ventricle. The diameter of the orifice is usually between 10 and 24 mm, but can be as small as 5 mm and as large as 40 mm. The volume of the LAA varies between 0.7 and 19 cubic centimeters (mL), and its length is between 16 and 51 mm.

The internal shape of the LAA varies considerably with a 2-lobe structure being the most common (54%), followed by a 3-lobe structure at 23%, a single lobe structure at 20% and a 4-lobe structure at 3%. Cardiac imaging has shown that the structure of the LAA can be visualized as "chicken wing" (48%), "cactus" (30%), "windsock" (19%), and "cauliflower" at (3%). A chicken wing structure is associated with the lowest risk of experiencing an ischemic stroke while the cauliflower structure is associated with the highest risk. [1-3]

The LAA has several important physiological functions [1-3]:

- As it is more distensible than the left atrium itself, it can act as a decompression chamber when left atrial pressure is high. Animal experiments have shown that eliminating access to the LAA results in an increase in the size and mean pressure in the left atrium.

- It helps regulate thirst response.

- It is a major endocrine organ and is the main producer of ANP (atrial natriuretic peptide) in the human heart. The ANP concentration is 40 times higher in the LAA walls than in the rest of the atrial free wall and in the ventricles. A study of patients having undergone the maze procedure and associated LAA removal found a significantly lower ANP secretion and a commensurate increase in salt and water retention.

Unfortunately, the LAA is also associated with two major problems of particular concern to atrial fibrillation patients.

- The edge of the orifice leading into the LAA and, to some extent, the internal walls of the LAA are home to a high concentration of rogue cells that can initiate atrial fibrillation especially in patients with persistent afib. Unfortunately, ablation of these rogue cells is frequently associated with a reduction of flow velocity in and out of the LAA resulting in blood stagnation and subsequent thrombus formation.

The LAA is a known incubator of blood clots (thrombi) that, if migrating to the brain, can cause an ischemic stroke or transient ischemic attack (TIA). It is estimated that close to 95% of all afib-related ischemic strokes involve thrombi released from the LAA. There is, however, evidence that afibbers without underlying heart disease and patients with atrial flutter are at low risk for thrombus formation in the LAA. [4, 5]

It is clear that the LAA can be a very problematical organ for atrial fibrillation patients with compromised heart function and thus not surprising that procedures have been developed for eliminating or occluding (blocking entrance to) the LAA.

Surgical removal/occlusion of the LAA

Surgical removal or occlusion of the LAA is performed by cardiac or cardiothoracic surgeons and is usually carried out as part of a maze procedure or other open heart surgery. In its simplest form it involves cutting off the LAA (excision) and closing the resulting wound with stitches. Other protocols involve closing of the LAA orifice with sutures or staples. Unfortunately, these surgical procedures are often unsuccessful with excision having the highest success rate at 73% while the success rates for suture exclusion and stapler exclusion are only 23% and 0% respectively. [6]

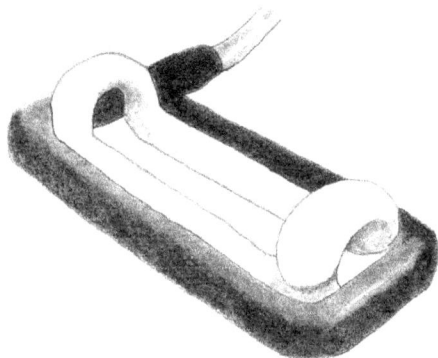

A less invasive procedure involves the use of an *AtriClip* device to squeeze the neck of the LAA tightly shut so as to prevent any movement of blood between the main left atrium and the LAA. The *AtriClip* (www.atricure.com) consists of two parallel, straight, rigid titanium tubes with elastic nitinol springs and a 90-degree angle at both ends of the tubes. The tubes are covered with a urethane elastomer and the whole clip is covered with a knit-braided polyester sheath. Clips are available in different sizes so as to fit a wide variety of LAA shapes. The *AtriClip* can be installed during open heart surgery or using thoracoscopic surgery (keyhole surgery).

Early experiments at the Cleveland Clinic indicated that the installation of *AtriClips* was quick, safe, and totally effective in closing off all blood flow between the left atrium and the LAA. NOTE: This study was supported by a grant from AtriCure. [7]

The first clinical trial of the *AtriClip* in atrial fibrillation patients was carried out in 2008 in University Hospital Zurich in Switzerland. The trial involved 34 atrial fibrillation patients scheduled for ablation and elective cardiac surgery (valve repair or replacement). Median age of the patients was 71 years, 58% were men, 42% had paroxysmal afib, 23% persistent, and 35% had permanent afib. Following pulmonary vein isolation and valve repair/replacement (open heart surgery on or off pump) *AtriClips* were installed as close as possible to the base of the LAA. If necessary, the clip was repositioned to obtain the best possible fit before releasing it from the positioning tool. Complete isolation of the LAA was confirmed with TEE (100% procedural success). NOTE: This study was supported by a grant from AtriCure. [8]

The trial participants were followed for 3.5 years. CT scans showed that the clips were still in their original position 3 years after the procedure, no intracardial thrombi were observed and none of the patients had a residual LAA (stump) more than 10 mm in depth. One patient experienced a transient ischemic attack (TIA) during follow-up and this was thought to be due to carotid plaque. No other patients experienced a TIA, stroke, or other neurological event during the follow-up period even though only 3 patients were still on warfarin. Of particular interest is the finding that complete electrical isolation of the LAA was observed immediately following clip placement. NOTE: This study was funded by AtriCure. [9]

The fact that no afib-related TIAs or strokes were recorded during follow-up and that the AtriClip procedure resulted in complete electrical isolation of the LAA could mean that successful placement of the clip would eliminate or vastly reduce two LAA-related problems: the initiation of atrial fibrillation by rogue cells in the LAA (particularly prevalent in persistent afib) and the formation and release of thrombi from the LAA.

The results of the EXCLUDE trial were reported in November 2011. This trial included 71 patients scheduled for elective open heart cardiac surgery at 7 cardiac centers in the US. Most of the trial participants (77.5%) underwent bypass surgery and 40% had aortic valve replacement. In addition, 35% of patients underwent a maze procedure (ablation or cut-and-sew). All study participants except one (LAA too small) had an *AtriClip* device inserted during or after cardiac surgery. The installation successfully eliminated blood flow between the LAA and the left atrium in 95.7% of patients as confirmed by TEE. No incidences of damage to the LAA or device migration from its original position were observed. At the 3-month follow-up 95% of patients showed complete isolation as measured by TEE or CTA (computed tomography angiography). At 12 months follow-up one patient had experienced a TIA (attributed to a hypertensive crisis) and one had experienced a stroke attributed to cholesterol plaque; at this point 30% of study participants were still on warfarin. NOTE: This study was funded by AtriCure. [10]

In July 2017 a group of Czech cardiac surgeons reported that the *AtriClip* could be successfully installed using a thoracoscopic approach. Their clinical trial included 101 patients undergoing cardiac surgery of which 57 patients underwent a maze (mini-maze) procedure carried out thoracoscopically and 7 had the *AtriClip* installed in a stand-alone procedure. Complete isolation of the LAA and a residual stump of less than 10 mm in depth was confirmed using Doppler echocardiography in 98% of *AtriClip* recipients. No TIAs or strokes related to LAA thrombi were recorded during a mean follow-up of 7 to 30 months. [11]

Percutaneous procedure is a medical procedure where access to the heart is achieved via a puncture of the skin, usually in the groin, followed by the threading of a carrier tube through the femoral vein to the inside of the heart.

Laparoscopic surgery (keyhole surgery) is a minimally invasive procedure carried out with the aid of a small video camera and one or more special, thin surgical instruments introduced into a body cavity through one or more small incisions. The surgeon uses the image transmitted by the video camera to guide the procedure which may be performed under general, spinal, epidural, or spinal-epidural anesthesia depending on the organ targeted.

Thoracoscopic surgery is laparoscopic surgery targeted at organs located in the chest cavity. Access is gained through incisions made between the ribs.

The Swiss team that performed the first clinical trial of *AtriClip* implantation in atrial fibrillation patients recently reported long-term follow-up data on 291 patients who had an *AtriClip* device implanted as part of an open heart surgery procedure. The majority (67%) of study participants had undergone a maze procedure or pulmonary vein ablation as part of their surgery. Twenty-three patients had long term CT scan data (5 to 8 year follow-up). The scans confirmed durable and complete LAA occlusion with no signs of substantial residual stump or changes of *AtriClip* position.

Two ischemic strokes occurred in the subgroup of 166 patients (average CHA_2DS_2-VASc score of 3.2) who were not on anticoagulants corresponding to an average incidence of 0.5%/year. This is well below the expectation for a group of 70-year-old healthy people and considerably below the 18 strokes which would be expected in a group with a CHA_2DS_2-VASc score of 3.2. The Swiss team conclude that LAA occlusion is an effective means of preventing afib-related stroke and discontinued prescribing post-procedure anticoagulants for patients having undergone successful *AtriClip* implantation after 2010. NOTE: This study was supported by a grant from AtriCure. [12]

In January 2018 a group of Czech cardiac surgeons reported on a trial involving 40 atrial fibrillation patients who underwent thoracoscopic ablation and installation of an *AtriClip* device. *AtriClip* installation was successful in 39 of the patients (procedural success rate: 97.5%). At follow-up 2-3 months after the procedure all devices in the 39 patients were stable without leaks, shifts, or thrombi formation. The average depth of the remaining LAA stump was 13 mm and the residual LAA volume was 3.6 mL. The Czech surgeons conclude that LAA occlusion with the *AtriClip* using the thoracoscopic approach is safe and as effective as occlusion carried out using open-chest surgery. [13]

The *AtriClip* device was approved by the FDA in 2009 for occlusion of the LAA. By 2017 close to 100,000 of the devices had been installed. [14]

Non-surgical occlusion of the LAA

Although the *AtriClip* is effective in occluding the LAA its installation requires cardiac surgery which may not be acceptable to some patients and their physicians. Thus the search for alternative, less invasive ways of closing off the LAA. The success and now routine acceptance of catheter ablation for atrial fibrillation spawned the idea of closing off the LAA from the inside of the heart rather than from the outside as is the case with the *AtriClip*. This concept involves catheterization of the heart in a procedure similar to that used for performing pulmonary vein ablation in which the ablation catheter is advanced into the left atrium through a tube inserted in the femoral vein at the groin. The difference being that instead of using the tube to advance an ablation catheter one would use it to advance an occlusion device to the mouth of the LAA and there expand it to tightly occlude the LAA. Currently the two favourite devices embodying this principle are the *WATCHMAN* device and the *Amplatzer Amulet*. Both devices are installed by specially trained electrophysiologists.

WATCHMAN system

The *WATCHMAN* device (www.watchman.com) was developed by Atritech (later acquired by Boston Scientific) and was first implanted in human beings in 2002. It received EU approval in 2005 and FDA approval in March 2015.

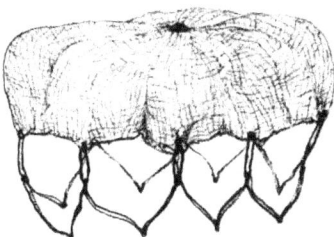

The device consists of a self-expanding nitinol frame shaped somewhat like an umbrella. The frame is covered with a PET (polyethylene terephthalate) membrane to prevent the outflow of thrombi from the LAA and to help promote endothelialization (growth of a skin of endothelial cells) covering the part of the device facing the atrium. The *WATCHMAN* comes in sizes ranging from 21 to 33 mm so as to fit LAA orifices of different diameters and is equipped with barbs around its perimeter to facilitate adherence to the inside of the LAA. Prior to implantation TEE is done to measure the dimensions and morphology of the LAA and to ensure that there are no thrombi in the LAA. The implantation of the device is performed with TEE guidance, takes 50 minutes or less and is done using local or general anaesthesia. Following completion of the procedure the patient is prescribed warfarin or one of the newer anticoagulants to be taken for 45 days to protect against stroke until endothelialization is complete.

In April 2007 an international group of electrophysiologists reported on their experience with implantation of a first (16 patients) and second (53 patients) generation *WATCHMAN* device in 75 atrial fibrillation patients with a mean CHADS$_2$ score of 1.9. Implantation was successful in 66 (88%) of the patients with the main reason for failure being an unsuitable LAA anatomy. Follow-up 45 days after the implantation procedure showed that the LAA had been completely closed in 54 of 58 patients (93%) with no significant flow of blood around the device. No strokes were reported during a 2 year follow-up period. However, 2 TIAs occurred during the six months following the implantation. At the end of the six months 91.7% of patients in the follow-up group had discontinued warfarin therapy. Adverse effects were more common in first generation implantations and included broken delivery wires, pericardial effusion, and thrombus formation on the device surface facing the atrium. [15]

The results of a large clinical trial (PROTECT AF) designed to compare the safety and efficacy of *WATCHMAN* implantation with standard warfarin therapy were reported in 2009. The trial involved 707 patients with non-valvular atrial fibrillation and one or more risk factors for ischemic stroke (average CHADS$_2$ score: 2.2). Intolerance to anticoagulation was an absolute cause for exclusion from the trial. Trial participants were randomly assigned to *WATCHMAN* implantation guided by fluoroscopy and TEE (463 patients) or to warfarin therapy (244 patients) with a target INR between 2.0 and 3.0. The *WATCHMAN* device was successfully implanted in 408 patients (88% of ITT population) while implantation was not attempted or failed in 55 patients.

Anticoagulation with warfarin in the *WATCHMAN* group was discontinued after 45 days if a TEE showed no or an acceptable degree of leakage around the device (jet less than 5 mm in width). At the 45 day mark warfarin therapy was discontinued in 86% of patients having undergone successful implantation. At the 1-year follow-up 92% of patients in the device group were no longer on warfarin. Antiplatelet therapy with once daily clopidogrel (75 mg) and aspirin (81-325 mg) was prescribed for use till the end of the 6-month follow-up period after which aspirin was prescribed to be taken indefinitely.

At 1588 patient-years of follow-up 3.0%/year of patients in the *WATCHMAN* group and 4.3% in the warfarin group had experienced stroke or systemic embolism or had died from cardiovascular causes (primary endpoint). This difference in outcome met the criteria for noninferiority using ITT analysis. The noninferiority criteria was also met in a PP analysis in which 2.1% of patients in the *WATCHMAN* group and 4.1% in the warfarin group had reached the primary endpoint. It is worth noting that the annual incidence of ischemic stroke was 1.9% in the *WATCHMAN* group versus 1.4% in the warfarin group which may indicate that the device tends to be less effective when it comes to protecting against ischemic stroke.

Serious adverse events (major bleeding, intracranial hemorrhage, pericardial effusion, and device embolization) occurred at a rate of 5.5%/year in the *WATCHMAN* group vs. 3.6% in the warfarin group. Most adverse events in the *WATCHMAN* group were periprocedural and included 22 patients with pericardial effusion requiring surgical intervention and 5 patients who suffered procedure-related strokes. The investigators involved in the trial concluded that *WATCHMAN* occlusion of the left atrial appendage is non-inferior to warfarin therapy and may be a viable alternative to chronic warfarin therapy. The FDA was less convinced of this and, citing the unacceptable level of procedural complications especially during installation, withheld final approval pending further trials. NOTE: This trial was funded by Atritech and the lead investigators had close financial ties to the company. [16, 17]

The conclusion reached in the PROTECT trial was challenged by researchers at McMaster University in Hamilton, Ontario who stated "No conclusive evidence exists to demonstrate that LAA exclusion reduces stroke in AF patients". They also pointed out that there is evidence that removing or isolating the LAA may decrease cardiac function, impair hemodynamic response to volume and pressure changes, impede thirst, and promote heart failure. Thus it is, by no means, certain that eliminating LAA function is a benign procedure. Furthermore, some studies involving surgical closure of the LAA have shown that stroke risk can actually increase if the LAA is not completely isolated.

In commenting specifically on the PROTECT trial they point out that 12.3% of patients experienced serious complications during the implantation procedure and that the rate of ischemic stroke during the follow-up period was actually 50% higher in the *WATCHMAN* group than in the warfarin group. Nevertheless, the total incidence of stroke (including hemorrhagic stroke), cardiovascular death, and systemic embolization was lower in the *WATCHMAN* group than in the warfarin group. Their final conclusion was, "the evidence of efficacy and safety is insufficient to recommend this approach for any patients other than those in whom long-term warfarin is absolutely contraindicated". [18]

The PREVAIL trial reported in July 2014 was instigated to alleviate concerns about serious complications during implantation of the *WATCHMAN* device in the PROTECT AF trial reported in 2009. The goal of the trial was to prove that the *WATCHMAN* device could be implanted safely and that it was no less effective than long-term warfarin therapy in preventing stroke, systemic embolism, and death from cardiovascular causes (primary endpoint). The trial involved 407 patients with non-valvular atrial fibrillation and one or more risk factors for ischemic stroke (average $CHADS_2$ score: 2.6). Patients were randomly assigned to *WATCHMAN* implantation guided by TEE and fluoroscopy (269 patients) or to warfarin therapy (138 patients) with a target INR of 2.0-3.0. The device was successfully implanted in 95.1% of the 265 patients in which an attempt was made to do so giving an ITT success rate of 93.6%.

After implantation, patients were prescribed warfarin and 81 mg/day aspirin for 45 days to prevent large thrombus formation on the device during its endothelialization. Anticoagulation was discontinued after 45 days if a TEE showed no or an acceptable degree of leakage around the device (jet less than 5 mm in width). At the 45 day mark warfarin therapy was discontinued in 92% of patients having undergone successful implantation. At the 1-year follow-up 99% of patients in the device group were no longer on warfarin. Antiplatelet therapy with once daily clopidogrel (75 mg) and aspirin (81-325 mg) was prescribed for use till the end of the 6-month follow-up period after which aspirin was prescribed to be taken indefinitely.

At 18 months follow-up 14 primary endpoint events had occurred in 5.3% of patients in the *WATCHMAN* group as compared to 4 endpoint events in 2.9% of warfarin-treated patients. The trial investigators conclude that *WATCHMAN* implantation is not non-inferior (i.e. it is inferior) to long-term warfarin therapy when it comes to protecting against stroke, systemic embolism, and death from cardiovascular causes. The incidence of procedure-related complications (cardiac perforation, pericardial effusion with tamponade, ischemic stroke, device embolization, and other vascular complications occurring in the first 7 days after implantation) decreased from 8.7% in the PROTECT AF trial to 4.2% in the PREVAIL trial. The *WATCHMAN* device was approved by the FDA in March 2015 for use to reduce the risk of stroke in patients with non-valvular atrial fibrillation.

NOTE: This trial was funded by Atritech/Boston Scientific and 7 out of the 8 investigators reporting on the trial had close financial ties to the company. [19]

Five-year combined outcomes for the PROTECT and PREVAIL trials performed in 100 centers in Europe and the USA were reported in December 2017.

5-Year Outcomes of *WATCHMAN* Trials

	WATCHMAN	Warfarin
Number of patients	732	382
Average CHADS$_2$ score	2.3	2.4
Efficacy *	2.8%/year	3.45%/year
Ischemic stroke	1.6%/year	0.95%/year
Hemorrhagic stroke	0.17%/year	0.87%/year
All-cause death	3.6%/year	4.9%/year

* Annual rate of stroke, systemic embolism, and cardiovascular death

The incidence of hemorrhagic stroke and all-cause death was significantly less in the *WATCHMAN* group.

The authors of the study conclude that the *WATCHMAN* device provides stroke prevention in non-valvular atrial fibrillation patients to a similar degree as anticoagulation with warfarin. In addition, the *WATCHMAN* device minimizes major bleeding and hemorrhagic stroke and thus results in less disability or death than warfarin. NOTE: This trial was funded by Atritech/Boston Scientific and all the 11 authors of this study had close financial ties to the company. [20]

Two studies have evaluated the extent of procedure-related complications associated with *WATCHMAN* implantation. One involved 3822 cases of implantation performed in the USA since FDA approval (Post-approval Study) and one involved 1021 patients who had a *WATCHMAN* device installed in centers in 13 European countries since October 2013 (EWOLUTION Study).

Procedural Complications during *WATCHMAN* Implantation

	Post-Approval Study	EWOLUTION Registry
Number of patients	3822	1021
Average CHADS$_2$ score	2.3	2.8
Implantation success	95.6%	98.5%
Procedure duration - minutes	50	N/A
Pericardial tamponade	1.02%	0.29%
Procedure-related stroke	0.08%	0.10%
7-day mortality	0.03%	0.29%

The authors of both studies conclude that procedural complication rates in *WATCHMAN* implantation are now acceptably low. NOTE: The EWOLUTION study was funded by Boston Scientific and 12 of the 20 authors of the reports presenting the results of the studies had close financial ties with Boston Scientific. [21, 22]

It is known that the risk of suffering an ischemic stroke increases substantially if surgical closure of the LAA is unsuccessful. Electrophysiologists at St. David's Medical Center report that gaps may develop between the periphery of the *WATCHMAN* device and the wall of the LAA thus allowing blood to flow into the left atrium and vice versa. Their study involved 58 atrial fibrillation patients who had a *WATCHMAN* device implanted between November 2008 and June 2010. The average age of the patients was 74 years, 64% were male, and 74% had a CHADS$_2$ score of 2 or higher. Transesophageal echocardiography (TEE) was used to guide the initial placement of the device. TEE was also used to check its position and look for gaps 45 days and 12 months after implantation. All patients were maintained on warfarin (INR between 2.0 and 3.0) for the first 45 days following implantation, after which, 55 (95%) discontinued anticoagulation.

Although TEE at the end of the insertion procedure showed tight closure and no gaps in 72% of patients, notable gaps were observed in the remaining 28%. At the 45-day TEE an additional 12% of patients had developed new gaps, but some of these had closed and others had opened at the 12-month TEE examination. All told, at the 12-month follow-up, 65% of patients had no visible gaps, while the remaining 35% had one or more. During 26 months of follow-up, one patient had a stroke (4.7 months after implantation). No device dislodgement occurred during follow-up. The investigators conclude that incomplete LAA closure with gaps between the *WATCHMAN* device and the LAA wall is relatively common. They recommend further trials to determine whether the presence, persistence, or variation in the size of the gaps is related to stroke risk. [23]

The protocol for anticoagulation used in such major *WATCHMAN* implantation trials as PROTECT AF and PREVAIL calls for warfarin to be administered prior to the procedure and for 45 days afterwards. This clearly poses a major obstacle for using the *WATCHMAN* device in patients who cannot tolerate anticoagulants. A US/European multicenter trial reported in June 2013 enrolled 150 patients with non-valvular atrial fibrillation and a contraindication for even short-term anticoagulation in the ASA Plavix Feasibility Study. The patients had an average $CHADS_2$ score of 2.8 and 93% had a documented history of major bleeding.

The implantation of the *WATCHMAN* device was carried out using heparin for anticoagulation and fluoroscopy and TEE for guidance. Following successful implantation patients were treated with clopidogrel or ticlopidine for 6 months and were then prescribed aspirin to be taken for life. Implantation success was 94.7% and average procedure time was 52 minutes. Thirteen patients (8.7%) suffered serious procedure- or device-related safety events including 5 patients with pericardial effusion, 3 with device embolization and 3 with hematoma relating to the femoral access.

The percentage of patients who reached the primary endpoint (stroke, systemic embolism, and death from cardiovascular causes) during a 177 person-year follow-up period was 4.6%/year. The incidence of ischemic stroke was 1.7%/person-year; this is well below the rate of 7.3% expected in a group of patients with a $CHADS_2$ score of 2.8 treated with aspirin alone. The trial investigators conclude that *WATCHMAN* implantation using post-procedural aspirin rather than warfarin is a reasonable alternative to consider for patients at high risk for stroke but with contraindications to systemic oral anticoagulation. NOTE: Boston Scientific provided financial support for this trial and six of the eight investigators had financial ties to Boston Scientific, the manufacturer of the *WATCHMAN* device. [24]

Embolization refers to the formation of a blood clot (embolus).

Endothelialization refers to the formation of endothelial tissue, for example, covering a stent or occlusion device.

Ligation refers to a surgical procedure in which a blood vessel or hollow organ in the body is closed with a ligature (string) or clip.

Amplatzer Amulet system

The *Amplatzer Amulet* system is manufactured and marketed by St. Jude Medical. It was first implanted in human beings in 2008 and received European CE approval in 2013. It is still awaiting approval by the FDA.

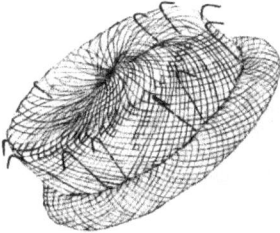

The *Amplatzer Amulet* is a three-part system consisting of a trans-septal access sheath, a delivery catheter, and the implant itself (a self-expanding nitinol cage covered by a polyester membrane). The *Amplatzer* cage distinguishes itself from the similar *WATCHMAN* cage in that it consists of two parts: a part equipped with hooks to ensure retention that is inserted into the left atrial appendage (the lobe) and an outer disc that seals the edges of the device against the atrium wall. The lobe is available in 8 different diameters from 16 to 30 mm. Prior to implantation TEE is done to measure the dimensions and morphology of the LAA so as to pick the optimum lobe diameter and to ensure that there are no thrombi in the LAA. The implantation of the device is performed with TEE and fluoroscopy guidance and is done using local or general anaesthesia. Following completion of the procedure patients are prescribed aspirin and clopidogrel for 1-6 months to protect against stroke until endothelialization is complete.

Between December 2008 and December 2009 137 atrial fibrillation patients underwent *Amplatzer* device installation at 10 European centers. Implantation was successful in 132 patients (96%). Patients with successful implantations were prescribed clopidogrel and aspirin for 1-3 months followed by just aspirin for 5 months or longer. Cardiac tamponade (a serious medical condition in which blood or fluids fill the space between the sac that encases the heart and the heart muscle) occurred in 5 patients, 3 suffered a stroke, and 2 experienced device embolization during the implantation procedure resulting in a procedure-related major complication rate of 7.3%. The comparable rate observed in the PROTECT AF trial was 6.7%. The study investigators conclude that implantation of an *Amplatzer Amulet* device is a feasible method for percutaneous occlusion of the LAA, but point out that the benefit risk/ratio of doing so in patients at low risk for ischemic stroke is likely to be negative. [25]

A separate trial carried out in Poland confirmed that implantation of the *Amplatzer* device can be done safely even in patients with a high risk of stroke and bleeding complications. This trial involved 21 atrial fibrillation patients with a mean age of 71 years, a mean CHA_2DS_2-VASc score of 4.4 and a HAS-BLED score of 3. The occlusion device was safely implanted in 20 patients (success rate: 95.2%). One major cardiac tamponade was observed during the implantation procedure yielding a procedure-related major complication rate of 4.8%. [26]

The first data regarding the efficacy and long-term safety of the *Amplatzer Amulet* was reported in July 2013 by a team of Canadian electrophysiologists. Their clinical trial, involving 7 cardiac centers in Canada, enrolled 52 patients with nonvalvular atrial fibrillation and contraindication to anticoagulation therapy. The mean age of the patients was 74 years (58% male) and median $CHADS_2$ score was 3. More than half (55.8%) had a history of ischemic stroke and 90% had a history of serious bleeding, mainly intracranial and gastrointestinal.

The *Amplatzer* device was successfully implanted in 51 patients (success rate: 98.1%). The incidence of serious procedural complications was 5.8% which compares favourably with the rate of serious procedural complications reported in other trials of percutaneous LAA occlusion. Antiplatelet therapy consisting of clopidogrel (75 mg/day) plus aspirin (80 to 325 mg/day) was given for 30 to 180 days following the procedure, after which single antiplatelet therapy was prescribed. During a mean follow-up of 20 months 1 cardiac tamponade, 1 stroke, 1 TIA, and 1 incidence of major bleeding were recorded yielding a total major complication rate of 4.7%/person-year. No cases of severe residual leak or device thrombosis were observed at the 6-month follow-up.

The trial investigators conclude that percutaneous closure of the left atrial appendage may be a therapeutic alternative to avoid thromboembolic events in patients with absolute contraindications to anticoagulation therapy. [27]

The results of a major observational study of the safety and efficacy of *Amplatzer* implantation in a "real world" population was reported in February 2016. The study included 1047 non-valvular atrial fibrillation patients (57% with permanent AF and 39% with a history of stroke/TIA) who had the device implanted between December 2008 and November 2013 at one of 22 European cardiac centers. The average age of the patients was 75 years and 62% were male. Average $CHADS_2$ score was 2.8 and average CHA_2DS_2-VASc score was 4.5. The patients had all been referred for LAA occlusion because of serious risk of bleeding. The average HAS-BLED score of the group was 3.1 which equates to an estimated annual risk of major bleeding of 5.4%.

The *Amplatzer* device was successfully implanted in 1019 patients (success rate: 97.3%). A TEE follow-up seven months after implantation found no significant leaks in 98% of implantees. There were 52 serious, procedure-related adverse events of which 8 were related to femoral artery access, 9 were strokes, and 13 were cardiac tamponades for a total incidence of serious, periprocedural events of 5%. Antiplatelet therapy consisting of clopidogrel (75 mg/day) plus aspirin (80 to 100 mg/day) was given for 1 to 3 months following the procedure, after which aspirin therapy was prescribed for at least another 3 months. During an average follow-up of 13 months (1349 patient-years) there were no device-related deaths, but 9 strokes, 9 TIAs and 31 cases of systemic thromboembolism were recorded for a total major complication rate of 4.1%/person-year.

The annual rate of systemic thromboembolism was 59% lower than expected for a group of patients with a CHA2DS2-VASc score of 4.5. The annual rate of major bleeding was 2.1% which is 61% lower than the rate expected for a group of patients with a HAS-BLED score of 3.1. Patients who were on aspirin monotherapy or no antithrombotic therapy at follow-up actually fared better than patients who were on more elaborate stroke prevention schemes. Annual incidence of thromboembolism was only 1.33% in the aspirin only group as compared to 4.28% in the other group. The risk of major bleeding was also significantly lower in the aspirin group with a reduction of 74.6% compared to 23.6% when compared to the risk estimated from the HAS-BLED score.

The study investigators conclude that LAA occlusion with the *Amplatzer Amulet* device showed high procedural success and a favourable outcome for the prevention of AF-related thromboembolism. NOTE: Twenty of the 27 authors of the study report had financial ties to St. Jude Medical. [28]

The most recent global, observational study involving LAA occlusion with the *Amplatzer Amulet* involved 1088 patients with non-valvular atrial fibrillation who were enrolled at 61 cardiac centers in Europe, Australia, Israel, Chile, and Hong Kong. The average age of the patients was 75 years and 64.5% were male. The vast majority (72.4%) had a history of major bleeding and 82.8% had contraindications to oral anticoagulation. This patient group was far from healthy with 84% having hypertension and 38% having a history of stroke or TIA. Mean CHA2DS2-VASc score was 4.2 and 77.5% of patients had a HAS-BLED score greater than 3.

The *Amulet* device was successfully implanted in 1077 patients resulting in a success rate of 99%. General anaesthesia was employed in 56.5% of procedures and conscious sedation in 41.2%. Major device-related adverse events occurring during the implantation procedure or within 7 days following the procedure were experienced by 35 patients (3.2%) with major bleeding being the most common event at 2.4% followed by hematoma at the femoral vein insertion site (0.4%), and stroke at 0.2%. Most patients (54.3%) were discharged on dual antiplatelet therapy with aspirin and clopidogrel, 18.9% were discharged on anticoagulant with or without dual antiplatelet therapy, and 16% were discharged on aspirin alone. In the 3 months following implantation (excluding the first 7 days post-procedure) 26 patients (2.4%) experienced a device-related major adverse event with ischemic stroke, systemic embolism, and cardiovascular death accounting for 1.4% and device embolization accounting for the remaining 1.0%.

Follow-up TEE results available for 673 patients showed adequate closure in 98.2%. However, device-related thrombus formation was observed in 10 patients despite antiplatelet or anticoagulation therapy. The incidence of major bleeding during the follow-up period (between 8 and 90 days post-implantation) was 4.0% and mainly related to gastrointestinal bleeding and anemia.

The study investigators conclude that the success rate for *Amplatzer* implantation is high and the risk of periprocedural complications low in a population with a high risk of stroke and major bleeding. NOTE: This study was funded by St. Jude Medical (now Abbott) and 12 out of the 16 investigators had financial ties to the company. [29]

Clinical trials of the *Amplatzer* device have involved mainly elderly atrial fibrillation patients with a history of serious bleeding and/or contraindications to oral anticoagulation. It was hoped that occlusion of the LAA with the *Amplatzer* would eventually (6 months or so after implantation) completely eliminate the need for anticoagulation and antiplatelet therapy. A study presented at the 2017 CARDIOSTIM conference in Vienna raises doubt that this hope will be realized.

The study (not industry-sponsored) involved 377 consecutive AF patients who underwent LAA occlusion in 7 French cardiac centers between March 2012 and September 2016. The average age of the patients was 75 years, mean CHA_2DS_2-VASc score was 4.5 and mean HAS-BLED score was 3.7. The estimated risk of suffering an ischemic stroke would be about 6%/year in this group and the annual risk of suffering a major bleeding episode would be about 7% with no antiplatelet or anticoagulation therapy.

There were 245 *WATCHMAN* devices and 115 *Amplatzer* devices implanted with a success rate of 96%. Patients were prescribed antiplatelet or anticoagulation therapy at discharge as follows:

Antithrombotic therapy on discharge	*Amplatzer*	WATCHMAN	Total
No therapy	14.9%	3.4%	8.1%
Single antiplatelet therapy	39.9%	30.9%	36.1%
Dual antiplatelet therapy	25.2%	20.3%	21.1%
Oral anticoagulation alone	18.5%	37.0%	28.9%
Anticoagulation + antiplatelet	1.7%	6.1%	5.8%

During a mean follow-up of 11 months a total of 75 major adverse events were recorded.

Major adverse event	Amplatzer	WATCHMAN	Total
Thrombus formation on device	8.6%	4.9%	6.1%
Ischemic stroke	-	-	2.8%
Major hemorrhages	-	-	5.0%
Cardiovascular-related death	-	-	1.3%

Older age and a history of previous ischemic stroke were the only independent predictors of thrombus formation. Being on single antiplatelet therapy or anticoagulation tended to be associated with a lower risk of thrombus formation although this association did not reach statistical significance. Patients with thrombus on the device had an 8 times greater risk of ischemic stroke than did patients without and thrombus on device was the only independent predictor of stroke during follow-up. [30]

During the actual presentation at the CARDIOSTIM conference, the presenter, Dr. Laurent Fauchier, added new data indicating that post-procedure antithrombotic treatment with aspirin + clopidogrel (dual antiplatelet therapy) may reduce the risk of on-device thrombus formation. Concluding his presentation, Dr. Fauchier emphasized the need to optimize antithrombotic management both during implantation and post-operatively in order to reduce device-related thrombus formation and incidence of ischemic stroke and TIA. [31]

It is of interest to note that most patients in the *Amplatzer* trials were discharged on aspirin alone or aspirin + clopidogrel rather than on warfarin or one of the newer oral anticoagulants. The reason for this is that a thrombus formed on a foreign device follows the intrinsic pathway in growing to a full-fledged thrombus whereas a thrombus formed in the LAA (cardioembolic thrombus) follows the extrinsic pathway. The key steps in the intrinsic pathway are platelet activation and platelet aggregation both of which are effectively halted by aspirin, clopidogrel and natural supplements such as vitamin B6, vitamin C, vitamin E, niacin, fish oils, garlic, ginkgo biloba, l-arginine, and resveratrol.

Unfortunately, the risk of major gastrointestinal bleeding is substantially increased both in patients treated with aspirin as well as in patients treated with dual antiplatelet therapy. A study involving 243 coronary heart disease patients with implanted drug-eluding stents reported a post-surgery incidence of serious gastrointestinal bleeding of 3.8%/year in patients treated with aspirin alone and 4.8%/year in patients treated with dual antiplatelet therapy. [32]

Endocardial Procedure: A medical [surgical] procedure where the heart wall is approached from the outside such as in the maze procedure.

Epicardial Procedure: A medical procedure where the heart wall is approached from the inside such as in catheter ablation.

Surgical/non-surgical occlusion of the LAA

LARIAT device

There is convincing evidence that introducing a foreign body into the blood stream, be it a stent or an LAA occlusion device, substantially increases the risk of thrombus formation and ischemic stroke. Thus the idea of squeezing the opening of the LAA shut from the outside of the heart rather than plugging it up from the inside with a foreign body intuitively makes eminent sense.

The *Atriclip* works on this principle of squeezing the LAA shut and so does the concept of squeezing it shut using a *LARIAT* suture delivery device.

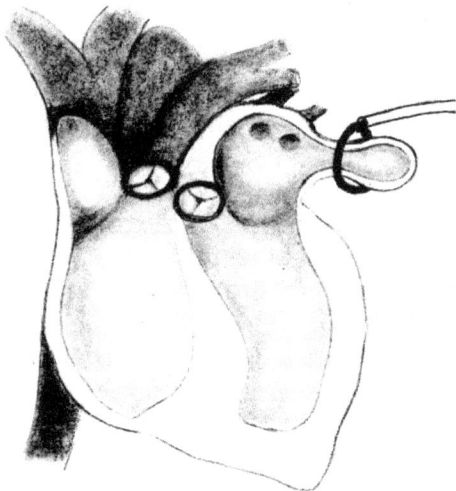

The *LARIAT* procedure employs a combination of thoracoscopic surgery and the technique used in catheter ablation to treat atrial fibrillation. A delivery tube is threaded through the femoral vein and used to advance a magnet-tipped wire through the right and left atria into the top of the left atrial appendage using TEE and/or fluoroscopy for guidance. Using thoracoscopic surgery a second magnet-tipped guide-wire is then inserted through a tiny hole below the breastbone and advanced to the top of the LAA where the two magnets join and form an uninterrupted guide-wire. The *LARIAT* (lasso) device is then advanced along the guide-wire until it comes to rest where the base of the LAA connects with the left atrium. The lasso is pulled tight thereby completely isolating (ligating) the LAA which, over time, atrophies. The *LARIAT* procedure is performed under general anaesthesia and takes 1-3 hours with the patient being released from hospital on the day following the procedure.

The *LARIAT* device is manufactured and marketed by SentreHEART, a California-based company. It was approved by the EU in October 2016, but has still to receive approval by the FDA for use in LAA occlusion.

The first installation of *LARIAT* devices in human beings was carried out in 2010 at the John Paul II Hospital in Krakow, Poland. It involved 11 patients undergoing concomitant catheter ablation for atrial fibrillation. The procedure was successful in 10 patients. [33]

The results of a clinical trial of the *LARIAT* involving Polish and American cardiac surgeons and electrophysiologists were reported in July 2013. The trial involved 89 patients with nonvalvular atrial fibrillation. The average age of the patients was 62 years, 57% were male, 66% had persistent afib, 94% were hypertensive and 94% were on warfarin. The mean $CHADS_2$ score of the group was 1.9, CHA_2DS_2-VASc score was 2.8 and HAS-BLED score was 2.4.

Immediate complete LAA closure (defined as a smaller than 1 mm jet of blood emanating from the LAA) was achieved in 85 patients (96% success rate). Total procedure time was 45 minutes and only three procedural complications arose, all related to pericardial or transseptal access. There were no significant changes in heart rhythm associated with the procedure. Post-operatively two patients developed pericarditis (inflammation of the heart lining) which was successfully treated. During the one year follow-up four patients experienced serious adverse events which were deemed to be unrelated to the *LARIAT*. Complete closure of the LAA was observed in 98% of patients having undergone a successful procedure. Fifty-five per cent of trial participants were still on warfarin therapy at the end of the first year. NOTE: Two of the 10 investigators involved in the trial have a close financial interest in the manufacturer of the *LARIAT* device. [34]

The results of a larger study involving 154 patients who underwent LAA ligation with the *LARIAT* device in 8 major US cardiac centers were reported in August 2014. Approximately two-thirds of the study participants had a history of major bleeding and 14% had suffered a prior intracranial hemorrhage thus making them less desirable candidates for continuing oral anticoagulation.

Average age of the patients was 72 years (62% male), mean CHADS$_2$ score was 2.8, CHA$_2$DS$_2$-VASc score 4.1, and HAS-BLED score 3.2. Prior to enrolling in the trial 60% of participants were on oral anticoagulant therapy, 28% were on antiplatelet therapy and 12% were on no antithrombotic therapy.

The *LARIAT* device could not be inserted in 9 patients two of whom required emergency surgery after right ventricular perforation. Among the 145 patients in which the device was delivered 138 (92%) demonstrated complete closure, 11 (7%) showed a residual leak less than 5 mm in diameter and one patient showed a leak greater than 5 mm by TEE. Procedural success was thus 94% with an average procedure duration of 77 minutes.

There were a total of 15 patients (10%) with at least one major periprocedural complication (death, heart attack, major bleed, or need for immediate cardiac surgery). Major bleed requiring blood transfusion occurred in 14 patients, 3 required emergency surgery. Significant pericardial effusion (escape of fluid into a body cavity) occurred in 16 patients and pleural effusion occurred in 4.

Most (55%) of study participants were discharged on aspirin monotherapy or dual antiplatelet therapy, but 23% were discharged on oral anticoagulants while the remaining 19% received no antithrombotic therapy. Two strokes and 2 cardiovascular deaths were recorded during follow-up (median 112 days) among 134 patients still followed in the study. TEE was performed in 63 patients at follow-up and indicated that there was complete closure in 79%, a leak smaller than 5 mm in 14% and a leak of 5 mm or greater in 6%.

The study investigators conclude that, given the incidence of procedural complications observed and the lack of long-term safety and efficacy data, *LARIAT* occlusion should be reserved for patients at substantial thromboembolic and bleeding risk. NOTE: This study was funded by SentreHEART, the manufacturer of the *LARIAT* device. [35]

A study by researchers at Scripps Clinic and University of Maryland provide further proof that complication rates associated with *LARIAT* use may be unacceptably high. Their analysis of the complications observed in five clinical trials involving 334 patients is shown below: [36]

Periprocedural adverse events*	14.7%
Pericarditis	8.3%
Significant pericardial effusion	7.5%
Pleural effusion	2.4%
Complication requiring surgical intervention	2.4%
LAA laceration	1.8%
Stroke or TIA	0.3%
Death	0.3%
Late adverse events	**10.6%**
Pericardial effusion	3.0%
TEE detected thrombus	2.2%
Pleural effusion	1.8%
Stroke or TIA	1.8%
Death	1.8%

*Events occurring prior to discharge not including pericarditis

NOTE: The incidence and severity of procedure-related pericarditis can be markedly reduced by giving patients colchicine prior to the procedure. [37]

Another study by medical researchers at five US hospitals/medical schools confirms the high rate of adverse events and conclude that "Formal, controlled investigations into the safety and efficacy of the device (*LARIAT*) for this indication (LAA occlusion) are warranted." [38]

In July 2015 the US Food and Drug Administration issued a safety communication to healthcare providers regarding 45 adverse events, including 6 deaths, associated with the *LARIAT* and associated devices. [39]

May 2016 saw the publication of a retrospective, multicenter study of 98 afib patients who had undergone a successful LAA ligation with the *LARIAT* device. Average age of the patients was 73 years (65% male), mean CHADS$_2$ score was 2.7, CHA$_2$DS$_2$-VASc score 4.1, and HAS-BLED score 3.2. Thirty-eight per cent of study participants had a history of stroke or TIA and 61% had a history of major bleeding. Periprocedural complications were 9% - mainly related to major bleeding. Half the patients were discharged on antiplatelet therapy and 35% on warfarin, rivaroxaban or dabigatran. At the 12-month follow-up 48% were still on antiplatelet therapy and 19% were still on anticoagulants.

At the end of the installation procedure 95% of patients exhibited no leaks and 5% had small leaks (less than 5 mm opening) as measured by TEE. At the 6-month follow-up 12 more patients had developed leaks (8 less than 5 mm and 4 at 5 mm or larger). These leaks were also apparent at the 12-month follow-up, but in addition another 4 small leaks and one large leak had developed. All leaks of 2.5 mm diameter or larger were closed with a septal occlusion device and anticoagulation resumed. During a mean follow-up period of 16 months 4 strokes and 1 TIA were recorded.

The study showed that 23% of patients had various degrees of leaks and the investigators conclude that leaks are a common feature of *LARIAT* ligation of the LAA and that the presence of leaks is likely to be associated with thromboembolic events. They also suggest that it may not be safe to discontinue anticoagulation for at least 12 months following the procedure unless inspection for leaks is done frequently preferably using 3D TEE. [40]

An earlier clinical trial indicated that secretion of atrial natriuretic peptide (ANP) dropped significantly after LAA removal as part of the maze procedure. This raised concern that ligation of the LAA might reduce both ANP and BNP (brain natriuretic peptide) resulting in detrimental changes in electrolyte and blood pressure. A study reported in September 2015 found that systolic blood pressure is reduced 24 and 72 hours following the *LARIAT* procedure and that the reduction persists, at least partially, 6 months after the procedure. A small reduction of sodium level was also observed 24 and 72 hours after the procedure, but this reduction was no longer present at the 6 month follow-up. [41]

More recently a study involving 66 afib patients undergoing *LARIAT* ligation reported that ANP and BNP levels did not change when comparing levels before the procedure (mean ANP level=249 pg/mL, mean BNP level=481 pg/mL) and 3 months after the procedure (mean ANP level=249 pg/mL, mean BNP level=495 pg/mL). The American and Polish researchers involved in the study conclude that the right atrial appendage takes over the production of ANP and BNP as the left atrial appendage atrophies. [42]

Combined ablation/LAA occlusion

Occlusion of the LAA with an *Atriclip* device is standard procedure when performing maze surgery be it via open heart surgery or thoracoscopically. In September 2012 Swiss cardiac surgeons reported that epicardial LAA occlusion with the *Atriclip* leads to complete electrical isolation of the LAA. They suggested that this may not only provide stroke prevention but may also reduce the recurrence of AF. [43]

Although catheter ablation of the left atrial appendage is sometimes successful in eliminating long-standing persistent afib, it is associated with a very real risk of reducing flow velocity through the orifice and thereby increasing the risk of ischemic stroke. About 50% of patients undergoing LAA ablation end up on life-long anticoagulation. Thus it is not surprising that the idea of combining catheter ablation and LAA occlusion in one procedure is gaining traction.

A group of electrophysiologists from Britain, the US, and Singapore report on the first trial of a combined procedure. Twenty-two patients with long-standing persistent atrial fibrillation (mean age: 68 years, 65% male, mean CHA$_2$DS$_2$-VASc score: 3.1) underwent a standard pulmonary vein antrum ablation followed by ablation of the LAA. Electrical isolation of the LAA was achieved in 20 patients with a mean ablation time of 25 minutes. At the end of a 60-minute wait period electrical isolation was checked again and re-isolation was performed as necessary (needed in 17 patients). The LAA was then occluded with a *WATCHMAN* device in the 20 patients with confirmed LAA isolation. Satisfactory occlusion was confirmed at the 45-day follow-up in 19 patients (95%) and at the end of three months these patients met the criteria for discontinuing warfarin. The trial investigators conclude that "Persistent AF ablation, LAA electric isolation, and mechanical occlusion can be performed concomitantly. This technique may improve the success of persistent AF ablation while obviating the need for chronic anticoagulation." NOTE: This study was funded by Boston Scientific. [44]

In an accompanying editorial Drs. Andrea Natale and Luigi Di Biase express concerns about the concomitant LAA ablation/occlusion approach suggesting that too early occlusion may affect the choice of the correct size of the *WATCHMAN* device and point out that a repeat LAA, should it be required, would be more difficult to perform with an occlusion device in place. They suggest that LAA occlusion should be performed as a separate procedure at a later date. [45]

Endocardial exclusion of the LAA (with the *Atriclip*) has been proven safe and effective in achieving complete electrical isolation of the appendage. A group of American and Polish electrophysiologists/cardiac surgeons report that the use of a *LARIAT* device is also not only effective in achieving complete electrical isolation of the LAA but also substantially increases the success of catheter ablation for persistent atrial fibrillation.

Their prospective, multicenter, observational study involved 138 patients with persistent afib half of which underwent a conventional AF ablation and half of which underwent the same procedure at least 30 days after having undergone a *LARIAT* procedure. The patients in the two groups (AF-only group and *LARIAT* group) were well matched with a mean age of 67 years (70% men) except in the case of stroke and bleeding risk which were higher in the *LARIAT* group. All patients were on antiarrhythmic drugs at the start of the study with flecainide, propafenone, and beta-blockers being the most frequently prescribed. Patients were also on warfarin (65%) or rivaroxaban (35%).

Study participants were followed for at least 12 months after their last procedure. The immediate success rate for *LARIAT* occlusion was 100%; however, at 3 months 10% had developed a leak ranging in diameter from 1 to 5 mm and 5% had experienced major complications. At 12 months follow-up 65% of patients in the *LARIAT* group and 39% in the AF-only group were free of atrial arrhythmias (tachycardia and fibrillation) after one ablation procedure without the use of antiarrhythmic drugs. These success rates increased to 77%

and 58% after repeat ablations. At 6 months following the ablation procedure 56% of patients in the *LARIAT* group had discontinued anticoagulation as compared to only 28% in the AF-only group. Although baseline left atrium volumes were comparable in the two groups (168 and 166 mL) the post-procedure LA volume was significantly smaller in the *LARIAT* group (129 mL vs. 149 mL). Two (3%) patients in the AF-only group suffered a TIA after discontinuing anticoagulation.

The authors of the study conclude that the success of ablation for persistent atrial fibrillation improves markedly if a *LARIAT* procedure is performed at least 30 days prior to the ablation procedure. [46]

Other researchers have found that *LARIAT* ligation on its own can terminate persistent afib in some patients. In a study reported in December 2016 thirteen of 162 patients scheduled for LAA ligation followed by catheter ablation converted to sinus rhythm on their own prior to the scheduled ablation. Eight of the patients converted during the procedure while the remaining 5 converted to sinus rhythm within 1-2 days. Six of the 13 patients subsequently underwent a pulmonary vein isolation procedure scheduled as part of a clinical trial. All 13 remained in sinus rhythm during a 16-month follow-up period. [47]

In a later study a team of American and Polish electrophysiologists/cardiac surgeons reported their findings regarding the effect of incomplete exclusion of the LAA on the success of subsequent catheter ablation. Of 91 patients who underwent the *LARIAT* procedure 11 (12%) showed incomplete exclusion as determined with contrast-enhanced CT scans. The observed leaks ranged in diameter from 1 to 5 mm. There was no difference in afib recurrence between patients with leaks and those without. Oral anticoagulation was discontinued in all patients with small leaks and in 2 patients with large leaks that had sealed up completely in follow-up imaging. There were no strokes or TIAs during a 12-month follow-up period. [48]

It is clear that LAA isolation significantly increases the success of ablation for persistent atrial fibrillation. What is less clear is: "Which isolation procedure is the best?"

Epicardial occlusion with the WATCHMAN or Amplatzer Amulet device has the advantage that it can be performed by electrophysiologists without the assistance of a cardiac surgeon. However, the rate of periprocedural complications is disappointingly high at about 5%. It also seems increasingly likely that patients having undergone occlusion procedures using either of these devices may have to remain on antiplatelet therapy for much longer than originally anticipated – perhaps for life – due to the now firmly established danger of device embolization inherent in placing a foreign object in the blood stream. While the WATCHMAN device was approved for use in LAA occlusion in 2015 the Amplatzer device is still awaiting such approval.

Installation of a Lariat device avoids the problem of device embolization but requires the input of both an electrophysiologist and a cardiac surgeon.

Clinical trials have shown that the development of leaks is fairly common and a 2015 analysis of five clinical trials involving 334 patients observed a 22% rate of periprocedural adverse events and an 11% rate of late adverse events. Although later trials have produced more favourable results the need for continued post-procedural anticoagulation is still not clear. The Lariat device is still awaiting FDA approval.

The Atriclip device is installed endocardially by a cardiac surgeon and was approved by the FDA for LAA occlusion in 2009. The installation procedure is quick, can be done thoracoscopically and is successful without periprocedural complications in at least 98% of cases. What is more, it is now routine practice to discontinue anticoagulation immediately after conclusion of the installation procedure or at least shortly afterwards.

In summary, it would seem that the optimum approach for safely achieving freedom from atrial fibrillation, off antiarrhythmics, anticoagulation, and antiplatelet therapy would be a catheter ablation, either epicardial or endocardial combined with LAA occlusion with the Atriclip or with the Lariat device when its safety and efficacy have been conclusively proven and FDA approval has been granted.

REFERENCES

1. Al-Saady, NM, et al. Left atrial appendage: structure, function, and role in thromboembolism. Heart, Vol. 82, 1999, pp. 547-55
2. Beigel, R, et al. The left atrial appendage: anatomy, function, and non-invasive evaluation. JACC Cardiovascular Imaging, Vol. 7 (12), December 2014, pp. 1251-65
3. Yaghi, S, et al. Left atrial appendage and stroke risk. Stroke, Vol. 46 (12), December 2015, pp. 3554-9
4. Blackshear, JL, et al. Appendage obliteration to reduce stroke in cardiac surgical patients with atrial fibrillation. Annals of Thoracic Surgery, Vol. 61 (2), February 1996, pp.755-9
5. Narumiya, T, et al. Relationship between left atrial appendage function and left atrial thrombus in patients with nonvalvular chronic atrial fibrillation and atrial flutter. Circulation Journal, Vol. 67 (1), January 2003, pp. 68-72
6. Kanderian AS, et al. Success of surgical left atrial appendage closure: assessment by transesophageal echocardiography. Journal of American College of Cardiology, Vol. 52 (11), September 9, 2008, pp. 924-9
7. Fumoto, H, et al. A novel device for left atrial appendage exclusion: the third–generation atrial exclusion device. Journal of Thoracic and Cardiovascular Surgery, Vol. 136 (4), October 2008, pp. 1019-27.
8. Salzberg SP, et al. Left atrial appendage clip occlusion: early clinical results. Journal of Thoracic and Cardiovascular Surgery, Vol. 139 (5), May 2010, pp. 1269-74
9. Emmert, MY, et al. Safe, effective and durable epicardial left atrial appendage clip occlusion in patients with atrial fibrillation undergoing cardiac surgery: first long-term results from a prospective device trial. European Journal of Cardiothoracic Surgery, Vol. 45(1), January 2014, pp. 126-31

10. Ailawadi, G, et al. Exclusion of the left atrial appendage with a novel device: early results of a multicenter trial. Journal of Thoracic and Cardiovascular Surgery, Vol. 142 (5), November 2011, pp. 1002-9

11. Kurfirst, V, et al. Epicardial clip occlusion of the left atrial appendage during cardiac surgery provides optimal surgical results and long-term stability. Interactive CardioVascular and Thoracic Surgery. Vol. 25 (1), July 1, 2017, pp. 37-40

12. Caliskan, E, et al. Epicardial left atrial appendage AtriClip occlusion reduces the incidence of stroke in patients with atrial fibrillation undergoing cardiac surgery. Europace, July 18, 2017.

13. Osmancik, P, et al. Residual echocardiographic and computed tomography findings after thoracoscopic occlusion of the left atrial appendage using the AtriClip PRO device. Interactive CardioVascular and Thoracic Surgery. January 18, 2018

14. Caliskan, E, et al. Interventional and surgical occlusion of the left atrial appendage. Nature Reviews – Cardiology. Vol. 14 (12), December 2017, pp. 727-743

15. Sick, PB, et al. Initial worldwide experience with the WATCHMAN left atrial appendage system for stroke prevention in atrial fibrillation. Journal of the American College of Cardiology. Vol. 49 (13), April 3, 2007, pp.1490-5

16. Holmes, DR, et al. Percutaneous closure of the left atrial appendage versus warfarin therapy for prevention of stroke in patients with atrial fibrillation: a randomised non-inferiority trial. Lancet. Vol. 374 (9689), August 15, 2009, pp. 534-42

17. Reddy, VY, et al. Percutaneous left atrial appendage closure for stroke prophylaxis in patients with atrial fibrillation: 2.3 Year Follow-up of the PROTECT AF (WATCHMAN Left Atrial Appendage System for Embolic Protection in Patients with Atrial Fibrillation) Trial. Circulation. Vol. 127 (6), February 12, 2013, pp. 720-9

18. Whitlock, RP, et al. Does left atrial appendage occlusion eliminate the need for warfarin? Left atrial appendage occlusion does not eliminate the need for warfarin. Circulation, Vol. 120 (19) , November 10, 2009, pp. 1927-32

19. Holmes, DR, et al. Prospective randomized evaluation of the WATCHMAN Left Atrial Appendage Closure Device in patients with atrial fibrillation versus long-term warfarin therapy: the PREVAIL trial. Journal of the American College of Cardiology. Vol. 64 (1), July 8, 2014, pp. 1-12

20. Reddy, VI, et al. 5-Year Outcomes after Left Atrial Appendage Closure: From the PREVAIL and PROTECT AF Trials. Journal of the American College of Cardiology. Vol. 70 (24), December 19, 2017, pp. 2964-2975

21. Reddy, VY, et al. Post-Approval U.S. Experience with Left Atrial Appendage Closure for Stroke Prevention in Atrial Fibrillation. Journal of the American College of Cardiology. Vol. 69 (3), January 24, 2017, pp. 253-261

22. Boersma, LV, et al. Implant success and safety of left atrial appendage closure with the WATCHMAN device: peri-procedural outcomes from the EWOLUTION registry. European Heart Journal, Vol. 37 (31), August 2013, pp. 2465-74

23. Bai, R, et al. Intraprocedural and long-term incomplete occlusion of the left atrial appendage following placement of the WATCHMAN device. Journal of Cardiovascular Electrophysiology, Vol. 23 (5), May 2012, pp.455-61

24. Reddy, VY, et al. Left atrial appendage closure with the WATCHMAN device in patients with a contraindication to oral anticoagulation. Journal of the American College of Cardiology, Vol. 61 (25), June 25, 2013, pp. 2551-6

25. Park, JW, et al. Left atrial appendage closure with Amplatzer cardiac plug in atrial fibrillation: initial European experience. Catheter Cardiovasc Interv, Vol. 77, No. 5, April 1, 2011, pp. 700-06

26. Streb, W, et al. Percutaneous closure of the left atrial appendage using the Amplatzer Cardiac Plug in patients with atrial fibrillation: Evaluation of safety and feasibility. Kardiol Pol, Vol. 71, No. 1, 2013, pp. 8-16

27. Urena, M, et al. Percutaneous left atrial appendage closure with the AMPLATZER cardiac plug device in patients with nonvalvular atrial fibrillation and contraindications to anticoagulation therapy. Journal of the American College of Cardiology, Vol. 62, No. 2, July 9, 2013, pp. 96-102

28. Tzikas, A, et al. Left atrial appendage occlusion for stroke prevention in atrial fibrillation: Multicentre experience with the AMPLATZER Cardiac Plug. EuroIntervention, Vol. 11, No. 10, Feb. 2016, pp. 1170-79

29. Landmesser, U, et al. Left atrial appendage occlusion with the AMPLATZER Amulet device: Periprocedural and early clinical/echocardiographic data from a global prospective observational study. EuroIntervention, Vol. 13, No. 7, Sept. 20, 2017, pp. 867-76

30. Fauchier, L, et al. Incidence, predictors and prognosis of thrombus formation on device in patients with atrial fibrillation after left atrial appendage occlusion for stroke prevention in a multicenter analysis. European Heart Journal, Vol. 38, Issue supplement 1, August 1, 2017, presentation 5718

31. Europace 2017 Cardiac Rhythm News: Thrombus formation on left atrial appendage devices strongly associated with higher risk of ischemic stroke. https://cardiacrhythmnews.com/europace-2017-thrombus-formation-on-left-atrial-appendage-occlusion-devices-strongly-associated-with-higher-risk-of-ischaemic-stroke/

32. Yasuda, H, et al. Upper gastrointestinal bleeding in patients receiving dual antiplatelet therapy after coronary stenting. Internal Medicine, Vol. 49, No. 19, 2009, pp. 1725-30

33. Bartus, K, et al. Feasibility of closed-chest ligation of the left atrial appendage in humans. Heart Rhythm, Vol. 8, No. 2, February 2011, pp. 188-93

34. Bartus, K, et al. Percutaneous left atrial appendage suture ligation using the LARIAT device in patients with atrial fibrillation: Initial clinical experience. Journal of the American College of Cardiology, Vol. 62, No. 2, July 9, 2013, pp. 108-18

35. Price, MJ, et al. Early safety and efficacy of percutaneous left atrial appendage suture ligation: Results from the U.S. transcatheter LAA ligation consortium. Journal of the American College of Cardiology, Vol. 64, No. 6, August 12, 2014, pp. 565-72

36. Srivastava, MC, et al. A review of the LARIAT device: Insights from the cumulative clinical experience. SpringerPlus, 2015 September 17; 4:522

37. Gunda, S, et al. Impact of periprocedural colchicine on postprocedural management in patients undergoing a left atrial appendage ligation using LARIAT. Journal of Cardiovascular Electrophysiology, Vol. 27, No. 1, January 2016, pp. 60-64

38. Chatterjee, S, et al. Safety and procedural success of left atrial appendage exclusion with the LARIAT device: A systematic review of published reports and analytical review of the FDA MAUDE database. JAMA Internal Medicine, Vol. 175, No. 7, July 2015, pp. 1104-09

39. FDA Announces Safety Issues with Lariat Left Atrial Appendage (LAA) Closure Device. Diagnostic and Interventional Cardiology, July 13, 2015 https://www.dicardiology.com/article/fda-announces-safety-issues-lariat-left-atrial-appendage-laa-closure-device

40. Gianni, C, et al. Clinical implications of leaks following left atrial appendage ligation with the LARIAT device. JACC Cardiovascular Interventions, Vol. 9, No. 10, May 23, 2016, pp. 1051-57

41. Maybrook, R, et al. Electrolyte and hemodynamic changes following percutaneous left atrial appendage ligation with the LARIAT device. Journal of Interv Card Electrophysiol, Vol. 43, No. 3, September 2015, pp. 245-51

42. Bartus, K, et al. Atrial natriuretic peptide and brain natriuretic peptide changes after epicardial percutaneous left atrial appendage suture ligation using LARIAT device. Journal of Physiology and Pharmacology, Vol. 68, No. 1, February 2017, pp. 117-23

43. Davtyan, KV, et al. Left atrial appendage occluder implantation for stroke prevention in elderly patients with atrial fibrillation: Acute and long-term results. Journal of Geriatric Cardiology, Vol. 14, No. 9, September 2017, pp. 590-92

44. Lakkireddy, D, et al. Left atrial appendage ligation and ablation for persistent atrial fibrillation: The LAALA-AF Registry. JACC: Clinical Electrophysiology, Vol. 1, No. 3, June 2015, pp. 153-60

45. Panikker, Sandeep, et al. Left Atrial Appendage Electrical Isolation and Concomitant Device Occlusion to Treat Persistent Atrial Fibrillation. Circulation. Arrhythmia and Electrophysiology, Vol. 9 (7), July 2016

46. Di Biase, L, and Natale, A. Left Atrial Appendage after Electrical Isolation: To Occlude or Not to Occlude, That is the Question. Circulation. Arrhythmia and Electrophysiology, Vol. 9 (7), July 2016

47. Badhwar, N, et al. Conversion of persistent atrial fibrillation to sinus rhythm after LAA ligation with the LARIAT. International Journal of Cardiology, Vol. 225, December 15, 2016, pp.120-122

48. Turagam, M, et al. Anatomical and electrical remodeling with incomplete left atrial appendage ligation: Results from the LAALA-AF registry. Journal of Cardiovascular Electrophysiology, Vol. 28 (12), December 2107, pp. 1433-1442

Appendix A

Glossary of Medical Terms

ADP Adenosine diphosphate
ANP Atrial natriuretic peptide
APC Activated protein-C resistance
BNP Brain natriuretic peptide
CRP C-reactive protein
LAA Left atrial appendage
INR International normalized ratio
PKC Protein kinase C
PVA Pulmonary vein ablation
PVI Pulmonary vein isolation
SEC Spontaneous echocardiographic contrast
tPA Tissue type plasminogen activator

Ablation
A procedure for destroying heart tissue that is creating abnormal electrical impulses.

ACE inhibitor
A pharmaceutical drug that inhibits the enzyme which converts angiotensin I to angiotensin II.

Acetylcholine
The neurotransmitter released at parasympathetic (vagal) nerve endings.

Adrenergic
Pertaining to the sympathetic branch of the autonomic nervous system.

Adrenergic LAF
Lone atrial fibrillation triggered by excessive sympathetic stimulation.

Adrenergic tone
The strength or vigour of the sympathetic branch of the autonomic nervous system.

Adenosine diphosphate [ADP]
A nucleotide stored in platelets involved in platelet aggregation

Antiarrhythmic
Pharmaceutical drug designed to prevent abnormal heart rhythms or to convert abnormal rhythms to normal sinus rhythm.

Anticoagulant
Pharmaceutical drug designed to prevent blood clotting.

Activated protein-C resistance [APC]
A condition caused by the presence of a mutation of blood coagulation factor V (factor V Leiden). APC is associated with an increased risk of venous thromboembolism.

Apoptosis
Self-destruction (suicide) of individual cells to avoid a threat to the survival of the organism as a whole.

Arrhythmia
An abnormal heart rhythm.

Atherosclerosis
The development of fatty plaque and scar tissue on the inner wall of the arteries – eventually leading to obstruction of blood flow and an increased risk of thrombosis.

Artery
A blood vessel that carries blood away from the heart.

Atria
The two upper chambers of the heart. The right atrium receives returning blood from the body and the left atrium receives oxygenated blood from the lungs.

Atrial appendages
Small pouches connected to the right and left atria. The left atrial appendage (LAA) is associated with the generation of blood clots during atrial fibrillation.

Atrial fibrillation
A chaotic movement of electrical impulses across the atria leading to a loss of synchrony between the atria and the ventricles.

Atrial flutter
An abnormal, sustained, rapid contraction of the atria. The rhythm is rapid, but regular as opposed to atrial fibrillation where it is rapid and irregular.

Atrial natriuretic peptide [ANP]
A hormone formed in the atria. ANP is involved in regulating blood pressure and salt and water balance in body fluids.

Autonomic nervous system [ANS]
The part of the central nervous system that is not under conscious control (involuntary). It controls the body's internal organs including the heart and digestive system and is responsible for regulating blood pressure.

Beta-blocker
A pharmaceutical drug which blocks the receptor sites for the neurotransmitters (catecholamines) used by the sympathetic (adrenergic) branch of the autonomous nervous system.

Bigeminy
An abnormal heart rhythm in which a normal heartbeat (originating from the SA node) is followed by an ectopic beat (originating outside the SA node) in rapid succession.

Bradycardia
An abnormally slow heartbeat.

Brain natriuretic peptide [BNP]
A hormone formed in the ventricles. BNP is involved in regulating blood pressure and salt and water balance in body fluids.

Calcium-channel blocker
A pharmaceutical drug that inhibits the flow of calcium ions through or across cell membranes. It is used in the treatment of stroke and certain heart conditions.

Cardiogenic emboli
Blood clots originating in the heart.

Cardioversion
The conversion of an irregular heart rhythm to normal sinus rhythm. Cardioversion can be done with drugs or through an electric shock administered to the chest area.

Catecholamines
A group of chemical compounds (amines) derived from tyramine and tyrosine. The group includes epinephrine,, norepinephrine, and dopamine.

Catheter

A tube designed to be inserted into a narrow opening or hollow organ such as the urinary bladder or a vein. The catheter is used to drain fluids or to allow the insertion of special instruments used for imaging or ablation.

Catheter ablation

Destruction of tissue by the application of electrical current, usually at radio frequencies, via a catheter threaded through a vein to reach the area to be ablated (AV node, pulmonary veins, "hot spots" in the atria).

Cerebrovascular event

See Stroke.

Coagulation (of blood)

Process whereby blood is converted from a liquid to a solid state.

Comorbidity

A disease condition accompanied by one or more unrelated disease conditions.

Congestive heart failure [CHF]

Failure of the heart to pump sufficiently strongly to prevent the accumulation of fluid in the lungs.

Coronary arteries

The arteries that supply the heart itself with oxygenated blood.

Couplet

An abnormal heart rhythm involving two ectopic beats in a row.

C-reactive protein

A blood marker for systemic inflammation.

Deep vein thrombosis [DVT]

A condition where a blood clot is formed in a deep vein, usually in the legs.

Diastolic

Pertaining to the time period between fillings of the ventricles. The diastolic pressure is the lower of the two readings reported when measuring blood pressure.

Echocardiogram

An ultrasound picture of the heart as it beats.

Ectopic beat

A heart beat that is initiated at a location other than the sinoatrial node. The junction between the left atrium and the pulmonary veins is a primary spawning ground for ectopic beats.

Edema

Swelling caused by an abnormal accumulation of fluid in body tissues.

Ejection fraction

The proportion of the blood volume in the left ventricle that is actually pumped out in each heartbeat. The proportion for a healthy heart is 50-60 per cent. A value of 40 per cent or below indicates ventricular dysfunction.

Electrocardiogram [ECG]

A recording of the electrical activity of the heart during contraction.

Electrolytes

Chemical substances that dissociate into two or more ions when dissolved in water.

Embolism
A condition in which a blood clot becomes lodged in an artery and obstructs the flow of blood [embolic].

Embolization
The formation of a blood clot [embolus] on a substrate.

Endocardial procedure
A medical [surgical] procedure where the heart wall is approached from the outside such as in the maze procedure.

Endothelium
The single layer of cells that line the heart, blood vessels and lymphatic vessels [endothelial].

Endothelialization
The formation of endothelial tissue, for example, covering a stent or occlusion device.

Epicardial procedure
A medical [surgical] procedure where the heart wall is approached from the inside such as in catheter ablation.

Epithelium
Membranous tissue that covers most internal and external surfaces of the body and its organs [epithelial].

Epinephrine
A hormone secreted by the medulla of the adrenal gland. Also known as adrenaline.

Factor V Leiden
A mutation in blood coagulation factor V that results in an increased tendency to blood clotting – especially deep vein thrombosis.

Fibrillation
Rapid and chaotic beating of the heart.

Fibrinolysis
The process by which blood clots are removed from the circulation. It involves digestion of insoluble fibrin by the endogenous enzyme plasmin [fibrinolytic].

Gastrointestinal
Relating to the stomach and intestines [gastrointestinal tract].

Heart failure
See Congestive heart failure.

Heart rate variability (HRV)
A measure of the beat-to-beat variability in heart rate.

Hematoma
A localized swelling of blood resulting from a break in a blood vessel.

Hemorrhagic stroke
See Stroke.

Holter monitor
A portable device for measuring heart rhythm over a 24-hour period.

Homocysteine
A sulphur-containing amino acid used by the body in cellular metabolism and the manufacture of proteins.

Hyperhomocysteinemia
An elevated blood level of homocysteine.

Hyperlipidemia
An excess of fats or lipids in the blood.

Hypertension
A blood pressure that is persistently above the upper limit of the reference range (140/90).

Hyperthyroidism
An overactive thyroid gland. The condition is characterized by increased metabolic rate, high blood pressure and a rapid heartbeat.

Hypocalcemia
An abnormally low blood level of calcium.

Hypokalemia
An abnormally low blood level of potassium.

Hypomagnesemia
An abnormally low blood level of magnesium.

Hyponatremia
An abnormally low blood level of sodium.

Hypotension
An abnormally low blood pressure.

Hypothyroidism
A condition caused by an underactive thyroid gland. The condition is characterized by fatigue, hair loss, feeling cold, constipation, and skin pallor.

ICD
Implantable cardioverter-defibrillator.

Idiopathic
Of no known cause.

Incidence
The extent or frequency of occurrence.

Infarction
Localized cell death (necrosis) resulting from obstruction of the blood supply.

International Normalized Ratio [INR]
A measure of the blood's tendency to coagulate (form clots) when on warfarin (Coumadin). A normal INR is 1.0. Warfarin dose is usually adjusted to give an INR between 2.0 and 3.0.

Intracellular
Situated or occurring inside a cell.

Intracranial
Within the head.

Ischemia
Inadequate blood flow to the heart or other body parts [ischemic].

Ischemic stroke
See Stroke.

Laparoscopic surgery [keyhole surgery]
A minimally invasive procedure carried out with the aid of a small video camera and one or more special, thin surgical instruments introduced into a body cavity through one or more small incisions. The surgeon uses the image transmitted by the camera to guide the procedure which may be performed under general, spinal, epidural, or spinal-epidural anesthesia depending on the organ targeted.

Left atrial appendage
See Atrial appendages.

Left ventricular dysfunction
Inadequate pumping capacity of the left ventricle. Characterized by a left ventricular ejection fraction below 40 per cent.

Ligation
The surgical procedure of closing of a blood vessel or hollow organ in the body with a ligature (string) or clip.

Maze procedure
A surgical procedure that involves the creation of a pattern of scar tissue to contain and channel the heart's electrical impulses and thereby prevent atrial fibrillation.

Medulla
The inner part of the adrenal gland. Epinephrine and norepinephrine are synthesized here.

Mitral stenosis
A narrowing of the opening of the mitral valve.

Mitral valve
A valve that allows blood to flow between the left atrium and the left ventricle while preventing back flow.

Mitral valve prolapse [MVP]
A usually benign abnormality of the mitral valve resulting in regurgitation (back flow) of blood from the left ventricle to the left atrium.

Monocytes
A variety of white blood cells whose purpose is to ingest foreign particles such as bacteria and tissue debris.

Mortality
Incidence of death in a given period.

Myocardial infarction [heart attack]
Destruction of heart tissue resulting from obstruction of the blood supply to the heart muscle.

Myocarditis
An acute or chronic inflammation of the heart muscle.

Myocardium
The middle of the three layers that form the wall of the heart. It is composed of muscle fibres.

Myocyte
A muscle cell.

Myxoma
Benign gelatinous tumour of connective tissue. Atrial myxoma most commonly involves a tumour in the left atrium.

Necrosis
Death of cells through injury, disease or obstruction of blood supply.

Nitric oxide [NO]
A colourless gas produced in cellular metabolism. It is involved in oxygen transport to tissues, the transmission of nerve impulses and the relaxation of blood vessel walls.

Non-valvular atrial fibrillation
Atrial fibrillation that is not caused by malfunctioning or damaged heart valves.

Norepinephrine
The neurotransmitter released at sympathetic (adrenergic) nerve endings. Also known as noradrenaline.

Normal sinus rhythm [NSR]
The normal rhythm of the heart when beats are initiated only at the sinoatrial node.

Occlusion
The blockage or closing of a blood vessel or hollow organ in the body.

Ostial PVI
A pulmonary vein isolation procedure where the ablation ring is placed in the left atrium around the

opening of the pulmonary vein rather than inside the pulmonary vein itself. The ostial procedure eliminates or sharply reduces the risk of pulmonary vein stenosis.

Oxidative stress
A condition that occurs when the body's natural antioxidant defences are overwhelmed by reactive oxygen species and other free radicals.

Pacemaker
An implanted device meant to provide small electric shocks to the heart to initiate heartbeats (contractions) at a predetermined rate.

Palpitation
A sensation of a rapid, irregular heartbeat.

Parasympathetic
Pertaining to the parasympathetic branch of the autonomic nervous system.

Paroxysmal
Occurring at intervals (intermittent).

Percutaneous procedure
Medical procedure where access to the heart is achieved via a puncture of the skin, usually in the groin, followed by the threading of a carrier tube through the femoral vein to the inside of the heart.

Peripheral arterial disease [PAD]
Atherosclerosis in arteries other than the coronary arteries. Intermittent claudication may occur if the atherosclerotic deposits are blocking the arteries feeding the legs.

Permanent LAF
Continuous atrial fibrillation that does not respond to cardioversion.

Persistent LAF
Atrial fibrillation episodes lasting more than seven days, but amenable to cardioversion.

Platelet
Blood cell involved in the initiation of blood clotting [thrombocyte].

Platelet inhibitor
A drug that prevents the aggregation of platelets.

Plaque
A build-up of cholesterol and fatty substances on the inner lining of arteries.

Premature atrial complex [PAC]
A premature heart beat originating in the atrium other than at the sinoatrial node.

Premature ventricular complex [PVC]
A premature heart beat originating below the atrioventricular node, often in the ventricular muscle itself.

Prevalence
The total number of cases of a disease in a given population at a specific time.

Proarrhythmic
Capable of inducing arrhythmia.

Protein kinase C [PKC]
An enzyme found in platelets that induces platelet aggregation and adhesion.

Prothrombin time
A measure of the blood's tendency to clot when medicated with warfarin. See INR.

Pulmonary embolism
A blood clot lodged in the pulmonary artery.

Pulmonary vein ablation [PVA]
Ablation of sources of ectopic heartbeats located at the junction of the left atrium and the pulmonary veins.

Pulmonary vein isolation [PVI]
Isolation of the pulmonary veins from the left atrium by ablating (generating scar tissue) a ring around each pulmonary vein.

Pulmonary veins
The veins draining oxygenated blood from the lungs to the left atrium.

Reperfusion
The restoration of blood flow to an organ or tissue that has had its blood supply cut off due to a stroke or heart attack. Reperfusion is associated with increased free radical activity.

Rheumatic heart disease
Heart disease caused by rheumatic fever.

Run
An abnormal heart rhythm characterized by four or more ectopic beats in a row.

Sinoatrial (sinus) node
The specialized (pacemaker) tissue that initiates a heartbeat. It is located near the top of the right atrium.

Sinus rhythm
See Normal sinus rhythm.

Spontaneous echocardiographic contrast [SEC]
A swirling pattern of blood flow observed by transesophageal echocardiography [TEE]. Dense SEC is associated with an increased risk of clot formation.

Stasis
Stagnation or cessation of flow; for example, of blood or lymph fluid.

Stenosis
A constriction or narrowing of a duct or passage; for example, pulmonary vein stenosis.

Stroke
An event that damages nerve cells in the brain. It is caused by an interruption of the oxygen supply to the brain due to a blood clot (ischemic stroke) or a burst blood vessel (hemorrhagic stroke).

Subcutaneous
Beneath the skin.

Supraventricular
Located above the ventricles, that is in the atria or atrioventricular node.

Supraventricular tachycardia (SVT)
A rapid, but regular heart rate caused by a fault in the conduction system around the atrioventricular node.

Suture
The closure of a wound or incision with material such as silk or catgut. The term is also used to describe the material used in closing the wound or incision.

Sympathetic
Pertaining to the sympathetic branch of the autonomic nervous system.

Systemic
Relating to or affecting the body as a whole.

Systolic
Pertaining to the time at which the ventricles contract. The systolic pressure is the higher of the two readings reported when measuring blood pressure.

Tachycardia
A rapid, but regular heart beat usually in excess of 100 bpm.

Thoracoscopic surgery
Laparoscopic surgery targeted at organs located in the chest cavity. Access is gained through incisions made between the ribs.

Thrombosis
A condition in which blood changes from a liquid to a solid state, i.e. forms a clot [thrombotic].

Thrombus
A blood clot.

Thrombolysis
The dissolution of a blood clot by the infusion of an enzyme, such as streptokinase, into the blood [thrombolytic].

Tissue type plasminogen activator [tPA]
A protein involved in the breakdown of blood clots.

Transesophageal
Through or across the esophagus. The term is often applied to a special form of echocardiography [TEE] used to check for blood clots in the left atrial appendage.

Transient ischemic attacks (TIAs)
A sudden, temporary loss of neurological function caused by blockage of small arteries supplying blood to the brain (mini-stroke).

Transthoracic
Through or across the chest. The term applies to the standard form of echocardiography.

Tricuspid valve
A valve that allows blood to pass between the right atrium and the right ventricle.

Trigeminy
An abnormal heart rhythm in which every third beat is ectopic (originating outside the SA node).

Triplet
An abnormal heart rhythm involving three ectopic beats in a row.

Vagal
Pertaining to the parasympathetic branch of the autonomic nervous system.

Vagal LAF
Lone atrial fibrillation triggered by excessive parasympathetic stimulation.

Vagal tone
The strength or vigour of the parasympathetic branch of the autonomic nervous system.

Vasodilatation
An increase in the diameter of blood vessels, especially arteries. It is brought about by a relaxation of vessel walls mediated, for example, by nitric oxide.

Vagus nerve
The tenth cranial nerve originating in the brain stem. It enervates the heart, gastrointestinal tract and larynx (voice box).

Vein
A blood vessel that carries blood towards the heart.

Vena cava
The large vein(s) that returns blood from the body to the heart (right atrium).

Ventricles
The two lower chambers of the heart.

Ventricular fibrillation
An often-fatal cardiac arrhythmia characterized by rapid, irregular fibrillation of the ventricles. Ventricular fibrillation is the main cause of sudden cardiac death (cardiac arrest).

Appendix B

REVIEW OF GUIDELINES

2016 ESC Guidelines for the Management of Atrial Fibrillation

These guidelines developed by the European Society of Cardiology are the most current and were prepared by a Task Force of 17 European EPs/Cardiologists and reviewed by a group of 50 of their peers. NOTE: The latest US guidelines were issued in 2006 and only partially updated in 2011 so are not up-to-date.

In 2010 more than 30 million people were living with atrial fibrillation [AF] worldwide and it is estimated that one in four middle-aged adults in Europe and the US will develop atrial fibrillation during their lifetime. Atrial fibrillation by itself is not a life-threatening condition, but, if accompanied by one or more common ailments such as atherosclerosis, hypertension, heart failure, and diabetes it is associated with a significantly increased risk of ischemic stroke. Thus the Guidelines place considerable emphasis on recommendations for effective stroke prevention. Highlights of these recommendations are:

- The risk of experiencing an ischemic stroke should be estimated using the CHA_2DS_2-VASc score.

- In male and female AF patients without additional stroke risk factors anticoagulant or antiplatelet therapy is not recommended for stroke prevention.

- Antiplatelet monotherapy is not recommended for stroke prevention regardless of stroke risk.

- Dual antiplatelet therapy (aspirin+clopidogrel) is not recommended for stroke prevention in AF patients as it has a negative benefit/risk ratio.

- There is strong evidence that men with a CHA_2DS_2-VASc score of 2 or more and women with a score of 3 or more benefit from preventive therapy with oral anticoagulants. There is less compelling evidence that men with a score of 1 and women with a score of 2 may also benefit.

- Bleeding risk factors such as hypertension, anemia, impaired liver or kidney function and the use of aspirin and NSAIDs should be identified and dealt with if possible before prescribing anticoagulants.

- Combinations of oral anticoagulants and antiplatelet agents increase bleeding risk and should be avoided in AF patients without another indication for platelet inhibition.

- When oral anticoagulation is initiated in a patient who is eligible for a novel oral anticoagulant (apixaban, dabigatran, edoxaban, or rivaroxaban) the patient should be prescribed the novel anticoagulant (NOAC) rather than warfarin. NOTE: NOACs are not recommended for AF patients with mechanical heart valves.

- Systemic thrombolysis with recombinant tissue plasminogen activator should not be used in acute ischemic stroke treatment if patients are on therapeutic anticoagulation.

Due to limited experience with occlusion and exclusion of the left atrial appendage levels of evidence for a proposed course of action are not "Grade A". However, the guidelines suggest that LAA occlusion/exclusion may be considered in the following cases:

- For AF patients with contra-indications to long-term anticoagulation (e.g. patients with a previous life-threatening bleed without a reversible cause).

- As an add-on procedure for AF patients undergoing cardiac surgery.

- As an add-on procedure for AF patients undergoing thoracoscopic surgery.

The Guidelines emphasize that the final decisions concerning treatment of an individual patient must be made by the responsible health professional(s) in consultation with the patient and caregiver as appropriate.

REFERENCE

Kirchof, Paulus, et al. 2016 ESC Guidelines for the management of atrial fibrillation developed in cooperation with EACTS. European Heart Journal, Vol. 37 (38), October 7, 2016, pp. 2893-2962.

Appendix C

Pharmaceutical Drugs for Stroke Prevention

Generic Name	Trade Names
Antiplatelet Agents	
Acetylsalicylic acid	Aspirin, ASA
Clopidogrel	Plavix
Ticlopidine	Ticlid
Dipyridamole	Persantine
Indobufen	Not available in the US
Glycoprotein inhibitors	Abciximab, Tirofiban
Anticoagulants	
Warfarin	Coumadin
Phenprocoumon	Marcoumar
Ximelagatran	Exanta
Enexoparin (Heparin)	Lovenox
Nadroparin (Heparin)	Fraxiparine
Novel Anticoagulants	
Apixaban	Eliquis
Dabigatran	Pradaxa
Edoxaban	Lixiana (Savaysa)
Rivaroxaban	Xarelto
Thrombolytic Agents	
tPA	tPA
Urokinase	Abbokinase
Streptokinase	Streptase
ACE inhibitors	
Captopril	Capoten
Perindopril	Aceon
Ramipril	Altace

Appendix D

Natural Supplements for Stroke Prevention

Common Name	Alternative Name
Vitamin B3	Niacin
Vitamin B6	Pyridoxine
Vitamin B12	Cobalamin
Vitamin C	Ascorbic Acid
Vitamin E	Tocopherol
Coenzyme Q10	Ubiquinone
Folic acid	Pteroylmonoglutamate
Lycopene	Lycopene
Magnesium	Magnesium (Mg)
Potassium	Potassium (K)
Fish Oil	Fish Oil (1)
Garlic	Allium sativum
Ginkgo biloba	Ginkgo biloba
L-arginine	L-arginine
Resveratrol	Resveratrol
Nattokinase	Nattokinase
Pinokinase (2)	Flite-Tabs

1) Also referred to as long-chain polyunsaturated omega-3 fatty acids. The active components are eicosapentaenoic acid and docosahexaenoic acid.

2) A proprietary mixture of nattokinase and pycnogenol.

INDEX

H

I-J

W

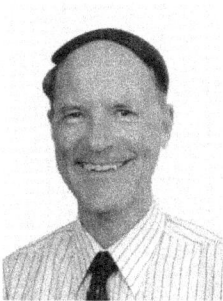

Hans Larsen is a Professional Engineer and holds a Master's degree in Chemical Engineering from the Technical University of Denmark. He developed a lifelong interest in biochemistry and nutrition through his early studies with Professor Henrik Dam, the Nobel Prize-winning discoverer of vitamin K. Later he honed his technical writing skills by abstracting for Chemical Abstracts then the world's largest abstracting service.

After having been diagnosed with atrial fibrillation and doing extensive research in the field of lone atrial fibrillation and stroke prevention Hans published *Lone Atrial Fibrillation: Towards a Cure* in December 2002 (A revised edition was published in November 2015) followed by *Thrombosis and Stroke Prevention* – a layman's guide to the causes and prevention of ischemic stroke published in 2007. (A third edition of this very popular book was published in April 2018).

www.ingramcontent.com/pod-product-compliance
Lightning Source LLC
Chambersburg PA
CBHW081459200326
41518CB00015B/2309